Physician Compensation Plans

State-of-the-Art Strategies

Physician Compensation Plans

State-of-the-Art Strategies

Bruce A. Johnson, JD, MPA

Deborah Walker Keegan, PhD, FACMPE

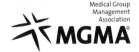

Medical Group Management Association
104 Inverness Terrace East
Englewood, CO 80112-5306
877.275.6462
Website: www.mgma.com

Production Credits

Editorial Director: Marilee E. Aust
Managing Editor: Marti A. Cox, MLIS
Copy Editor: Dianne Nelson
Fact Checker: Mary S. Mourar, MLS
Proofreaders: Larry Beckett, Mara Gaiser, and Scott Vickers – InstEdit
Page Design, Composition, and Production: Boulder Bookworks, Boulder, CO
Cover Design: Andrew Gayer, LabMercury

LIBRARY OF CONGRESS CATALOGING-IN-PUBLICATION DATA

Johnson, Bruce A., 1958-
  Physician compensation plans : state-of-the-art strategies / Bruce A. Johnson, Deborah Walker Keegan.
  p. ; cm.
  Includes index.
Summary: "A guide to physician compensation plan analysis, development, and implementation processes in medical group practices. Addresses plan methods and architectures, legal and regulatory compliance, industry trends, consensus-building, and plan evaluation. Presents case examples for different types of health care organizations, including private (physician-owned), hospital-affiliated, and academic medical practices"—Provided by publisher.
  ISBN 1-56829-275-9 (hardcover)
  1. Medicine—Practice. 2. Medical economics. 3. Managed care plans (Medical care)   I. Keegan, Deborah Walker. II. Title. [DNLM: 1. Physicians—economics—United States. 2. Salaries and Fringe Benefits—United States. 3. Fees, Medical—standards—United States. 4. Group Practice—organization & administration—United States. W 79 J66p 2006]
  R728.J64 2006
  610.068'1—dc22
                                                                                        2006007365

Item 6451

ISBN 1-56829-275-9 (hardcover)

Printed in Canada
10 9 8 7 6 5 4 3 2 1

CPT® is a trademark of the American Medical Association.

The Medical Practice Management Core Learning Series is a structured approach to help medical practice managers and their staffs build the fundamental knowledge and skills required for success in their jobs and careers. The series was developed by the Medical Group Management Association (MGMA) with its certification body, the American College of Medical Practice Executives (ACMPE). Focusing on the competencies identified in The ACMPE Guide to the Body of Knowledge for Medical Practice Management, the series includes seminars, Web-based education programs, books and online assessment tools. These resources provide a strong, expansive foundation for managing the myriad job responsibilities and challenges medical practice managers face every day. For more information, go to *Professional Development* at www.mgma.com.

Contact Information:

Bruce A. Johnson, JD, MPA
MGMA Health Care Consulting Group
Faegre & Benson, LLP
TEL: 303.607.3620
bajohnson@faegre.com

Deborah Walker Keegan, PhD, FACMPE
Medical Practice Dimensions, Inc.
TEL: 828.651.9709
dwalkerbwa@msn.com

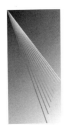

Contents

PART I   Physician Compensation Plan Development

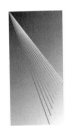

List of Exhibits

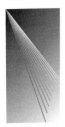

Introduction

Why would medical directors or practice executives decide to champion a new compensation plan for their medical practice? Just the mere thought of tackling the complex, emotionally laden, legal minefield of physician compensation puts fear in the hearts and minds of otherwise rational beings. It is fully recognized that the process of changing a physician compensation plan may not be top on the list of career-enhancing events.

This book presents both the "art" and "science" of physician compensation plans. By "physician compensation plans," we mean the method by which income is determined and paid to physicians in a wide variety of health care organizations – group practices, academic medical centers, hospitals, and integrated delivery systems.

We present innovative approaches to physician compensation – its development, the method of allocating practice revenue and expenses, compensation plan architectures, compensation plan mechanics, implementation methods, and legal and regulatory compliance issues – the "science" of compensation plan development

Equally important, however, is the "art" of plan development – the importance of process – developing, understanding, and reaching consensus on a compensation plan, evaluating the pros and cons of various plans, and employing methods to achieve physician buy-in during plan development and implementation.

The focus of this book is to inform medical practices about "what to do" and, perhaps most important, to show them "how to get from here to there" – to move the organization forward and embrace "state-of-the-art" compensation plans. The development, transition, and implementation of compensation plans are just as important as the plan methodology for a medical practice's long-term success. If physicians are not actively engaged in the process, it will be extremely difficult to reach consensus on a new plan, and any new plan that may be implemented may be largely short-lived.

HISTORICAL CONTEXT

Historically, compensation plans for physicians were not all that complicated. For partnerships of physicians, the compensation plan simply consisted of an equal share (or predominantly equal share) of profits after payment of practice expenses. For these typically small, single specialty practices, this distribution of physician income – combined with peer pressure – seemed to work just fine to ensure equitable levels of work and production. The compensation plans for hospital-employed physicians were equally simplistic, consisting of "negotiated" or straight salary arrangements that often involved some disagreement regarding the level of "negotiation" that took place.

Medical practice ownership was also not as complicated as it is today. The shingle was passed from a senior physician to junior physicians when the right time came along. Physicians crafted their compensation plans on the basis of perceived fairness, and everyone worked equally hard (or at least made the valiant attempt) to achieve success.

Perhaps most important, in the old days, plenty of money seemed to be paid to each element in the health care service chain, and physicians were generally compensated well for their efforts. They were able to focus on caring for their patients, not on capturing upstream and downstream revenue to contend with an ever-shrinking reimbursement pie.

TODAY'S MEDICAL PRACTICE ENVIRONMENT

Today, the business of medicine is increasingly prominent as sophisticated health care delivery systems are crafted to capture new revenue sources and to provide low cost, high quality care to patients. Compensation and other management coordination systems in today's health care environment are being aligned to promote these objectives. Hospitals and medical practices are working to align themselves to care for their communities. Medical practice compensation plans are being aligned to focus physicians' attention on the practice's strategic and organizational goals, along with performance outcomes and quality.

Today's medical practices are highly varied and complex. Each seeks to align compensation within the group practice and at the same time encourage productivity and performance. The medical practices of today tend to be heterogeneous. They include:

- ► Large "mega" practices or health system networks involving a myriad of specialties that are affiliated with hospitals, health plans, and other key constituents in the health care delivery system in a simultaneously competitive and collaborative relationship;

- ► Midsize medical practices often consisting of individual practices that have simply been co-located rather than being "true" group practices, with physicians continuing to exercise significant autonomy in regard to practice style, personal time, and otherwise; and

- ► Small medical practices often comprised of physicians with competing goals and objectives – some favoring entrepreneurship and others seeking to maintain the status quo.

With the growth of integration and managed care in the 1990s, the medical practice may also consist of hospital-employed physicians or a group of physicians working in an HMO. Or the practice may involve academic faculty members organized into one or more practice plans as they work to balance clinical service, teaching, and research commitments in a health care environment where the true "triple-threat" academic physician is increasingly rare.

Today's medical practice isn't your grandparents' practice, nor are the challenges facing it the same.

EXTERNAL CHALLENGES

In today's health care environment, sophisticated business strategies involving new revenue streams require compensation plans to take multiple revenue sources and expenditure types into account. In addition, many physicians are essentially "locked into" their health plan contracts; thus, physician exit strategies are different than in the past, and they impact physician recruitment, retention, and compensation plans.

Recent regulatory changes in the health care environment have had a tremendous impact on physician compensation plans. Compensation plans now need to be analyzed with a legal and regulatory lens involving the Stark self-referral law, the federal anti-kickback statute, laws covering tax-exempt organizations (501)(c)(3), and others.

In today's health care market, money is tight, malpractice costs are high, legal challenges are great, and physician compensation is complicated, laden with emotion and situated in an environment with significant business challenges and risk.

INTERNAL CHALLENGES

If the systemic issues referenced above are not enough to challenge medical practices today when they embark on developing the "right" physician compensation plan, virtually every practice faces generational issues involving physicians of different ages with different life priorities. In many practices, the physicians are working together to meet the health care needs of their communities within the framework of a single physician compensation plan that was designed at one point in the past to meet goals that may be inconsistent with contemporary physician values and work/life priorities. The combination of physician demographics and generational issues that are predominant in many medical practices has led to a focus on compensation mechanics, practice buy-in and buy-out, and the development of retirement, work slowdown, and other forms of "transition" strategies.

Of course, when faced with declining revenue, medical practices are more likely to face compensation plan–related issues. When money gets tight, physicians may question practice operating costs, the work hours and practice styles of their colleagues, how expenses are distributed, or all of these. In doing so, questions are commonly raised regarding the current compensation plan rather than engaging physicians in constructive conversations regarding ways to enhance revenue and/or reduce expense.

As these examples demonstrate, the challenges facing medical practices and their compensation plans are as varied and complex as the practices themselves.

THE AUTHORS

The authors bring two complementary perspectives to the design and implementation of physician compensation plans.

Bruce A. Johnson is a consultant with the Medical Group Management Association (MGMA) and special counsel in the health care and nonprofit organization practice group of the international law firm of Faegre & Benson LLP. In addition to his education and work experience in law, Mr. Johnson has a master's degree in public administration and blends his education and skills in management and law in support of client health care business activities.

Mr. Johnson spends much of his time working with physician practices, academic practices, and hospital-affiliated systems in developing physician compensation and incentive systems that support the organization's goals. His background and work experience enable him to provide a focused assessment of various legal issues on compensation and incentive systems. Mr. Johnson has conducted research on compensation systems used in MGMA better-performing practices and has unique practical expertise regarding the legal challenges presented by the Stark, anti-kickback, and tax-exempt organization laws to physician compensation arrangements. He is the developer and manager of MGMA's Stark Compliance Solutions product (www.stark compliance.com), a web-based physician compensation and Stark law-compliance resource.

Deborah Walker Keegan is president of Medical Practice Dimensions, Inc. With more than 25 years of experience in health care, including positions as a practice administrator and consultant, Dr. Keegan has developed special expertise in enhancing management coordination systems to improve business operations critical for success. She assists medical practices and health care organizations to reduce administrative costs, improve productivity and efficiency, and develop physician compensation and performance incentive systems.

Dr. Keegan received her master's degree in business administration from the Anderson Graduate School of Management at the University of California, Los Angeles, and her doctorate degree from the Peter F. Drucker and Masatoshi Ito Graduate School of Management. She is a Fellow of the American College of Medical Practice Executives. She has authored numerous articles on medical practice operations and incentive compensation plans and is co-author of the best-selling books *The Physician Billing Process: Avoiding Potholes in the Road to Getting Paid* and *Rightsizing: Appropriate Staffing for Your Medical Practice*. She is a leading practice management consultant, author, and keynote speaker.

OVERVIEW OF THIS BOOK

This book presents a detailed blueprint to guide the physician compensation plan development and implementation process in any medical practice. In Part I, we define what we mean by "physician compensation plan" and share a methodology to permit medical practices to determine whether or not they need a new compensation plan. We present a 12-step process for a compensation planning committee to undertake as it develops a new compensation plan. That process emphasizes the importance of actively engaging physicians in compensation plan development. The notion of a compensation plan life cycle is also introduced so that practices can anticipate impacts to the compensation development process and can assess their administrative readiness for change. We review the process needed to communicate compensation plan issues and to achieve buy-in on a new plan, and we discuss various implementation strategies that can be used to transition from the current plan to a revised or new plan.

State-of-the-art strategies – including structures, plan dimensions, and industry trends – are presented in Part II, with a pro-and-con analysis of various compensation plan architectures by reference to a compensation plan matrix. By situating a medical practice's current compensation plan on the matrix, practices can readily see the plan options available to them as they work to improve and revise their current plan. We describe how to measure physician work and effort and how to benchmark these measures for compensation planning purposes. We discuss the alignment of compensation with reimbursement strategies – specifically, pay-for-performance (P4P) – and provide examples of ways to reward specific clinical activity and practice efficiency.

We also explore the legal issues associated with physician compensation, including the Stark self-referral law, anti-kickback statute, and laws that govern tax-exempt organizations. Of course, given the numerous legal and regulatory issues associated with the development and implementation of physician compensation plans, every medical practice must consult with its legal and other advisors.

Special issues in compensation – including determining base compensation levels, rewarding nonclinical production activities such as leadership and administrative roles, developing compensation plans for new physicians, and determining appropriate rewards for activities that may fail to generate high clinical production, yet are important to a medical practice's overall strategic plan (e.g., outreach programs, satellite practice sites, and new programs) – are described. In Part II, we also discuss the key issues involved in developing physician transition plans to address generational issues in the practice and to address part-time, work slowdown arrangements, and/or retirement.

In the final chapter in Part II, we discuss industry trends related to compensation that include sophisticated and emerging compensation strategies that are aligned with the changing health care environment.

In Part III, we share case examples of compensation plans by organization type:

- ► Private group practices (physician-owned);
- ► Hospital-affiliated medical practices (either direct employees or employees of a hospital-affiliated group practice); and
- ► Academic practices.

And while the plans are grouped along host organization lines, different features of the plan examples can be mixed and matched to develop numerous alternatives, and virtually any alternative can be adapted and adopted in private, hospital-affiliated, and academic practice settings.

We also discuss special considerations for hospitals, academic practices, and tax-exempt organizations, including the application of compliance issues that are generally pertinent to these contexts.

The development of a physician compensation plan presents a unique challenge for a medical practice. The future of a medical practice depends upon its ability to develop a compensation plan that the physicians in the practice can "live with." At the same time, the plan needs to be aligned with the practice's future direction and strategy and with the changing demands of the external environment. Compensation plan development is indeed both an "art" and a "science."

Physician Compensation Plan Development

"For the enterprise is a community of human beings. Its performance is the performance of human beings. And a human community must be founded on common beliefs, must symbolize the cohesion in common principles. Otherwise it becomes paralyzed, unable to act, unable to demand and to obtain efforts and performance from its members."

PETER F. DRUCKER

"The fundamental question is 'how do you design management systems to manage work in light of human nature?'"

JOSEPH A. MACIARIELLO
The Peter F. Drucker and Masatoshi Ito Graduate School of Management

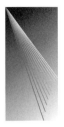

ONE

Do You Need a New Compensation Plan?

L et's begin with a definition of what we mean by the phrase "physician compensation plan." Fundamentally, a physician compensation plan involves a method of allocating revenues and expenses in a medical practice and determining payment to the practice's physicians for their services. But a compensation plan is also a component of a medical practice's overall incentive and performance feedback system, and a tool to encourage – or discourage – performance in furtherance of the practice's goals.

A physician compensation plan can also be viewed as a communication tool. It communicates what is expected of physicians and what behaviors or activities are particularly valued by the medical practice. Compensation plans help to focus and communicate practice values and culture as applied to physician productivity, expense of practice, quality, and other key components of a medical practice. The definition of a physician compensation plan is presented in Exhibit 1.1.

EXHIBIT 1.1   Definition of a Physician Compensation Plan

- ► Method of allocating revenues, expenses, and of determining pay for services
- ► Component in overall *incentive and performance feedback* system
- ► Tool to encourage (or discourage) performance in furtherance of goals
- ► Communication tool

A PRACTICE BAROMETER

In light of the tremendous challenge for a medical practice when it embarks upon the development of a new physician compensation plan, a practice barometer is useful to help determine whether a medical practice truly needs a new plan. That barometer can be viewed as a continuum. At one end of the continuum are those practices that simply have no choice in the matter; they must revise their current compensation plan in order to survive or remain financially viable. On the other end are those practices that voluntarily consider to change their plan as part of an overall alignment strategy as they work to effectively position their medical practice due to the changing internal and external environments. Exhibit 1.2 further illustrates a "practice barometer."

EXHIBIT 1.2   **A Practice Barometer**

		BAROMETRIC INDICATORS			
	LEVEL	**Perceptions**	**Productivity**	**Financials**	**Comp Levels**
No Choice	Level 3	Group fractionates: veiled or overt threats, "demergers," and competition	Personal and professional imbalance	The bank knows you too well	Downward trend
In the Middle	Level 2	Highly productive physicians complain: "I work harder"	A few outliers	Some borrowing	Fluctuations
Seeks Alignment	Level 1	Isolated complaints: "Unfair"	Consistent styles	Acceptable operating margin	Stable

© 2006 Johnson & Walker Keegan

The medical practices in the middle of the continuum have the toughest decision, because the answer to the question of whether a practice should consider a new plan will have no black-and-white answer. Would a change in the compensation plan benefit a practice financially? Would a change better position a practice for the future? Is physician behavior aligned with the practice's goals and objectives? Thoughtful reflection and detailed calculation are required by practices in this latter category as they decide whether or not a change is in the best interests of the practice, its physicians, and its patients.

▶ MEDICAL PRACTICES THAT HAVE NO CHOICE

Some practices simply do not have a choice. These practices find themselves either no longer able to sustain past compensation levels or no longer able to maintain a financially viable position. For these practices, the journey to a new physician compensation plan is at times easier than for those practices on the fence post in the middle. Faced with declining reimbursement, increased expenses, declining physician compensation levels, physician departures, and/or recruitment challenges, these medical practices have no choice but to pursue a new compensation strategy. Physicians in these practices tend to understand the need to embark upon the journey to a new compensation plan, and they know the challenge is time-sensitive. The leverage for change is internal to the practice as it fights to maintain its current position or, at times, fights for its very survival.

▶ MEDICAL PRACTICES THAT SEEK ALIGNMENT

Other practices routinely ask questions regarding the alignment of their current physician compensation plan with changing strategic and tactical goals, market position, reimbursement environment, and other key practice changes that occur. To ensure that the current plan is not misaligned, medical practice leaders periodically evaluate the compensation plan and determine if incremental tweaking or adjustment is needed. For these practices, a revised (or at times, new) compensation plan is part of the "natural order" of things as the medical practice continuously adapts to the complex health care environment. These practices may not develop a new compensation plan for "yesterday, today, and tomorrow," but instead they systematically – and with purpose – analyze their current compensation strategy to determine appropriate alignment, both internally within the medical practice and externally with the health care environment.

▶ MEDICAL PRACTICES IN THE MIDDLE

For the vast majority of medical practices, the decision to embark on the journey to a new compensation plan represents a conscious choice. They are not in a situation where their very survival depends upon it, nor have they embraced systematic alignment. Rather, practices in the middle have concerns regarding whether the present plan is optimal for the organization as it faces current challenges or as it positions itself to achieve its strategic goals.

When should medical practices or other organizations pursue this journey? Experience shows that the leading indicators relate to four core issues: (1) physician perceptions; (2) production changes; (3) financial realities; and (4) changes in compensation levels.

1. Physician Perceptions

The first indicator relates to physician perceptions of the plan and "the problem."

Level 1: Individual Complaints

The first sign that a plan may not be having its intended effect is if one of the practice's physicians complains that the plan is "unfair" to him or her. For example, an individual physician could conceivably view a compensation plan that allocates revenues and expenses based on individual production as a percentage of total practice production as being "unfair." This physician may speak to the medical director, a practice executive, or other practice leader to voice his or her concerns. However, the complaint is isolated and not shared by the majority or even a significant faction of the practice's physicians.

Level 2: "I Work Harder"

This type of complaint is typically voiced by highly productive physicians and therefore moves the barometer upward. "I work harder" is commonly a precursor to what we term "the rise and fall of a partnership." At this juncture, if the most productive physicians in the practice do not feel they are adequately compensated, their actions may lead to one of two outcomes: (1) a change in their productive behavior to that of the "status quo" or "mean" of the practice; or (2) a fight-or-flight response. A decline in productivity to the mean presents problems for practices that have set their performance floor too low, because if all physicians revert to the floor level of production or performance, the practice may be unable to meet its commitments to pay practice expenses (including expected levels of physician compensation) or to service health plans and patients. A fight-or-flight response tends to negatively impact relationships, leads to trust deficits, and is generally accompanied by heated debates. Hearing complaints of "I work harder" may be the first sign that the long-term future of the current compensation plan (and potentially the practice) is not assured.

Level 3: The Practice Fractionates

When a group of physicians in the practice complains about the plan with veiled or overt threats to fractionate the group, then the compensation plan issue has been raised to a very high or "red alert" level. By the time this level has been broached, it may be too late to address the deteriorating relationships in the practice via a simple change to the physician compensation plan. Instead, more dramatic changes to compensation and, frequently, to practice governance, culture, and relationships will be required. Without a change, individual physicians or entire factions of a practice's physicians may "de-merge" to form their own practice and actively compete with their former colleagues in the marketplace.

2. Productivity Fluctuations

The second indicator relates to changes in physician production and performance.

Level 1: Relatively Consistent Practice Styles

For practices at Level 1, the approaches to patient access and work productivity are fairly consistent among the practice's physicians. A culture that supports group practice prevails.

Level 2: A Few Outlier Physicians

Level 2 involves a few outlier physicians who either peak in their performance or fall short of performance levels that are the norm for the rest of the practice. Physician autonomy in behavior takes precedent over group practice goals.

Level 3: Personal and Professional Imbalances

For medical practices at Level 3, variation in performance and polarized practices of physicians at the extremes provide a ripe environment for change. Such polarization commonly involves one subset of physicians that emphasizes personal time and may seek reduced work hours, take a high number of vacation days, or seek other changes to support a lifestyle choice. These physicians work less, so their productivity is less. Another subset of physicians commonly focuses on improving patient access and productivity. These physicians may be working harder and generating more money.

Entrenched behaviors by relatively large subsets of physicians in medical practices that are in personal/professional imbalance create obstacles to governance, decision-making, and other key organizing influences. Such polarization is also a sure sign that a new compensation plan may need to be developed as part of a broader strategy to help refine the group culture (or alternatively, develop a plan with direct linkages to physician work and effort) and get the practice back on course.

3. Financial Realities

This indicator focuses on the practice's overall financial health.

Level 1: Acceptable Operating Margin

A medical practice with an acceptable operating margin may not feel a need to embark upon a new compensation plan. The practice is financially sound and meets budgetary goals, and physicians believe they are fairly compensated – all is well with the world.

Level 2: Some Borrowing

With a line of credit at the bank, at Level 2 the medical practice finds itself in a position where it borrows a few times during the year in order to make payroll and/or meet physician compensation levels.

Level 3: The Bank Knows You Too Well

At Level 3, the medical practice finds that it cannot sustain its current operations without a major change in financial performance. Its level of borrowing is a concern for the medical practice's leaders, and it is evident that the organization needs to make dramatic changes in revenue and/or expenditure performance. In these practices, physician compensation may be "out of sync" with issues concerning changing payer mix, changing health plan reimbursement strategies, and/or the rising costs of the practice. At Level 3, a change to the compensation plan may permit the group to realign its revenues and expenses to achieve financial health.

4. Compensation Levels Fluctuate

This final barometric indicator relates to the changes and variations in physician compensation levels themselves.

Level 1: Stable Compensation Levels

For practices at Level 1, compensation levels are fairly stable and are within physicians' expectations of what constitutes "fair" reimbursement for their work and effort. For example, if the practice has a large portion of compensation based on productivity, the productivity fluctuations are within acceptable levels and hence, physician compensation does not fluctuate greatly from month to month or quarter to quarter.

Level 2: Compensation Levels Fluctuate

At Level 2, physicians are not able to rely upon a consistent level of compensation, and this is impacting their ability to make personal financial decisions. This is voiced as a serious concern by a number of physicians, with discussion of potential physician departures if this trend continues its current progression.

Level 3: Compensation Is on a Downward Trend

At Level 3, the practice has experienced declining compensation levels over the past three to six months. It is apparent that without significant changes, problems in physician recruitment and retention are assured.

Of course, the issue of legal compliance effectively "trumps" each of these four barometric pressures. A medical practice may recognize that its current compensation plan is in violation of legal and/or regulatory issues associated with its legal status or treatment of ancillary services (e.g., designated health services). Or, the practice may employ plan features that are inconsistent with the changing legal environment surrounding physician compensation. Such practices will have no choice but to immediately embark on a new compensation plan.

RECOMMENDED ACTION FOR MEDICAL PRACTICES

Evaluate your medical practice using the barometer in Exhibit 1.2, then periodically reassess your practice to watch for movement over time.

► PRACTICES AT LEVEL 1

If a majority of your responses indicates a Level 1 for your practice, continue to evaluate your practice at periodic intervals to ensure external and internal alignment. Changes to the physician compensation plan may not be needed at this time.

► PRACTICES AT LEVEL 2

If a majority of your responses are at Level 2 for your practice, it is probably time to have a discussion regarding the goals of the current compensation plan and to revisit whether the current compensation plan is aligned with the practice's strategic and operational goals and financial realities. This can be accomplished via a number of avenues, including scheduling a physician retreat to discuss the current state of the practice and determine whether a new compensation plan can assist in better positioning the practice for the future, or actively engaging the executive board of the medical practice regarding the compensation conundrum. In this latter scenario, the board will make a recommendation to the physicians concerning whether or not to work on the development of a new compensation plan.

▶ PRACTICES AT LEVEL 3

If your practice has a number of Level 3 ratings, it is probably time to formally embark upon a new compensation plan for the practice in order to ensure a viable entity for the future. Frankly, if the medical practice has reached Level 3 status in all four barometric categories, the tenor of the group is likely pretty miserable. For some medical practices, it may even be too late to change the trajectory and salvage the practice. It is likely that beyond changes to the physician compensation plan, governance, structure, and other changes may also be warranted.

If you conclude that you are ready to embark on the development of a new (or revised) compensation plan, the next chapter outlines the detailed work of the Compensation Planning Committee and a 12-step process for compensation plan development and implementation.

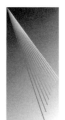

TWO

The Compensation Plan Development Process

The development of a new (or revised) compensation plan requires careful attention to the "art" of compensation plan development. The process through which a plan is developed, communicated, and implemented will impact physician perceptions, trust among practice members, and physician acceptance of any new plan.

PROJECT SPONSORSHIP

While a medical practice may seek outside assistance from consultants, attorneys, accountants, or other advisors to assist with developing a new compensation plan, it is important that the plan development process itself be physician-led. The president, medical director, department chair, or combination of other physician leaders must reasonably support the cause and assist in communicating the need for a new compensation plan to physicians in the practice. It is not enough that a hospital director, practice administrator, or consultant champion the cause.

When compensation issues are discussed, there is typically a heightened awareness and interest on the part of physicians. This is natural. In fact, physicians *should* be concerned about their income. From our experience, if the overall process is not physician-led – meaning that key physicians are truly behind and involved in the plan development and change process – plan implementation and long-term success will be difficult, if not impossible. This is not to say that advisors such as practice administrative leaders and/or external consultants won't need to be relied upon for technical expertise and other forms of "heavy lifting" related to a new plan, but that this assistance must be in support of physician leadership, not take its place.

COMPENSATION PLANNING COMMITTEE

While there are a number of compensation development options (see Exhibit 2.1), in all but the smallest medical practices a compensation planning committee is formed to develop the new compensation plan that will be proposed and recommended to the practice's physicians. A smaller committee effort permits focused attention on the issues involved in compensation plan design and development.

EXHIBIT 2.1   Compensation Development Options

OPTIONS:

1. Compensation Planning Committee – Elected or appointed; representative of the medical practice

2. Top Down – Board or "management" decision

3. Bottom Up – Physicians elected or appointed to investigate options

4. Consultants – Physician-led or consultant-led

5. Combination Options

© 2006 Johnson & Walker Keegan

► COMMITTEE COMPOSITION

The compensation planning committee itself is typically comprised of a cross-section of the practice's members – physician leaders and nonleaders, senior and junior associates, primary care and specialty physicians, high and low producers, and others. Even within a single specialty practice, the compensation planning committee will typically include a balance of the subspecialties within the practice. For example, a cardiology practice may have a five-person compensation planning committee that includes an interventionalist, an invasive cardiologist, a noninvasive cardiologist, an electrophysiologist, and the practice administrator. Of these subspecialists, an effort is typically made to include a balance of seasoned and junior physicians and physician leaders and nonleaders. Likewise, in a practice with no subspecialization, it will be important to ensure a good cross-section of the practice – for example, a good mix of high, medium, and low producers; a good mix of young, middle-age, and older physicians; a good gender mix; and other similar balancing attributes.

While there is no "typical" size for a compensation planning committee, we recommend that it be relatively small – generally in the range of five to seven members. This permits the committee to meet as frequently as needed to work on the compensation plan design process.

► CHARGE TO THE COMPENSATION PLANNING COMMITTEE

The charge to a compensation planning committee should be specific and well-defined. The charge should be communicated to the practice's physicians so that they understand the role and activities that are expected of committee members. An example of a charge issued to a compensation planning committee is provided in Exhibit 2.2.

EXHIBIT 2.2

Charge to the Compensation Planning Committee

1. Determine goals and design principles for a new compensation plan.
2. Educate regarding compensation plan alternatives and the strengths and weaknesses of alternative compensation plan architectures.
3. Define preferred plan architecture or framework to be used.
4. Define performance measures and incentives.
5. Evaluate alternatives and define specific details within the agreed upon architecture.
6. Reach consensus on a proposed plan design.
7. Consider implementation issues and develop an implementation plan.
8. Present the proposed plan design to practice physicians and facilitate decision making.

© 2006 Johnson & Walker Keegan

COMPENSATION PLAN DEVELOPMENT TIME LINE

The time line for the development of a new compensation plan will depend upon the leverage points currently at play in the medical practice. For example, if the medical practice is currently unable to make its payroll, or is faced with a series of actual or imminent physician departures or legal compliance issues, then a "rapid cycle" or revolutionary redesign process will likely ensue.

If the medical practice is relatively small and not in a crisis situation, then the plan design process will typically take from three to six months. During that period, the practice should assess physician views, select a preferred architecture and methodology, design and model plan alternatives, communicate with physicians, and achieve consensus on the new plan. Beyond the three- to six-month period, the medical practice will also need to fully implement the plan via a defined process. That process of transition and implementation may add additional months or sometimes even years for the new plan to be adopted in its final form. A sample compensation plan development time line is provided in Exhibit 2.3.

Unless the medical practice is extremely large and/or highly complex, practices that find themselves engaged in a plan development process that is substantially in excess of six months (e.g., nine months or more) should generally view the length of the process as a wake-up call that the process may not be proceeding as it should. Compensation plan development is typically a demanding, conflict-inducing process for any medical practice or other organization attempting to address physician com-

EXHIBIT 2.3 Compensation Plan Development Time Line

Month 1:	Collect and review pertinent data: current compensation plan(s), employment contracts, compensation, production, and performance data for physicians.
	Appoint a Compensation Planning Committee.
Month 2:	Perform benchmarking analysis and assessment of current compensation system based on available data.
	Submit survey instrument to physicians; conduct confidential interviews with physicians.
	Hold educational sessions with physicians regarding the current compensation plan and the need for change.
	Convene the Compensation Planning Committee. Share findings from the interview process. Educate committee members regarding state-of-the-art compensation plans.
Months 3-4:	Convene Compensation Planning Committee (typically three to five meetings).
	Identify compensation plan goals and design principles.
	Identify plan architecture.
	Identify methodological alternatives.
	Conduct financial modeling.
Month 4:	Communicate with physicians and achieve consensus, buy-in, and acceptance.

© 2006 Johnson & Walker Keegan

pensation issues. As a result, long-term engagement in such a process, without resolution, may lead to its own problems, challenges, and pathology that may stretch beyond the central issue of compensation.

Practices that spend considerable time developing a plan without reaching resolution should consider whether external assistance is required. Likewise, in circumstances where plan development is being undertaken with external assistance, the lack of solid progress and/or decision making after a long period of focused development efforts – again, in the six- to nine-month range – may be a sign that the external assistance is not working as it should. In either circumstance, consideration should be given to changes that might be required to jump-start the process and get it moving again in order to redirect efforts to achieve resolution.

Of course, rough estimates regarding typical time frames are just rules of thumb. Some processes can and should take longer; however, in *all* circumstances, if a sense of progress and action is limited or absent, then the compensation plan development process may need a "wake-up call" and redirection.

ROLE OF A CONSULTANT IN PLAN DEVELOPMENT

When a consultant is hired to assist in the compensation plan development process, the consultant's role typically includes facilitating the activities of the compensation planning committee. For such purposes, a consultant can be virtually any third party who is asked to assist in the process, including administrators, health care consultants, accountants, lawyers, and others. This facilitation typically includes:

1. Assisting in identification of current system strengths and opportunities;

2. Providing relevant background education regarding compensation plan arrangements and alternatives;

3. Working with the practice to define goals and design principles for a new plan;

4. Exploring compensation system options, including compensation plan architectures and technical dimensions;

5. Working with the practice to conduct financial modeling of potential compensation plan alternatives;

6. Preparing communication materials and conducting formal presentations of the recommended plan; and

7. Facilitating decision making.

COMMITTEE OPERATING AGREEMENT

The compensation planning committee process itself consists of a number of meetings to progress through the issues associated with compensation plan design and development. The compensation planning committee members should identify a committee chair and outline the steps in compensation plan development that it will undertake. The committee should identify specific dates and times for meetings and assign action items to responsible parties – with deadlines – in order to keep the planning process on track.

It is also helpful for the committee to identify an operating agreement or "ground rules" by which it will govern. Issues such as confidentiality, candor, communication, and other topics should be addressed at the first meeting, and as needed thereafter. This is important so that committee members feel comfortable sharing their ideas and concerns in a confidential fashion during meeting forums. In their combined roles as physician representatives, ambassadors, and physicians who are personally impacted by the plan, committee members must have a free and open ability to ask questions and present "creative" options and ideas during committee meetings. The concept that no idea is too foolish to at least submit to the committee will frequently encourage the participants to think "outside the box," while also adding useful perspectives to the process that can sometimes open up new ideas, options, or opportunities.

COMMUNICATION PLAN

While free and open communication is essential in the confines of the committee's discussions, equally important is a communication plan that is developed at the end of each meeting. That plan should define what information can, and will, be shared outside of the committee process. The purpose of such a communication plan is not to create "secrecy" around the process of developing a new compensation plan, but to ensure that committee work is shared with the rest of the practice in a systematic and appropriate fashion, and at the appropriate time.

A structured communication strategy is required, because just as creative ideas and candid discussion are to be encouraged in the context of the committee meetings, it should also be recognized that not every creative idea will be adopted and implemented. The objective with the communication process is, therefore, to highlight the process and the key points about which the committee has reached some general consensus.

The communication plan will typically be expressed in written communication to include memos to update physicians and other stakeholders and a useful list of key points that can be used by committee members in their discussions with practice physicians who seek to learn more about the committee's work while it is in process. That communication will tend to focus on the status of the compensation process (e.g., interviews have been conducted and benchmarking results reviewed), the results to date (e.g., agreed upon plan goals and a description of the basic architecture), and the next steps (e.g., when modeling will be performed and when a written summary of the recommended plan is expected to be provided).

While communication is essential at various stages in the committee process, information might not yet be ready to be publicly aired, as the committee may be in a formative stage of plan development, or it may be grappling with specific plan details. In these instances, the communication memo to physicians should indicate the types of activities that are currently in progress, absent the details. The details will obviously be shared when the committee is ready to go forward with a recommended plan or when it has completed specific steps in the plan development process.

A sample of a memo that communicates a compensation planning committee's actions is provided in Exhibit 2.4. This type of communication should be provided at regular intervals throughout the committee's deliberations and should contain the information that the committee is ready to share with physicians in the practice.

Physicians should also receive oral updates regarding the status of plan development to promote understanding, acceptance, and buy-in of any new plan. They should be encouraged to talk with members of the planning committee to address their goals, issues, concerns, and fears. It may also be appropriate to hold special forums to share information and obtain feedback from physicians at critical junctures in the plan development process.

EXHIBIT 2.4

Physician Communication Memo – Status of Committee Activity

TO: Physicians, XYZ Medical Practice

FROM: Physician Compensation Planning Committee

RE: STATUS OF COMPENSATION PLAN DEVELOPMENT

This memo summarizes the work conducted at the Compensation Planning Committee meeting of May 19. We will continue to provide communication updates to you throughout the planning process.

The agenda for the meeting was to review the role of the committee, share findings associated with the interview process, and provide education regarding various compensation plan architectures. The following summarizes key areas of findings and discussions at the meeting:

- ▶ **Role of the Committee**: Work with consultants to review current strengths, weaknesses, and opportunities associated with the current plan; work with consultants to understand differences in compensation plan architectures; develop goals and design principles; develop revised compensation plan consistent with goals; recommend compensation plan for consideration by physicians.

- ▶ **Strengths of Our Current System**: The strengths identified through the interview process included: easy to administer; avoids internal competition for patients; encourages outreach activity; has the potential to promote teamwork; results in compensation levels that are generally satisfactory; encourages a team philosophy.

- ▶ **Weaknesses of Our Current System**: Equal compensation for unequal work; does not measure quality; no sense of ownership in the group; no clear performance criteria or expectations.

- ▶ **Compensation Plan Architectures**: The consultants provided education regarding different compensation plan architectures and their strengths and weaknesses.

- ▶ **Goals of a Compensation Plan**: Goals of a new compensation plan were developed. These include: Promote group viability; reward and encourage work; support physician recruitment and retention; promote areas beyond clinical production; promote personal responsibility and accountability.

- ▶ **Next Steps**: The next committee meeting will be held in late May. The agenda for that meeting will be to prioritize the goals of the plan, understand legal and regulatory issues associated with plan development, and continue discussion of potential plan architectures and design features of a new plan.

If you have any questions regarding the compensation planning process, please feel free to contact any member of the Compensation Planning Committee.

THE 12-STEP COMMITTEE PROCESS

The precise process adopted by the compensation planning committee will frequently vary somewhat depending upon the type of organization and the physician-organization relationship involved. For example, hospital-affiliated practices, integrated delivery systems, and very large medical practices, including academic practices, will also require an intervening step (or series of steps) involving review and approval by the appropriate leadership and/or governing body. Nonetheless, the basic process outlined below is relevant to physician-owned practices, as well as to these other types of practices, since the specific steps are critical to plan development, physician engagement, and physician acceptance of any plan that is ultimately developed.

There are 12 distinct steps in the compensation planning committee process (see Exhibit 2.5). We recommend that the committee progress through each of these steps – in order – to ensure that committee members attend to each of the key elements in plan design. Again, we cannot over-emphasize that the **process** of plan development is as important as the final **outcome** of the plan itself.

1. ASSESS THE EXTERNAL ENVIRONMENT AND OBTAIN PHYSICIAN INPUT

A compensation plan needs to be aligned not only internally within the medical practice, but with the external health care environment as well. For example, it needs to be consistent with changes in reimbursement methods and levels, and with the financial

EXHIBIT 2.5

The 12-Step Committee Process

1. Assess the external environment and obtain physician input.
2. Determine compensation plan goals.
3. Develop design principles.
4. Understand state-of-the-art compensation plans.
5. Benchmark key indicators.
6. Identify compensation plan architecture(s).
7. Determine compensation plan methodology(ies).
8. Perform financial modeling.
9. Evaluate alternative models.
10. Develop transition and implementation plans.
11. Recommend new (or revised) plan to physicians.
12. Achieve practice consensus on a new (or revised) plan.

© 2006 Johnson & Walker Keegan

realities of the practice. Additionally, it needs to ensure that physicians receive a competitive wage that is consistent with the market in order to support physician recruitment and retention. Importantly, it also needs to be structured to ensure that physicians work to evolve the medical practice consistent with the changing patient population and needs of the community in which it resides, including an analysis of the current number and specialty mix of physicians. Thus, in Step 1 of the committee process, an assessment of the "fit" of the medical practice and its current compensation plan with the external environment needs to be conducted.

Beyond this assessment, it is essential for the compensation planning committee to actively engage other practice physicians in developing a compensation plan at Step 1 of the committee's process. The committee needs to consider the perspectives of the medical practice's physicians and other leaders and stakeholders.

If the medical practice is designing its compensation plan with internal resources only, then we recommend that a written confidential survey instrument be used to obtain input from practice physicians and other key stakeholders. If an external consultant has been engaged to work with the compensation planning committee, then feedback may be obtained via confidential surveys and/or one-on-one interviews between the consultant and all or a subset of the practice's physicians and other leaders.

With either scenario, it is important that the physicians and other stakeholders have time to prepare their thoughts regarding the current compensation plan and issues related to a future plan. It is also essential that they be encouraged to think beyond their own visceral goals with respect to the new plan. That is, physicians will typically have a "gut" reaction or personal goal related to the plan development process; for example, they would like to earn more money, they want to make sure they don't take a pay cut, or they want money set aside to ensure the practice's (and their) future. Yet an effective process requires the physicians and others involved to go beyond those preferences and goals and focus on organization-wide goals and perspectives, including those related to the optimal goals of the new plan. Physicians need to assume an organizational lens to focus on questions such as, "what are we trying to accomplish by developing a new plan?" and "what outcomes are we looking for through a new plan that are not being achieved through the current plan?"

A survey instrument that can be used to obtain physician input to the compensation planning process is provided in Exhibit 2.6. Physicians and other interviewees (e.g., representatives from administration, the hospital, school of medicine, or faculty practice plan) should be given the survey in advance of any interview process, or the survey can be used to obtain written confidential feedback when an interview process is not employed.

The survey instrument asks physicians to identify the goals they are looking for in a compensation plan and to outline the strengths and weaknesses of the current plan. In addition, issues and concerns regarding a future plan and any "deal breakers" are solicited to assess perceptions regarding the compensation plan development process and the new plan itself.

EXHIBIT 2.6 Survey Instrument

<u>Goals</u>: Please list the top three goals that should be promoted through the compensation plan.

1. _____

2. _____

3. _____

<u>Current Plan Strengths</u>. What is good or positive about the *current* compensation plan?

<u>Current Plan Weaknesses</u>. What do you view to be the primary weaknesses or problems with the current plan?

<u>Issues/Concerns</u>. What issues or concerns, if any, do you have regarding the development of a new or revised compensation plan?

<u>Deal Breakers</u>. Are there any "deal breakers" or issues you would find unacceptable related to the development of a new compensation plan?

<u>Other Issues</u>. What other issues should be examined or addressed as part of this process?

© 2006 Johnson & Walker Keegan

It should be noted that one-on-one confidential interviews often elicit information not readily provided on a written survey, regardless of the level of anonymity that is assured. Discussion of physician compensation tends to raise a host of other issues beyond the mechanics of the plan and the levels of compensation to be paid. Perceptions of fairness tend to arise, and very often, concerns regarding personal autonomy, lifestyle, and self-worth emerge. In addition, at the time a compensation plan is discussed, many other issues tend to rise to the surface, such as trust deficits that may be present in the medical practice, either real or perceived. These more visceral reactions are difficult to glean from a written survey, yet they can have significant impacts on the compensation plan development and implementation processes.

For example, physicians typically indicate that they want a compensation plan that is "fair." Unfortunately, the perception of "fairness" is highly individualistic. For many physicians, the compensation plan will be judged as "unfair" if it results in a reduction in compensation level; yet the only way for everyone's compensation to get bigger is for the pot of money that is used for compensation to grow larger. By holding individual meetings with physicians, the perceptions of fairness expressed by a physician can be translated to specific goals or design features that he or she wants to see in any new plan; for example, a plan that is consistently applied and easily understood, or a plan that permits a "fair" transition from the current plan, or a plan that does not result in large compensation changes from one year to the next. Probably the best we can hope for when we strive for "fairness" is a plan that will make everyone just a little bit uncomfortable (thus, there are no distinct winners and losers), but a plan they can "live with." From our experience, this type of discussion is best conducted on a one-to-one basis with the physicians who will be impacted by the new plan.

2. DETERMINE COMPENSATION PLAN GOALS

The second step in the compensation plan development process is to define the overall goals of the plan. An effective compensation plan is linked to and promotes important, agreed upon goals. The goals are medical practice-specific and reflect the culture of the medical practice – both where it is today and what is desired for the near future.

Thus, the committee members need to articulate specific overarching goals for the physician compensation plan. That is, they need to define the desired outcome of changes to the current plan. When designing the compensation plan, the committee should then use these agreed upon goals to: (1) evaluate alternative plan models; and (2) assess whether a particular new plan is consistent with these goals. A plan that achieves a pragmatic goal of quieting the most vocal critic of the current plan, but that cannot be looked at and evaluated as being consistent with, and in furtherance of the practice's overall goals, will commonly have a relatively short life.

For example, a compensation planning committee might determine that the goals of the plan are to: (1) enhance productivity; and (2) promote quality care. Or, it might determine that the desired outcome of the plan is to: (1) grow market share; (2) align compensation with reimbursement; and (3) provide greater physician responsibility and accountability for revenues and expenditures. While the committee is developing the new plan, it should compare the technical dimensions of the plan (its basic architecture and more specific methodology) at frequent intervals to ensure that the plan is consistent with the identified goals.

Effective compensation plans typically promote many of the goals listed below. By "effective," we mean plans that seem to meet the needs of the physicians in the medical practice, while at the same time meeting the needs of the business of medicine and promoting high quality clinical care. Effective plans will:

► Encourage and reward productivity and work;

► Recognize and reward diverse activities (e.g., professional services, ancillary contributions, outreach activities, leadership roles, etc.);

► Promote group practice cohesiveness and teamwork;

► Ensure fiscal responsibility;

► Clarify performance expectations and requirements;

► Facilitate physician recruitment and retention; and

► Align compensation with reimbursement methods (e.g., fee-for-service, capitation, pay-for-performance [P4P], etc.).

3. DEVELOP DESIGN PRINCIPLES

The third step in the plan development process focuses on design principles – the overall features of the compensation plan design itself. The key question to be asked of compensation planning committee members is: *What characteristics should optimally be present in any new compensation plan?*

Based on our experience, "better-performing" compensation plans exhibit the following design features:

1. Objective measures (to the extent possible);
2. Relatively few performance measures;
3. Clear definitions, consistently applied;
4. Openness and transparency;
5. Simplicity and ease of understanding;
6. Relatively "stable" income;
7. Balance of individual and team responsibility;
8. Fair and reasonable transition from the current plan to a future plan;
9. Fiscal responsibility; and
10. Legal compliance.

Obviously, these last two measures – "fiscal responsibility" and "legal compliance" – should be part of any plan design. The business risk associated with compensation plan development, from both a fiscal and legal standpoint, needs to be carefully evaluated and considered in the design process. The legal challenges and factors affecting compensation plan development are further explained in Chapter 9, "The Legal Element," and, as noted earlier, consultation with a medical practice's legal counsel is highly recommended.

Some medical practices do embark on a compensation plan change because "their lawyer made them do it" due to legal compliance conditions. We wholeheartedly agree that every organization should ensure that its internal compensation system complies with all applicable legal requirements. Yet, a compensation system that only promotes legal compliance – without consideration of other goals – will be ineffective in the long term.

At least the following ingredients, in addition to legal compliance, are essential to an effective physician compensation plan:

- ► A clear linkage to practice and individual physician goals;
- ► Physician "buy-in" regarding plan goals and the overall methodology; and
- ► A recognition that no compensation system is perfect.

By assessing the environment, obtaining physician input, and articulating the goals and design principles for the compensation plan in Steps 1 through 3 of the 12-step process, the committee provides the foundational elements for an aligned compensation plan (see Exhibit 2.7).

4. UNDERSTAND STATE-OF-THE-ART COMPENSATION PLANS

The fourth step in plan development involves committee education to "state-of-the-art" compensation plans – including structures, dimensions, and trends. That is, the compensation planning committee needs to understand the types of compensation plans being used by similar medical practices, the performance measures that have been

EXHIBIT 2.7   The Aligned Compensation Plan

EXTERNAL ALIGNMENT	INTERNAL ALIGNMENT	
Alignment with Environment	**Alignment with Goals**	**Alignment with Design Principles**
What changes to reimbursement methods, health plan products, and other financial vehicles have taken place?	What behaviors and/or values within the organization should the compensation plan encourage, promote, and reward?	Technical/Methodological Characteristics: ► Objective measures ► Few performance measures ► Clear definitions, consistently applied
What are current market rates for physician compensation by specialty and subspecialty?		► Openness and transparency
	What is a desired outcome of changes to any plan?	► Simplicity and ease of understanding ► Relatively "stable" income
Has the patient population or patient demand for the practice's services changed?		► Balance of individual and team responsibility
	What objective criteria can be used to evaluate any new compensation plan that may be proposed?	► "Fair" transition from current plan ► Fiscal responsibility ► Legal compliance

© 2006 Johnson & Walker Keegan

adopted for incentive payment, and other factors related to compensation plan architecture, methodology, measurement, and implementation.

If a consultant is hired to assist in plan development, he or she should be able to educate and provide support to the committee regarding key aspects of the compensation plan development process. A consultant should give examples of other compensation plans, discuss the pros and cons of various approaches to compensation, provide relevant benchmarks for compensation plan design, and be able to respond to questions and concerns voiced by members of the compensation planning committee related to different alternatives.

If the practice is designing its own compensation plan with internal resources, then either all committee members or a subset (e.g., committee chair, medical director, and the practice administrator) should be charged with gathering relevant articles and examples of compensation plans used by other practices. This will allow them to further their education regarding compensation plans and to identify features they may want to consider when developing their own compensation plan. The information gathered should be shared and evaluated in an objective fashion, meaning that the plan alternatives should be described and evaluated by reference to perceived strengths and weaknesses, and by reference to the goals and design features of the new plan identified in Steps 2 and 3 of the committee process described earlier.

The educational process is important, as many of the medical practice's physicians may have experienced only one or two plans during their tenure as practicing physicians. New, more innovative strategies may not be recognized without this focus on education.

Also, keep in mind the distinctions between education and advocacy at this stage of the process. The information collection and education process will commonly result in one or more participants advocating their own "preferred" model option. That selection might be based on their own objective evaluation of the plan methodology, or, in some instances, a particular model will be viewed as the "right," "best," or "fairest" model because it is being used by another respected physician or medical practice. However, the objective of gaining education is to obtain ideas regarding potential alternatives – not to seize on the "correct" or "right" methodology that will then be advocated throughout the remainder of the plan development process.

It is important to keep in mind that the process (and the journey) of developing a compensation plan is just as important as the outcome. The educational process is designed to collect useful information related to alternatives and to identify a variety of "good ideas." But another essential feature of the development process is for committee members to consider a number of alternatives, and to rule out those that are not acceptable for one reason or another. That process of exploring ideas, ruling out alternatives, and gradually narrowing the plan alternatives will yield a better-informed committee that will, in turn, typically lead to enhanced levels of physician buy-in and acceptance of the plan that is ultimately approved. After all, there is no one "perfect" compensation plan; therefore, the educational process itself must acknowledge that fact by encouraging committee members to reasonably and objectively evaluate potential alternatives, coupled with developing a plan from the ground up.

5. BENCHMARK KEY INDICATORS

Benchmarking is an essential component of the physician compensation plan development process. It involves the systematic comparison of key financial, productivity, quality, and other indicators for one physician or practice, to those of other "representative," similar, or like physicians or practices. Benchmarking should generally occur at two broad levels: (1) at the level of the individual physician; and (2) at the practice or organization-wide level.

At the individual physician level, benchmarking can provide useful information and perspective regarding key questions, such as:

- ► Is a particular physician paid at, above, or below the median level of compensation for peers in that physician's specialty?

- ► Is a particular physician's production (measured by net collections from professional services, work relative value units (WRVUs), weeks worked, or other measures) at, above, or below that of his or her peers based upon market data?

- ► Where does each physician stand in relation to his or her peers in the practice on these and other measures?

At the organizational level, benchmarking will also provide useful information regarding the financial health, productivity levels, and other aspects of the enterprise. This information may include how the organization's performance compares to that of similarly situated organizations and practice entities. Important questions to ask in connection with organizational performance are:

- ► Does the practice have a problem with collections of insurance and guarantor accounts (e.g., as reflected in its aged accounts receivables)?

- ► Is the practice's payer mix the same, better, or worse than that of similar practices?

- ► Does the practice's payer mix rely more heavily on one reimbursement strategy (e.g., fee-for-service or capitation)?

- ► Is the practice's operating cost at an aggregate level and at individual department levels (e.g., by specialty) at, above, or below that of other practices in the marketplace?

- ► Is the practice demonstrating performance outcomes (e.g., clinical and quality indicators and practice efficiency) that are at, above, or below those of other practices with which it competes?

Benchmarking is not an end unto itself. It is merely performed as part of the compensation plan development process in order to provide useful perspective and understanding regarding productivity and performance, and how that performance relates and translates into compensation for individual physicians. Benchmarking is also undertaken in connection with legal compliance efforts, as discussed in Chapter 7, "Measuring Physician Work and Effort," and in Chapter 16, "The Special World of Hospital and Academic Practices – Assessing Reasonableness and Promoting Compliance." However, the benchmarking undertaken in connection with plan development is primarily intended to provide an understanding of how individual physician and medical practice performance relates to that of similarly situated peers.

Benchmarking offers perspective. That perspective will frequently help individual physicians develop a better understanding of whether they are being treated fairly or unfairly through a practice's compensation system. It may also be essential in opening up a more objective view regarding the need for change in a compensation plan and the particular direction of that change.

For example, in most physician practice settings, an ultimate stated goal of the physician compensation plan development process is to develop a plan that is perceived to be "fair." At the level of the individual physician, perception of what is "fair" will typically relate to the physician's perceptions regarding the amount of work that physician engages in and the associated level of compensation that he or she receives.

Benchmarking can provide objective information to help assess whether or not individual physician perceptions are realistic, and whether or not the ultimate level of compensation earned by individual physicians is, in general, at, above, or below that of their peers. In doing so, benchmarking contributes useful perspective and helps to open eyes and minds regarding the need for change in a practice's compensation plan. It can also provide data and useful information on the potential direction or result of that change.

6. IDENTIFY COMPENSATION PLAN ARCHITECTURE(S)

Step 6 in the compensation planning process is to select the compensation plan architecture. This is a broad framework or typology for the plan, such as a base salary plus incentive system, a productivity-based system coupled with cost allocation, or the like. As is true with any framework, the plan architecture should be viewed as a rough outline of what the plan will likely look like and how it will work in a general sense. Chapter 6 provides more details on the broad types of compensation plan architectures.

The selected architecture (or potential architectures) should generally consist of a plan design that is viewed as consistent with the goals identified in Step 2 of the committee process. This means, for example, that if the stated goals underlying the plan include making individual physicians more responsible and accountable for their own work and production levels and associated expenses, the plan architecture should have features that promote those goals. In this example, a productivity-based system with some level of cost allocation might fit the bill, while a plan promoting a pure salary or a 100 percent equal share of practice profits would not.

The basic combinations of design features and compensation architectures are outlined in Chapter 6. Keep in mind that the compensation plan "architecture" is initially expressed at a high level – without significant detail. The remaining steps of the plan development process will be used to define those details and, where appropriate, compare and evaluate competing architectures in order to settle on the preferred plan, along with all the associated and required plan mechanics and technical dimensions.

7. Determine Compensation Plan Methodology(ies)

Once the overall plan architecture is determined, the committee needs to define the technical dimensions or plan methodology(ies). To guide this process, five key questions must be addressed. These questions are detailed in Exhibit 2.8 and are summarized below:

1. How should physicians be compensated for work performed?
2. What types of behavior and performance should be rewarded?
3. At what level should physicians be evaluated and rewarded?
4. What portion of compensation should be earned and paid through incentive systems?
5. How does compensation link to overall funds flow and the strategic direction of the medical practice?

At this step in the planning process, decisions are made regarding the level of autonomy that departments or specialties will have in methodological aspects of the compensation plan. For example, a decision could be made in a multispecialty practice that the overall plan architecture will be consistent across departments or specialties; however, the actual methodologies, such as the exact performance measures to be employed or whether or not to use a team-oriented incentive pool, may vary by specialty.

If one common methodological design is intended, then the committee identifies the funds flow model, the measures that will be used to determine physician performance and other important aspects of the plan's technical dimensions. It is at this step in the planning process that the compensation planning committee delves into the details of plan design. Detailed plan designs are provided in Chapters 13 to 15 of this book.

8. Perform Financial Modeling

Step 8 of the committee's work involves financial modeling of the compensation plan architecture and its methodology. Internal, practice-specific data are used to model both historical and projected future levels of compensation. In addition, relevant benchmarks are often used in the financial modeling process to ensure market relevancy of compensation plan levels, productivity indices, and other performance measures. In some contexts, benchmarking is also used as part of legal tests related to the "reasonableness" of compensation for physician services.

Typically, the medical practice's accounting and finance staff perform financial modeling as directed by the committee (or in conjunction with compensation plan

EXHIBIT 2.8

Key Design Questions

1. How should physicians be compensated for work performed?	► Clinical ► Teaching ► Research ► Service
2. What types of behavior and performance should be rewarded?	► Productivity ► Outcomes and quality ► Managed care ► Patient satisfaction ► Clinical resource management ► Teaching ► Research ► Leadership
3. At what level should physicians be evaluated and rewarded?	► Individual ► Specialty ► Practice ► Some or all
4. What portion of compensation should be an incentive?	► Fixed vs. variable ► Portion "at risk"
5. How does compensation link to the overall funds flow and to the strategic direction of the medical practice?	► Degree of financial support – clinical, teaching, research, service ► Expenses – individual, specialty, practice

© 2006 Johnson & Walker Keegan

consultants). The financial modeling usually involves the development of multiple scenarios responding to "what if?" situations. Financial modeling is essential if the practice is to ensure a physician compensation plan that is fiscally responsible for the medical practice. Thus, from the practice's perspective, the modeling must demonstrate that the plan will not spend more money than is available or undermine the practice's financial margin targets or requirements.

Of course, the modeling must also demonstrate that the plan is realistic from the individual physician's perspective. In other words, the modeling must generally demonstrate that shifts in compensation for individual physicians or subsets of physicians in the practice under a proposed alternative compensation plan are both reasonable and rational. Financial modeling of any proposed compensation plan will typically use historic and/or projected data to model how compensation levels would change under a new plan architecture and methodology, and the modeling will reflect those changes in "bottom line" financial terms. Such modeling will always show shifts in income, but those shifts should generally be in a direction and a magnitude that are rational and justified based on benchmarking findings and/or in a direction that is more consistent with the new plan's underlying goals. All new plans will result in changes in individual physician income, but new plans that truly are able to be implemented must result in changes that can be justified and supported on various grounds (e.g., due to physician production levels, changes in expense allocation, practice philosophy, etc.).

It is very important that the financial modeling *not* be conducted too early in the compensation plan development process. This is because once numbers are affixed to the compensation plan architecture on a per physician basis, objectivity tends to get a bit "muddled." Therefore, sharing the model results in a blinded manner (without physician names) is recommended, at least initially. It is paramount at this step to ensure that individual physician interests do not take priority over the interests of the medical practice as a whole.

Equally important is that the confidential nature of the committee process be protected; at this stage in the compensation plan design process, the committee is not yet ready to communicate its recommendations. The financial modeling provides an opportunity to see how the plan that was considered to be a "good idea" at a theoretical level actually works using the medical practice's own numbers on an individual physician basis. The compensation plan will frequently need to be revised depending upon the outcome of the modeling to ensure: (1) fiscal appropriateness; and (2) consistency of the plan with the goals and design features that were identified by the committee in Steps 2 and 3 of the planning process.

9. EVALUATE ALTERNATIVE MODELS

A key step in the compensation plan development process involves considering potential plan architectures and methodologies, coupled with a systematic ruling out of different options. The end result is typically a narrowing of alternatives and, eventually, closure (e.g., agreement) on a single recommended compensation plan. The evaluation of plan alternatives is an essential step in this process. The exact number of models that might be evaluated will frequently range from a few (e.g., six to ten permutations of a basic architecture) to many (e.g., 40 to 60 alternatives of two to three different architectures).

The evaluation process is intended to lead to an assessment of potential methodologies by reference to the practice's agreed upon goals and design principles for the new compensation plan. It must also include, however, an assessment by relation to certain pragmatic realities – that is, the magnitude of change and the level of physician compensation under one or more particular models.

The plan evaluation process itself should involve at least two broad steps:

First, a particular plan architecture and plan methodology should be evaluated by reference to the agreed upon goals driving the plan development process. The compensation planning committee should evaluate the model at a conceptual level – *without* reviewing financial modeling results. This means, for example, that the committee reviews the specific goals and design features identified for a new plan and evaluates a particular architecture and methodology by using those particular goals and design features as the committee's guideposts.

Of course, few committee members will feel comfortable making an ultimate decision regarding a plan without "seeing the numbers." Nonetheless, it should also be noted that, in terms of human behavior, financial modeling results will frequently tend to skew perceptions regarding an otherwise desirable (or undesirable) compensation plan. Therefore, the committee should be encouraged, if not required, to take a "straw vote" regarding whether a particular compensation plan appears to meet the committee's goals at a conceptual level, before the financial impact of the plan is examined at the level of the medical group and individual physicians.

Second, the committee should review actual financial data in a *blinded fashion*. By "blinded," we mean that identifying information of individual physicians is removed. Here, too, an acknowledgement of the reality of human behavior is in order. Although all committee members will be charged with thinking "for the good of the organization" in connection with plan design, it is at times difficult to divorce personal feelings from an evaluation of a particular model. Therefore, steps to sanitize the data and present them in such a manner as to allow for a reasonably objective evaluation of the plan "on the merits" are of critical importance.

This evaluation process will result in a series of activities involving conceptual models and financial information. Through this process, the compensation planning committee typically settles on either a single preferred model or two to three alternatives that can be submitted to others in the organization for ultimate review, consideration, and adoption. The process of reviewing and evaluating multiple plan alternatives will itself involve a "rule out" process that is akin to that used in medical diagnosis and decision making. Likewise, that process will lead to a more informed compensation planning committee and will typically result in greater consensus and shared understanding of the relative strengths and weaknesses of any compensation plan option that is ultimately settled upon.

10. DEVELOP TRANSITION AND IMPLEMENTATION PLANS

Once the financial modeling has been completed and the committee has agreed on the new plan (or plan options) that it will recommend to practice physicians and others, it is important that the terms and conditions of plan transition and implementation be outlined. For example, if the medical practice has six months until the plan is implemented, a plan that takes the practice from its current compensation plan to the new plan is needed.

In some practices, the implementation process may encompass a one- to two-year process of successive, incremental changes to the compensation plan architecture. Likewise, if new performance measures (e.g., WRVUs) are to be used in the new compensation plan, the practice may want to provide the data to physicians for a six-month period prior to plan implementation. This will give physicians the opportunity to fully understand the data, help to improve upon data capture and reporting, and make "course corrections" as needed. See Chapter 4 for a detailed discussion of implementation plans.

11. Recommend New (or Revised) Plan to Physicians

At Step 11, a proposed compensation plan is now ready to be shared with the practice's physicians. Typically, this communication is in the form of a written narrative describing the plan goals and methodology, coupled with face-to-face communication and question-and-answer sessions performed at a retreat-type format or over a series of meetings. The objective of this communication is to educate practice physicians regarding the plan methodology and to take physicians through aspects of the committee process in order to ensure that they understand the plan and its components and how the committee reached its option(s) and recommendation.

The medical practice should provide a number of avenues for physicians to share questions and concerns; for example, meetings with the president, medical director, or practice executive; e-mail communications; physician forums; and other methods. Again, it is important to recognize that the process or "art" of compensation plan development is important if physician buy-in and acceptance of a new plan are to be achieved.

12. Achieve Practice Consensus and Decide on a New (or Revised) Plan

The final step is to achieve consensus on the new plan – at least to the extent possible. The governing documents of the medical practice typically impose requirements for the adoption of a new compensation plan, as do employment contracts and other documents that lay out the method by which a new compensation plan is introduced. If outside consultants have assisted in plan development, they can facilitate the decision-making process. It is important that physicians do not feel that they are being "railroaded" into a new plan. At this step in the plan development process, the committee is hoping to get physicians to agree that, while the new plan may not be "perfect" (since no plan is), they can "live with it."

If the committee has followed a systematic process, such as the 12-step committee process outlined above, the actual decision-making process at this final step is generally not all that contentious. If the physicians understand the need for a new plan, if they have received regular communication updates regarding the plan process, if they have had the opportunity to provide feedback and ask questions, and if they understand the steps that have been taken by the committee, the resulting decision is typically one of confirmation rather than heated debate. If a well-defined process (or "art") of plan development has been undertaken, there are typically no surprises at this last step, when the new compensation plan itself (the "science") is presented for physician confirmation.

THREE

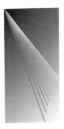

The Life Cycle of Compensation Plan Change

The 12-step process outlined in the previous chapter provides a detailed road map for progressing through the compensation plan design process. Implicit in the road map are assumptions regarding the underlying change process in a medical practice related to physician compensation. An understanding of that change process in a more explicit fashion is essential to understanding the "art" of developing a new compensation plan.

Compensation plan change will always result in some winners and some losers, along with potentially dissatisfied and unhappy physicians for one reason or another. For this reason, the "best" plan for a particular medical practice is typically viewed to be the one that makes every physician "a little bit unhappy."

On the surface, this statement sounds like a medical practice has to "settle" for a plan with which everyone is dissatisfied, rather than working to develop an "optimal" plan. That is not what we mean. While there will be "winners" and "losers" with any plan, the gap between these two groups should not be too great. It is also for this reason that the development of a new compensation plan should generally occur at the right time and for the right reasons – as opposed to being proposed and implemented because it just seems like the "right thing to do." As we discussed in Chapter 1, a medical practice should evaluate its current level on the practice barometer to determine whether or not the practice actually needs to embark on new plan development.

Medical practices – ranging from the smallest two- or three-physician practice that is privately owned and operated to the largest networks that are privately owned or affiliated with a hospital or health system – are collectives of human beings that tend to have their own unique organizational culture and life cycle. Like other organisms, medical practices tend to go through their own cycles of growth, development, maturity, decay, and regeneration. So, too, the compensation plans in a medical practice change and evolve over time.

LIFE CYCLE PHASES

The compensation plan life cycle is akin to a roller coaster. As with a roller coaster, it is rather fun to watch, but if you are on the ride it can be energizing or gut wrenching. Some may want to get off in the middle of the ride. There are three distinct phases of

EXHIBIT 3.1

The "Roller Coaster" Model of Change

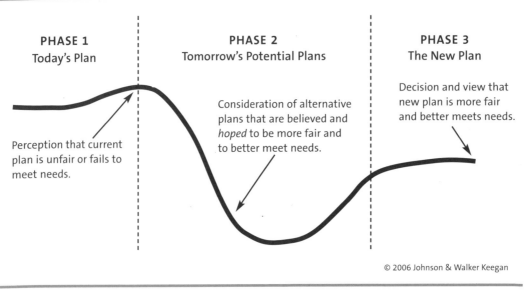

© 2006 Johnson & Walker Keegan

a compensation plan's life cycle during the change process: Phase 1 – Today's plan, Phase 2 – Tomorrow's potential plans, and Phase 3 – The new plan. Exhibit 3.1 outlines this roller coaster scheme of today's plan, tomorrow's plan, and the new compensation plan change process.

► PHASE 1 – TODAY'S PLAN

In a steady-state environment, the compensation plan that was created when an organization was small and had limited complexity may work for a long period of time. Yet, over time, additional forces and changes inevitably occur through the addition and departure of physicians, increased subspecialization, practice outreach activities, changes in reimbursement, market changes, financial pressures, and others. As a result of these and other factors, in Phase 1 of the change process, pressures on the "fairness" of the practice's existing compensation plan will frequently increase. The current or existing plan that is reflective of "the way we've always done it" may become subject to pressure and stress. An increasingly large number of physicians in the practice or, in some circumstances, certain powerful physicians in the practice, will come to view the plan that has heretofore always worked as being less than desirable and eventually unacceptable.

The result of the above activities will frequently manifest itself in one of four ways: (1) a call for the development of a new plan; (2) the threatened departure of physicians if a new plan is not developed; (3) a conscious decision by the organization to consider alternatives and develop a "better" compensation plan; or (4) a "decision" to do nothing at all.

► PHASE 2 – TOMORROW'S POTENTIAL PLANS

Once the decision has been made to develop a new plan, individual physicians or subsets of physicians within the practice will often have an opportunity to test and evaluate their own plan "favorites." In many instances, favorite plans for one physician or one group of physicians will be viewed as less than desirable or suboptimal for one reason or another to other physicians or groups. This shouldn't come as a surprise, given that medical practices are comprised of diverse physicians.

Through the plan development process, often the "favorite" plan of one physician or subset of the practice will be found to be wholly undesirable by that physician, subset, or the group as a whole once it is examined in greater detail. More commonly, the favorite plan of a single physician or subset of physicians will be viewed as a "practice breaker" in that if the favorite plan were implemented, higher levels of physician dissatisfaction would more likely ensue. As a result, Phase 2 of the change process involves an evaluation of desired alternatives, coupled with a ruling out of many, if not most, of those alternatives and ultimately settling on the plan that works reasonably well for the practice as a whole – but which is not, by any means, "perfect."

► PHASE 3 – THE NEW PLAN

The third phase of the change process involves its own level of stability for a period of time. The new plan that was designed to address the perceived inequities and problems of the past will be implemented and will stay in place for a period of time. In some practices, that period of time will be as short as three to five years, in others it may be considerably longer, and in a few it may be considerably shorter.

The length of time that the compensation plan will be viewed to be acceptable will depend on a number of factors specific to the external and internal environments of the medical practice and the physicians within it. This means that a plan may need to be changed sooner or later due to the same combination of internal and external changes discussed previously; for example, declining reimbursement or changing methods of reimbursement, changing payer mix, market changes, physician departures due to a perception that they can make more money elsewhere, recruitment and retention challenges, mergers, acquisitions, and other events.

Not surprisingly, as the compensation plan ages, so do the physicians who participate in it. Along with that aging will frequently come a modification of physician perceptions, values, and needs. Thus, the compensation plan that worked just fine for a particular physician at one point in his or her career may no longer work quite as well as that physician's personal goals, desires, and outlooks evolve.

Unfortunately, there is no universal definition of a "fair" compensation plan. The combination of individual physician perceptions, along with external and internal factors, will come together to shape perceptions related to the compensation plan, the need for change, and the adequacy of the plan that currently exists. In this context, the new plan developed in Phase 3 of the change process eventually becomes the foundation for the emergence of a new Phase 1, and the change process begins anew.

THE COMPLEXITY OF CHANGE

Change in any organization will frequently be rather messy. Despite the best efforts to structure, manage, and objectify the compensation plan development and change process, unexpected events can and generally will occur. The change process may be linear or circular and/or incremental or revolutionary. This means, for example, that where a particular practice will go in terms of its future compensation plan, will, of course, be based in part on the practice's current plan. But that current plan need not define precisely what the future plan will look like.

Indeed, many practices will set out on the compensation plan development process with the stated objective of incrementally modifying or "tweaking" the plan to better address particular goals, desires, or needs. The practice's pragmatic objective may be to make a small adjustment or tune-up to the basic plan that addresses a perceived goal or problem, a particular constituency within the practice, or all of these. In many instances, such an incremental adjustment will be possible, but in other instances, the planned evolutionary change leads to more dramatic or revolutionary modifications.

Conversely, in some practices, individual physicians or subsets of the physician community commonly seek revolutionary changes to the compensation plan in an effort to better meet their own desires or needs. Here also, despite what may be commonly viewed as a "consensus" for revolutionary change, the ultimate result may be one of incremental modification that is viewed as better meeting the overall desires of the practice as a whole.

The complexity of change is further realized by evaluating the generational issues that may be at work in a medical practice and the different goals and perspectives of the physicians based on their own personal situations. Each physician will naturally bring his or her own specific circumstances to the table during new compensation plan development, and a recognition of these differences among the practice's physicians is another element that must be addressed as part of the change to a new compensation plan.

It would be incorrect to say that slavish devotion to the 12-step process for the work of the compensation planning committee outlined in the previous chapter will allow a medical practice to ride the waves of change without risking injury from all the bumps. It would also be incorrect to say that an incremental, revolutionary, or middle-ground form of change is appropriate in all circumstances and for all medical practices.

For the most part, compensation plans should operate in the background of a medical practice akin to a silent operating system that reflects, reinforces, and promotes the practice's goals and overall culture. The plan will always be noticed, and complaints will frequently occur, but in most instances, those complaints will not require immediate action, nor will they be a sign of an impending crisis.

Yet, like the canary in the mine shaft, attention to the plan and the dynamics surrounding it will also be critical to the medical practice's survival. Once the issues regarding the plan reach a fevered pitch and change starts to occur through physician departures, backroom modeling of potential alternatives, or veiled and not so veiled threats, the time for action should be clear.

ADMINISTRATIVE READINESS FOR A NEW COMPENSATION PLAN

The inherent reality is that much of the data that are tracked, monitored, and reported in a medical practice can be improved. Rarely have we found a medical practice entirely pleased with its data elements and management reporting. When a new compensation plan is developed in a medical practice, the best-case scenario would be to take the time to improve the data and information processing in the medical practice prior to implementing any new plan. Unfortunately, this best-case scenario is not very realistic. More commonly, medical practices add data elements and improve the data concurrent with the development of a new compensation plan. In fact, improvements to data tracking, monitoring, and reporting are likely to occur on an ongoing basis in a medical practice.

If the data are not at least reasonably accurate, then lack of confidence in the data by physicians will create additional plan development and implementation hurdles. Thus, a new compensation plan may dictate the need for changes to information technology and operational priorities to ensure data capture, accuracy, completeness, and timeliness. Again, however, rather than wait for the data to be perfect, more typically, the data "catch up" with the compensation plan and are continuously reviewed and updated as they are improved.

Medical practices need to address ongoing practice management and implementation issues throughout the life of a compensation plan by asking questions such as those listed below:

1. Does the current practice management system provide the type and level of data needed for the new plan?

2. Is the information processing, capacity, and reporting at acceptable levels?

3. Does the data pass the "reasonableness" test for completeness and accuracy?

4. Are management reports provided to physicians at regular intervals so that physicians are aware of their performance?

5. Are physicians able to understand the data that are shared?

6. Do physicians make a meaningful connection to the data – for example, have data been translated into information (such as by reflecting internal and external benchmark comparators, providing physicians with education or methods to alter their behavior, or others)?

Equally important is to develop appropriate administrative avenues for physicians to air their issues, concerns, and grievances related to the compensation plan, data measurement and monitoring systems, and other key aspects of compensation plan implementation. Policies and procedures for physician feedback and grievances should be developed. It is also important to establish a future date when the compensation plan will be reviewed to ensure that it is meeting its intended goals.

We would not expect a medical practice to design a new compensation plan every year. Our goal, when we assist medical practices to develop a new plan, is to develop a consistent plan architecture that may permit variable performance measures to be adopted (from year to year if necessary). Even with multispecialty group practices, our initial strategy is to determine if one common plan architecture for the group will meet its needs; however, there commonly will be variable performance measures and thresholds for performance based on specialty.

The life cycle of compensation plan change and the messiness of the change process inherent in compensation plan development are realities for most of today's medical practices. Once this is understood, it may not make designing the compensation plan any easier, but it serves as a useful "reality check" when it comes to understanding the behaviors and issues surrounding physician compensation.

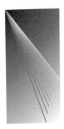

FOUR

Compensation Plan Decision and Implementation

The issues discussed in this chapter relate to *process* and are important if consensus on a new compensation plan is to be achieved. Deciding on new plan adoption constitutes the final step in the 12-step compensation planning process that we presented in Chapter 2. But before that decision is made, a checklist tool will help the compensation planning committee ensure that it is ready to proceed to this last and final step in the plan development process.

COMPENSATION PLAN CHECKLIST

Prior to putting the compensation plan to a vote or making a decision regarding its adoption and implementation, the compensation planning committee will want to make sure that it has completed its charge. The use of a checklist allows the committee to determine if all key areas of an effective compensation plan have been addressed and that committee members understand their position on each of these areas so that they can adequately address any questions or concerns raised by physicians.

A sample compensation plan checklist is provided in Exhibit 4.1. The checklist elements in this example summarize key areas that should be considered with any compensation plan:

- ► Is the new plan linked to the mission and goals of the medical practice?

- ► Is the description of the new plan clear and concise?

- ► Are performance expectations and performance measures clearly defined?

- ► Would others view the plan as simple, understandable, and explainable?

- ► Does the plan permit information and data to be openly shared and transparent?

- ► Does the plan balance individual and team responsibilities?

- ► Is the new plan fiscally responsible?

- ► Is the new plan legally compliant?

Once the committee is satisfied that these areas have been appropriately addressed, it is ready to proceed with the decision-making process.

EXHIBIT 4.1

Compensation Plan Checklist –
Features and Considerations Related to Effective Compensation Plans

1. Alignment with Mission and Goals
    - ► Are compensation plan goals and objectives defined?
    - ► Does the compensation plan reward mission, vision, values, goals (and for academic practices, are all mission components rewarded, or just one or a few)?
    - ► Does it achieve balance (and for academic practices, does it balance components of the academic mission)?

2. Clarification of Performance
    - ► Does the plan clarify performance expected of physicians?
    - ► Are minimum performance standards defined (e.g., time commitment, production, timeliness of service or clinic, on-call, business policies [coding, charge completion])?
    - ► Is there linkage to administrative responsibilities (and, for academic practices, teaching and research)?

3. Fiscal Responsibility
    - ► Are safeguards provided in the event of deficits?
    - ► Does the plan consider funds flow (and, for academic practices, tithing and revenue definitions for inclusion)?
    - ► Are future needs considered (e.g., practice development, cash flow, and reserves)?
    - ► How will shortages be dealt with (e.g., reduction of base salary or supplement, equal-percentage, equal-dollar, formulas, or discretion, etc.)?

4. Legal Compliance
    - ► Has the methodology been assessed for compliance with the Stark law and other applicable laws?
    - ► Is the plan documented, and is the documentation current?
    - ► When applicable, is compensation consistent with fair market value, and is it reasonable?

5. Clear Definition and Consistent Application
    - ► Is the plan in writing?
    - ► Does it involve specific rules (rather than open-ended discretion)?
    - ► Is there structure to areas of discretion (e.g., clearly rests with medical director or chair, pursuant to committee recommendations, etc.)?

6. Simplicity, Ability to Be Understood and Explained
    - ► Is it likely that physicians can explain the plan to others?

7. Openness, Transparency, Consistent Application
    - ► Does the plan involve a "common set of rules"?
    - ► Does the plan document include examples? Can the math be replicated?
    - ► Are management, productivity, and other reports included as part of the plan?

8. Balance of Individual and Group Responsibility
    - ► Does the plan promote group practice and teamwork, or does it view each physician as his or her own unique and independent practice? Or in combination?

THE DECISION-MAKING PROCESS

The human element is very directly involved during the decision-making process for a new compensation plan. At the time physicians are asked to endorse a change to the current plan or a new compensation plan, organizational politics may heighten and there may be a general angst among physicians in the practice. But the decision-making process really does not have to be as contentious as all that.

The decision-making process for a new compensation plan should not be structured as a "major event." Rather, it should take place in incremental steps.

We have previously noted the importance of engaging physicians in the plan development process and providing multiple communication channels for physicians to air their concerns and issues regarding compensation. This cannot be overemphasized. By the time the medical practice is ready to make a decision on a new plan, the following should have already taken place:

1. **Education regarding the need for a new compensation plan.** Physicians should understand the reasons why the practice is embarking on a transition to a new plan, the strengths and weaknesses of the current plan, and the current external environmental issues impacting the practice. Physicians should not be questioning the need for a new plan at the time they are being asked to vote on one.

2. **Education regarding the progress of the compensation planning committee.** The physicians should have received regular updates from the committee regarding its process and progress. At the time of a formal vote on a new plan, physicians should have already known, for example, the goals that have been decided for a new plan, and they should have had an opportunity to provide feedback on those goals. Physicians should already have known the design principles used in plan development, and again, should have been solicited for their input and feedback on the design principles.

3. **Evaluation of the architectural alternatives.** In the weeks and months leading up to the decision-making process itself, the compensation planning committee should have evaluated the universe of plan architectures, with a repetition sequence involving consideration and elimination until the "best" plan (or plan alternatives) has been identified for the medical practice. The committee should have communicated the different plan architectures it has considered, the strengths and weaknesses of the architectures, and the committee decisions to eliminate various architectures from consideration and for what reasons. Thus, at the time a vote is called, the physicians should already be familiar with the architectural elements of the new plan.

4. **Discussion of the measures of physician performance.** In the months of committee deliberation, the specific measures of physician work should have been discussed. Physicians who are unfamiliar with specific measures (e.g., work relative value units [WRVUs]) should have had an opportunity to understand their

own performance in relation to the measures that will be selected for the plan's methodology.

If the compensation planning committee has followed the 12-step process of plan development, it has been working to achieve physician and cultural readiness for a new plan to include:

- ► Soliciting physician input and feedback;
- ► Sharing the reasons for the development of the new plan;
- ► Educating physicians regarding weaknesses of the current plan;
- ► Educating physicians to "state-of-the-art" compensation plans;
- ► Providing regular communication updates;
- ► Developing open communication channels; and
- ► Conducting consensus-building activities.

Without a cultural readiness for change, a compensation planning committee's best efforts at developing a new plan may be met with entrenchment behavior from the practice's physicians. The physicians may not agree that a new plan is needed. They may argue for incremental changes to the current plan rather than be open to a newly developed plan. They may not feel that their voices have been "heard," or that the plan that they think would work has been considered, either directly or indirectly. Cultural readiness relates to "state of the mind," or the "art" of plan development, a key behavioral ingredient for successful compensation plan development and implementation.

In summary, by the time the compensation plan is put to a vote by physicians (or alternatively, presented as the leading plan for physician feedback), there really should be no surprises. The physicians in the practice should have had ample opportunity to understand the need for a new compensation plan, to provide feedback, and to understand the incremental decisions that the compensation planning committee has made regarding compensation plan alternatives. This is why we believe that the decision-making process regarding a new compensation plan itself is an incremental process. It should not be positioned as a war of political wills. It is essentially the culmination of a process of sequentially considering and eliminating – from a variety of alternatives – and finally deciding on the one "right" plan for the medical practice.

When physicians are up-to-date regarding the committee's deliberations, the decision-making process itself is relatively straightforward. While there are typically no real surprises at this stage, the actual procedure used for this decision making will vary based upon the organizational type of the medical practice.

► DECISION MAKING IN PRIVATE MEDICAL PRACTICES

In private, physician-owned medical practices, the physicians will typically meet and, based upon their bylaws, either a super-majority or majority vote will be needed to change the compensation plan. Typically, before the vote is called, the plan has been well communicated and the concerns and issues advanced by the physicians in the group have been addressed. If the vote does not carry the new plan, then the group may still want to pursue development of performance expectations, investigate legal issues that might impact the current plan, and other factors, as appropriate.

Once the physicians and practice are ready to make a decision, the decision-making process itself should proceed in a stepwise fashion. At each step, there is closure so that by the last step, the decision has been reached by the practice's physicians.

A sample of a decision-making process for a new plan involving this stepwise approach is outlined below. It is often used by physician-owned medical practices as part of an incremental decision-making process to a new compensation plan.

> **Step 1: Narrative Description.** Physicians should be provided with a narrative description of the current plan, the need for a new compensation plan, and a description of the proposed plan, including goals and design principles intended for the new plan. They should be formally asked to endorse the goals and design principles at this step.

> **Step 2: Plan Example.** Physicians should be presented with an example of the plan architecture, absent financial data. At this step, the physicians should be asked to vote on whether the architecture meets the stated goals and design principles.

> **Step 3: Financial Details.** The next step is to present the financial modeling of the plan architecture that has been voted upon. At this step, the numbers should be blinded; that is, there should be no physician-identifying information in the financial modeling. Also at this step, the physicians should again be asked to vote on the methodological design of the plan.

> **Step 4: Individual Financial Detail.** By Step 4, the goals, design principles, plan architecture, and plan methodology have been agreed to. At this step, each physician should be given his or her own personal production and financial information under the new plan in a confidential fashion (e.g., in a sealed envelope).

➤ DECISION MAKING IN HOSPITAL-AFFILIATED OR HOSPITAL-EMPLOYED PRACTICES

In hospital-employed medical practices or medical practices that are closely affiliated with a hospital, the ultimate decision making regarding the plan will typically rest with the hospital board. Nonetheless, a group of hospital and physician leaders will be actively involved in plan development, and the plan development, decision making, and implementation processes will commonly be similar to those outlined above in the private practice context. This is because a successful plan will require adequate levels of physician understanding, acceptance, and buy-in regarding plan design. Accordingly, the physician leaders who are involved in plan design will need to take active steps to ensure that the physicians' issues are heard by the compensation planning committee and by leaders of the delivery system. A compensation plan that is not accepted by a majority of the physicians, for example, will create ill will among the key players in the delivery system and may lead to physician recruitment and retention problems. The plan should be shared with physicians, and the physicians should have appropriate time and avenues with which to provide their comments.

► DECISION MAKING IN ACADEMIC PRACTICES

Similar to the hospital setting, in academic practices, the overall faculty practice plan may be decided by the board, the regents, the dean, the department chair, or other party, yet faculty members must still understand, accept, and buy in to the plan design. Here, too, the process outlined above will commonly be essential for understanding and buy-in, although the particular level of faculty involvement in plan development and ultimate decision making may vary. Faculty members should be given sufficient time to review the plan and its details, and again, channels to permit communication of issues and concerns should be established.

A BALLOT APPROACH TO DECISION MAKING

An example of a decision-making approach that can be used by medical practices as they decide on a new compensation plan is provided below. Descriptive materials summarizing the proposed plan alternatives (narrative form with examples of mathematical calculations but *without* practice-specific financial modeling results) would accompany this balloting approach.

A sample communication memo to the medical practice's physicians is provided in Exhibit 4.2. The actual memo may be more extensive and detailed by providing a summary of the plan options, sample calculations (using hypothetical data), and related information. This memo can also be accompanied by a formal ballot. A sample ballot used for this purpose is provided in Exhibits 4.3 and 4.4. In this example, the balloting involves a two-part process. In Part I, the physicians are asked to evaluate each plan option with respect to the compensation plan goals. In Part II of the balloting, physicians are asked to rank-order their preferred options. In this example, three discrete options are presented for consideration. In most instances, the financial results of multiple options are generally similar; therefore, the true focus will be on the plan philosophy and mechanics rather than on the bottom-line financial results. In many cases, however, the plan development process will result in only one truly recommended plan – in which case the ballot process will be designed to promote an objective evaluation of the recommended option rather than an assessment of how one option compares to another.

Through the use of such a formalized approach, physicians have the opportunity to provide feedback and share their preferences before putting the compensation plan to a formal vote process. This feedback is typically taken into consideration in the

EXHIBIT 4.2

Physician Compensation Memo – Decision Making Regarding New Plan

To: Physicians, Medical Practice Anywhere
From: Compensation Planning Committee
RE: Decision Making Regarding Compensation Plan Options

As you are aware, the Compensation Planning Committee was charged with identifying three compensation plan options for physician consideration. The purpose of this memo is to obtain your feedback regarding the identified plan options.

Compensation Plan Goals

The goals that were identified for the new compensation plan and that have previously been shared with you are summarized below:

- ▶ Have a fair system.
- ▶ Have income be allocated appropriately.
- ▶ Allow equitable distribution of overhead based on resource utilization.
- ▶ Avoid competition for cases between divisions and specialties.
- ▶ Maintain current practice culture.
- ▶ Have a flexible system that can change over time.
- ▶ Promote responsibility and accountability for revenue and expense.
- ▶ Have a plan that is simple, understandable, and easy to administer.
- ▶ Have a transparent and objective system.
- ▶ Promote the practice's long-term success.

Additional Comments and Concerns

Other concerns that were expressed by physicians included a need to compensate physicians fairly for outreach activities and to ensure that differential payer mixes among physicians do not negatively impact compensation levels.

Compensation Plan Options

Three compensation plan options are outlined on separate attachments. The options range from largely "individualistic" to more "team-oriented" plans.

Option I involves significant levels of specialty, location, and physician-specific cost accounting of revenues and expenses.

Option II involves more of a team-oriented plan involving the allocation of overhead costs on a combined or equal share basis, combined with separate allocation methods of the net amount available for compensation.

Option III involves more of a team-oriented plan involving allocation of a small portion of practice revenues across the group as a whole, combined with the use of equal share compensation in all divisions.

Consider the following questions in connection with your review of each of the three plan options:

1. Which of the compensation plan goals are promoted (or not) through the option?

2. Does the option address (or not address) the "other comments" and concerns referenced above?

3. What's good and bad about the option – both from an individual physician and group (or division) perspective?

4. In what other ways does the option promote, or potentially detract from, the goals that have been identified?

Rank the three options using the ranking sheet provided, and using the goals identified above as ranking criteria. Your rankings should not be viewed as "making a final decision" on the plan options at this time, but will provide a sense of the practice's collective views to help inform and guide discussions and ultimate decision making.

© 2006 Johnson & Walker Keegan

EXHIBIT 4.3 Decision-Making Ballot for a New Compensation Plan – Part I

Part I – Evaluate each option using the following scale

4 = Strongly Agree (e.g., this option does an excellent job of meeting this goal)

3 = Agree

2 = Disagree

1 = Strongly Disagree (e.g., this option does a very poor job of meeting this goal)

0 = Don't Know

Goal Statement	Ranking Option I	Ranking Option II	Ranking Option III
1. Fair system			
2. Appropriate allocation of income – no subsidies			
3. Equitable distribution of overhead based on resource utilization			
4. Avoid competition for cases between divisions and specialties			
5. Maintain current practice culture			
6. Flexible (not static) system that can change			
7. Promote responsibility and accountability – income and expense			
8. Simple, understandable, and easy to administer			
9. Transparent and objective system without nitpicking			
10. Promote group's long-term success			

© 2006 Johnson & Walker Keegan

committee's deliberations to determine if additional committee work or communication vehicles are required prior to a formal vote on the new compensation plan.

We cannot overstate the importance of attending to the key "process" elements in compensation planning. The combination of communication and incremental decisions over time will typically yield a final voting process that is nonadversarial or, at the very least, that will ensure that the practice is not blindsided with respect to physician issues and concerns at this last and final step of the compensation plan journey.

EXHIBIT 4.4   Decision-Making Ballot for a New Compensation Plan – Part II

Part II – Based on your knowledge and understanding of the plan options described here, rank your preferences of the plan options (circle one preference per line).

Most preferred – I like this one	Option I	Option II	Option III
Second most preferred	Option I	Option II	Option III
Least preferred – I dislike this one the most	Option I	Option II	Option III

© 2006 Johnson & Walker Keegan

IMPLEMENTATION PLANS

Implementation plans are a way of "getting from here to there." An implementation plan typically outlines steps that the medical practice will take to get to the end result – the final compensation plan that has been developed. The length of time it takes to implement a new compensation plan will depend upon a number of factors, including:

- ➤ Financial solvency of the practice;
- ➤ Leverage for change;
- ➤ Current data systems and organizational readiness;
- ➤ Magnitude of change from current compensation methodology;
- ➤ Magnitude of projected change from current compensation levels; and
- ➤ Physician readiness.

Some implementation plans are essentially "turnkey"; that is, there is really no transition or interim plan. A turnkey approach is typically taken when there are financial and/or legal imperatives requiring change – the medical practice simply has no choice but to transition its compensation plan "overnight."

In other medical practices, plans that will provide for plan implementation over a relatively short period of time (e.g., three to six months), or a more gradual implementation over a one- or two-year period, will be outlined to help get the physicians engaged in the new process, provide time to collect and monitor new data, foster physician understanding of the plan's approach to performance measurement, and provide some transition with regard to changing or fluctuating compensation levels under any new plan.

There are three distinct types of plan implementations that can be used to move the medical practice from today's plan to tomorrow's plan: (1) incremental; (2) blended; and (3) segmented.

► INCREMENTAL ADOPTION

Under this approach, new compensation plans are adopted at a strategic (e.g., system-wide) level but are implemented with respect to individual physicians in an incremental manner (e.g., as contracts are renewed). This approach is often used if there is a wide diversity of existing compensation plan arrangements, as is common in many hospital-affiliated and academic practices (but less common in physician-owned group practice settings). The use of this approach permits time for physicians to understand the common vision and approach taken by a new compensation plan architecture.

► BLENDED ADOPTION

A blended approach moves the medical practice incrementally forward to its new compensation end state by blending portions of the current plan and the new plan over time. For example, if a medical group has historically been compensating physicians based on gross charges from professional services and now seeks compensation based on net collections from professional services, the implementation plan could involve a "blending" of the measures over a defined time period. An example of this blended approach to compensation plan implementation is depicted in Exhibit 4.5. This example illustrates a fairly lengthy implementation process. Implementation over a shorter time period (e.g., one to two years) may also be in order, depending upon the circumstances.

► SEGMENTED ADOPTION

The segmented approach involves implementing portions of the plan in distinct segments over time. The specifics of compensation implementation plans are typically highly detailed due to the importance of these plans in assisting the medical practice

EXHIBIT 4.5   Blended Approach to Plan Implementation

Year 1:   75% gross charges/25% net collections

Year 2:   50% gross charges/50% net collections

Year 3:   25% gross charges/75% net collections

Year 4:   100% net collections

© 2006 Johnson & Walker Keegan

EXHIBIT 4.6   Segmented Approach to Plan Implementation

Year 1:   Continue negotiated salary levels; however, provide data to reflect new compensation plan as if it were in effect.

Year 2:   Continue negotiated salary levels; however, place 15% "at risk" and pay the at-risk portion consistent with the new plan.

Year 3:   100% base plus incentive plan.

to "move from here to there." For example, if a medical practice historically has been compensating physicians via a negotiated salary arrangement, a base plus incentive plan that puts compensation "at risk" will typically require some sort of transition arrangement. Exhibit 4.6 illustrates an example of this segmented approach to plan implementation. Here, too, a shorter or longer implementation process may be in order, depending upon the circumstances.

Key elements for any compensation implementation plan include the actual measurements and computations for the new compensation plan, identification of responsible parties for each element of the plan's implementation, the assigned role of physicians in the implementation process, availability of data and reporting formats provided to physicians, and a defined process by which compensation and/or measurement can be contested by physicians.

In developing implementation plans, it is important to ensure that the time line to achieve the end-state plan is not drawn out beyond that which is absolutely necessary. As we have described, the life cycle of the compensation plan changes over time, as do the specific circumstances in which the medical practice resides. A combination of time and circumstance can derail a new compensation plan's implementation as medical practices continually seek to balance change with readiness. A well-documented implementation process, coupled with a relatively tight time line, is preferable to one that languishes over time.

State-of-the-Art Strategies

"The future cannot be known. The only thing certain about it is that it will be different from, rather than a continuation of, today."

PETER F. DRUCKER

INTRODUCTION

In Part II, we discuss state-of-the-art strategies for physician compensation plan development. Part II is organized into three separate subsections. We first present a discussion of compensation plan options, situating each option on a compensation plan matrix representing an array of compensation plan architectures. We then progress to detailed dimensions of compensation plan design. The five chapters in this subsection on state-of-the-art strategies discuss benchmarking for compensation plan purposes, pay-for-performance (P4P) reimbursement and compensation strategies, legal and special issues in compensation plan design, and finally, the development and implementation of transition plans to address compensation issues for physicians in part-time, slowdown, and similar statuses. We conclude this part of the book with a discussion of state-of-the-art industry trends and their impact on physician compensation planning and development. The key industry trends are a direct result of the significant challenges and changes facing medical practices today.

Part II of the book is organized as follows:

1. **State-of-the-Art Structures**
   Chapter 5: Compensation Plan Options – The Compensation Plan Matrix
   Chapter 6: Compensation Plan Architectures

2. **State-of-the-Art Dimensions**
   Chapter 7: Measuring Physician Work and Effort
   Chapter 8: Pay-for-Performance (P4P) and Physician Compensation
   Chapter 9: The Legal Element
   Chapter 10: Special Issues in Physician Compensation
   Chapter 11: Physician Transition Plans – Physicians in Part-Time, Slowdown, and Similar Status

3. **State-of-the-Art Trends**
   Chapter 12: Industry Trends in Physician Compensation

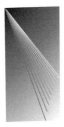

FIVE

Compensation Plan Options – The Compensation Plan Matrix

Our experience in working with numerous physician compensation plans over the years has led us to identify a number of core "truths" related to physician compensation.

First, there is no perfect compensation plan – only alternatives that are more or less imperfect.

Second, no two compensation plans are precisely the same. For example, two "production-based" plans will commonly differ in how production is measured, how expenses are allocated, how outside income and personal expenses are treated, and in other ways. In physician compensation plans, the details matter.

Third, all plans relate to and influence the medical practice itself – its goals, its physician practice styles, and its overall culture.

And finally, every plan must deal with and address the most basic of financial realities involving practice-related revenues and expenses.

Of these four "truths," the last two are the most important and the most interrelated. They relate to the culture of the medical practice and its financial realities.

CULTURE AND COMPENSATION

The medical practice's compensation plan will help to determine – and can either promote or detract from – the practice's goals and its desired culture. In most medical practices, the culture is most tangibly reflected in the compensation plan – whether that culture is an "all-for-one-and-one-for-all" culture of mutual support, a competitive "dog-eat-dog" culture, or something in-between. The culture of the medical practice is apparent by simply reading its compensation plan and its plan mechanics. It is easy to determine whether the medical practice is simply a collection of individual physician practices or a true group practice based on the plan architecture and measures that are used. In some medical practices, a new compensation plan is viewed as a useful vehicle to help change the practice culture by promoting and rewarding certain practice goals that have heretofore not been at the forefront of physician focus, attention, and/or behavior.

FINANCIAL REALITIES AND COMPENSATION

Regardless of the setting or situation, revenues and expenses must be considered – either directly or indirectly – as part of any compensation plan. This is the financial reality of medical practices (and, indeed, of most businesses). In every medical practice, the compensation plan must take into account the financial realities of the medical practice, the reimbursement environment in which it functions (e.g., fee-for-service, capitation, pay-for-performance [P4P]), the types of services that the physicians perform (e.g., professional services, ancillary services, outreach activities, leadership roles), the money that is available, the cost of practice operations, and the pragmatic reality that, in the end, the only way for each physician to receive more money is for the funds available for compensation to increase.

These last two truths involving a practice's culture and finances are dynamically interrelated, and they bring us to our final "truth." As long as there is plenty of money to go around, even the worst plan can look like a winner. Conversely, when the pot of money is too small, even the most methodologically artful plan will be an utter disaster. Effective compensation plans truly meld the practice's financial realities with the practice's culture to promote success. Thus, understanding these two compensation plan dimensions – culture and finances – can help us to better understand current compensation plans and inform the development of a new compensation plan for a medical practice.

COMPENSATION PLAN DIMENSIONS

There are literally hundreds of different compensation plans that are used in different medical practice settings. While no two plans are exactly the same, it is possible to understand the plans by reference to the cultural and financial truths related to compensation plans.

Because issues of culture and financial mechanics are so fundamental to any physician compensation plan, it will be useful to understand how these dimensions are perceived and how they interrelate. These dimensions are depicted in Exhibit 5.1, which shows the two separate axes or dimensions of compensation. The horizontal or X-axis of Exhibit 5.1 reflects the culture and practice style that are promoted through the compensation plan. The Y-axis reflects the financial dimensions of compensation plans in terms of revenue and expenditure treatment. These dimensions can provide a solid foundation for a more useful (and complex) framework or matrix for understanding how compensation plans work, and how these concepts can be combined to create an almost infinite number of plans. Before moving on to that more sophisticated matrix, however, we will quickly review some basics.

EXHIBIT 5.1 Compensation Plan Dimensions

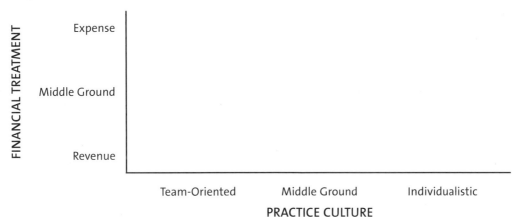

© 2006 Johnson & Walker Keegan

➤ THE CULTURAL X-AXIS:
TEAM-ORIENTED TO INDIVIDUALISTIC PLANS

As depicted in Exhibit 5.1, at one end of the cultural (horizontal) X-axis are plans that recognize and reward "team-oriented" activity. We use the concept of "team" in this context to represent the fact that the practice's physicians engage in and support some level of sharing and teamwork, or compensation is based on and is more directly linked to overall medical practice (as opposed to individual physician) performance.

At the opposite extreme of the cultural X-axis are "individualistic" plans, which tend to adopt an individual physician focus, recognizing and rewarding productivity and performance of each physician. Not surprisingly, in practices in which such an individualistic approach to compensation is used, the level of "group practice" orientation and teamwork is typically less than in other settings. The individualistic vs. team orientation of a medical practice is reflected in its compensation plan, and, in turn, in its practice culture.

Of course, the cultural "middle ground" that falls between these two extremes is enormous. In fact, most medical practices use a compensation plan methodology that promotes a culture that combines some level of teamwork with individual physician performance.

► THE FINANCIAL Y-AXIS: REVENUE-TO-EXPENSE TREATMENT

The vertical Y-axis reflects the medical practice's approach to financial issues, or, simply put, how the math works in the context of the compensation plan. In physician compensation, as in any business, two financial dimensions are addressed:

- ► How **revenues** are measured and allocated in connection with the compensation plan; and
- ► How **expenses** of the practice are measured, allocated, and considered as part of the plan.

As with the cultural dimension, this financial dimension also has extremes that are reflected in different compensation plans. Some plans have a decided revenue focus in that the plan methodology focuses physician attention – at the individual or some other level – on revenue generation, production, or work. Other plans focus on practice expenses – sometimes to an extreme level.

The financial Y-axis also has large "middle ground" models that consider both issues of revenue and expense allocation in compensation plan design.

These basic concepts, as reflected on the X- and Y-axes illustrating compensation plan dimensions, lead to descriptions of general compensation plan "typologies" or "architectures" that are reviewed throughout the rest of this book. These architectures incorporate these core cultural and financial dimensions and range along the horizontal axis from (1) team-oriented plans through (2) middle ground plans to (3) individualistic plans. Before going much further, let's review the dimensions of these three basic stops.

► TEAM-ORIENTED PLANS

Not surprisingly, team-oriented plans tend to place a cultural focus on the performance of the "team" or the practice as a whole, minimizing the focus on individual physician performance. Team-oriented plans generally recognize and pay practice expenses "off the top," out of all available practice revenues, to create a compensation pool that is then allocated among practice physicians. The compensation plan focuses on distributing the compensation pool rather than focusing attention on how practice expenses are allocated. In this regard, team-oriented models tend to treat the *practice* as a single economic unit and involve some level of "sharing" rather than simply functioning as a collection of separate profit-and-loss centers of individual physician practices, as is found in individualistic compensation plans. Examples of team-oriented plans are those involving equal share or partnership compensation models and straight salary plans.

Advantages of Team-Oriented Plans

- ► Recognize the reality of a single economic unit and "group practice";
- ► Promote a collaborative work ethic;

▸ Permit production orientation (even with a significant equal share methodology);

▸ Are simple and straightforward;

▸ Can be linked to market levels of compensation; and

▸ Can include clear messages regarding performance expectations.

Disadvantages of Team-Oriented Plans

▸ Are more difficult to sustain with large variations in production and work levels between physicians;

▸ Lack direct responsibility for costs and/or resource utilization;

▸ Enable some physicians to shirk responsibilities absent a strong group culture or explicit performance expectations; and

▸ May not provide sufficient reward for "working harder."

➤ INDIVIDUALISTIC PLANS

Individualistic plans place a cultural emphasis on the performance of individual physicians in the practice rather than on a more global group practice orientation. They do so by treating each individual physician as a largely separate profit-and-loss center for compensation plan purposes. These types of compensation plans typically involve a specific allocation of a portion of group practice revenues to individual physicians, along with an explicit allocation of a portion of the practice's expenses, in order to determine physician compensation.

Examples of individualistic plans include allocation of revenue based on individual production combined with cost accounting or similar expense allocation methods. Thus, the financial model of individualistic plans typically addresses both revenue and expense allocation. Because questions of both revenue and expense allocation are addressed in individualistic plans, there are two broad areas in which physicians can have differing views (and disputes) regarding what is a "fair" and appropriate approach to such issues in the compensation arrangement.

Advantages of Individualistic Plans

▸ Can allow for an "eat-what-you-kill" or "eat-what-you-treat" format to reward individual physician effort and work;

▸ Promote a sense of individual responsibility for costs;

▸ Are arguably easy to administer;

▸ Can include a clear message regarding expectations; and

▸ Are consistent with an intuitive view of how income is determined (i.e., revenues minus expenses).

Disadvantages of Individualistic Plans

► May undermine a group practice perspective;

► May lead to behaviors associated with the "dark side" of productivity; for example, patient theft or churning (scheduling patients for more visits when not necessary);

► May permit expense allocation fights to emerge; and

► Can permit expense micromanagement and a desire to shift expenses.

► MIDDLE GROUND PLANS

Middle ground plans are those that blend aspects of team-oriented and individualistic approaches. These plans frequently involve any number of mixed methodologies, which is understandable given that these models sit in between the extremes of team-oriented and individualistic compensation plans. These plans generally consider and address the allocation of both practice revenues and practice expenses in determining physician pay, but they also typically involve different degrees of either explicit or implicit "sharing" within the compensation plan.

For example, one type of middle ground plan that tends to have a team orientation is a base plus incentive plan. In this plan, there is typically a base or guaranteed level of compensation that is predicated on physician performance of a basic set of expectations. An additional incentive can be earned, with that incentive itself frequently awarded based on productivity and/or profitability thresholds or targets at the individual physician level, at the specialty level, at the department level, at the practice level, or in combination. This base plus incentive model combines team-oriented features (i.e., a largely guaranteed base salary) with a more individualistic dimension (i.e., a productivity-based incentive component).

THE COMPENSATION PLAN MATRIX

While our basic discussion regarding compensation plan dimensions is helpful, it only tells part of the story. It provides a general perspective regarding how the cultural and financial dimensions of compensation are interrelated – but it is limited as a tool that can be used to describe or understand the numerous compensation plans existing today. Moreover, it does not provide much of a framework to help readers determine where their current compensation plan resides and where they might go in terms of alternative compensation plans.

However, a more expanded version of our basic discussion regarding compensation plan dimensions in the form of a more formal compensation plan "matrix" will fit the bill. Our compensation plan matrix, depicted in Exhibit 5.2, uses the basic X (cultural) and Y (financial) axes previously referenced – but it provides more detail to help describe the alternatives and options that can be combined to represent different basic types of compensation plan architectures through its definition of **nine basic plan "elements."** These elements can be used, either independently or in combination, to describe virtually the full range of compensation plans that are used and/or available to a particular medical practice.

EXHIBIT 5.2 The Compensation Plan Matrix

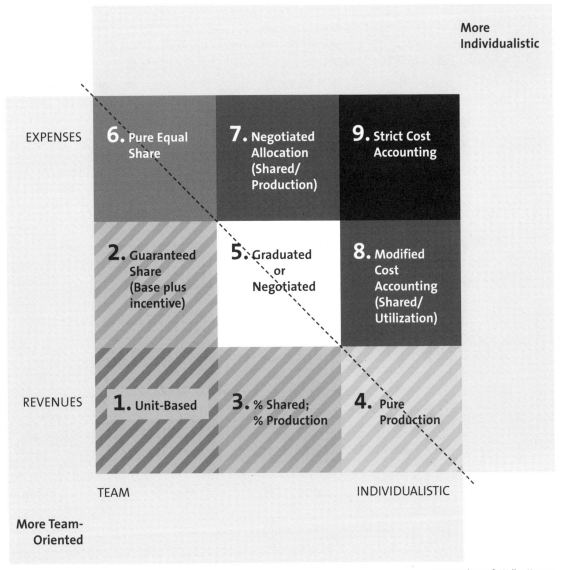

© 2006 Johnson & Walker Keegan

The nine basic plan elements consist of four revenue elements, four expense elements, and one mixed element (encompassing both revenue and expense treatment). These elements serve as the basis for most compensation plans, although other features (including additional incentive measures linked to quality, P4P, or similar measures) may also be layered onto or incorporated directly into the architectures that can be developed through the use of these elements. In Exhibit 5.2, the four revenue elements are depicted in varying shades of light gray with diagonal lines, while the expense elements are represented by darker shades of gray to black.

Revenue Elements 1 through 4 address how practice revenues or income are treated as part of a physician compensation plan. These revenue-oriented elements generally involve more of a positive cultural focus. In Exhibit 5.2, the most team-oriented element (Revenue Element 1) is represented by medium gray with diagonal lines. The most individualistic of these elements (Revenue Element 4) is represented by a lighter gray with diagonal lines. More precisely, these elements consist of the following:

► **Revenue Element 1**: Unit-based allocation of revenues or income (e.g., equal share and straight salary plans, or even plans that pay a defined dollar amount for each work relative value unit [WRVU]).

► **Revenue Element 2**: Guaranteed share of revenues (e.g., base salary plus incentive plans), plus other incentive measures (e.g., addressing qualitative issues).

► **Revenue Element 3**: Combined equal share and production-based allocation of revenues or income (e.g., 50 percent equal share, 50 percent production-based revenue allocation).

► **Revenue Element 4**: Pure production-based methods used to allocate revenues or income.

Expense Elements 6 through 9 express the expense portion of the matrix; these elements are represented by even darker shades of gray to black. These four darker squares (6 through 9) represent different approaches to expenses. The most team-oriented approach to expense treatment (Expense Element 6 – pure equal share) is depicted in a medium gray; the most individualistic approach to expense treatment (Expense Element 9, involving "strict cost accounting") is represented by the color black. The four elements on our matrix addressing expense treatment consist of the following:

► **Expense Element 6:** Equal share expense allocation (e.g., with expenses expressly divided on an equal share basis, and that equal share being included in a mathematical calculation that is used to determine physician compensation).

► **Expense Element 7:** Negotiated expense allocation with a production-based component (e.g., 50 percent equal share, 50 percent production-based expense allocation).

► **Expense Element 8:** Modified cost accounting involving utilization-based expense allocation systems (e.g., expense allocation methods in which practice expenses are divided into broad categories of "direct" [physician-specific], "fixed" [or equal share], and "variable" [utilization-based]).

► **Expense Element 9:** Strict cost accounting expense allocation based entirely on utilization (to the extent possible).

Squarely in the middle of our matrix is **Element 5**, in which revenues and/or expenses may be negotiated or graduated. Examples of compensation arrangements using this type of methodology include:

► Graduated payments per WRVU (e.g., $25 per WRVU for the first 3,000 WRVUs, $28 for the next 2,000 WRVUs, $30 for the next 2,000 WRVUs, etc.); and

► Plans that apply different "overhead" assessments or "taxes" to physician-generated revenues on a "tiered" basis (e.g., 60 percent of the first $400,000; 55 percent of the next $200,000, etc.).

This is a true middle ground element in that it frequently involves a variety of "blended" approaches to revenues and expenses as part of the plan methodology.

Exhibits 5.3 through 5.5 summarize the nine elements that comprise the compensation plan matrix – encompassing matrix revenue elements, matrix expense elements, and the matrix middle ground element – and provide examples of these elements.

► PLAN "ARCHITECTURES" BASED ON THE NINE ELEMENTS

The nine elements in the compensation plan matrix can be used to represent and describe the universe of compensation plan architectures. By "architectures," we refer to the basic approach or framework that is used in a compensation plan. That framework effectively considers and addresses the cultural and financial dimensions of compensation. Specifically, the matrix elements can be used, either individually or in combination, to describe 18 distinct architectures, with each falling on different points on an array of team-oriented to individualistic model architectures. The various combinations of revenue and expense elements are illustrated in Exhibit 5.6.

The specific architectures referenced in Exhibit 5.6 will be examined in greater detail in Chapter 6. For present purposes, it is important for medical practices to understand their current compensation plan by reference to the compensation plan matrix and the array of architectures referenced on Exhibit 5.6, as this serves as a useful starting point for compensation plan discussion.

For example, if the practice uses a base plus incentive plan (using Revenue Element 2 on the matrix), and the practice does not include an explicit overhead or expense assessment as part of its methodology, then the practice has a heavily team-oriented plan at the present time (Architecture B on the array referenced in Exhibit 5.6). As will be described later on, if the practice has determined that one of the goals of a new compensation plan is to make physicians more responsible and accountable for the costs associated with their practice, then any number of compensation architectures would

EXHIBIT 5.3-A   Matrix Revenue Elements

6	7	9
2	5	8
1	3	4

REVENUES

Element 1 – Unit-based

► Dollars per WRVU, equal share, straight salary, hourly

Element 2 – Guaranteed share (base plus incentive)

► Market-based salary plus incentive

► Quality, citizenship, and other incentive pools

Element 3 – % Shared and % production

► 50/50, 25/75, (or other split) with production portion

Element 4 – Pure production-based

► Actual professional services net collections or percent of production (measured by professional services gross charges, WRVUs, etc.)

Element 5 – Graduated/negotiated

► Graduated and "tiered" percentage of professional services gross charges or net collections or dollars per WRVU

Examples of Matrix Revenue Elements

Revenue Dimension	Examples
Element 1 – Unit-based share of revenues or income	► Straight salary ► 100% equal share ► Compensation per unit of work, measured by WRVUs, percentage of professional services gross charges, net charges, net collections, etc. ► Hourly rates
Element 2 – Modified sharing of revenues or income (e.g., base plus incentive) plus other incentive	► Base salary plus incentive ► Market-based salary plus incentive ► Nonclinical production-based incentive determined by qualitative, patient satisfaction, or other measures
Element 3 – Combined equal share and production-based allocation of revenues or income	► 70% equal share of net income with 30% production-based incentive (or other percentage combinations)
Element 4 – Pure production-based allocation of revenues or income	► Total net income allocated 100% based on individual physician net collections ► Total net income allocated based on each physician's percent to total production (with production measured by professional services gross or net charges, WRVUs, or other measures)

© 2006 Johnson & Walker Keegan

EXHIBIT 5.4-A   Matrix Expense Elements

EXPENSES

Element 5 – Graduated or negotiated

► Percent to total net collections, market-based, or graduated/tiered expense allocation

Element 6 – Pure equal share

► Explicit equal share expense allocation

Element 7 – Negotiated allocation (shared/production)

► 50/50, 25/75, or other percentage combinations; based on production (higher production incurs greater portion)

Element 8 – Modified cost accounting

► Fixed (shared), variable, and direct based on estimated utilization (higher utilization incurs higher portion)

Element 9 – Strict cost accounting

► Microlevel cost allocation based on utilization

EXHIBIT 5.4-B Examples of Matrix Expense Elements

Expense Dimension	Examples
Element 6 – Equal share expense allocation	▶ Expenses allocated on pure equal share basis, and explicitly as part of formula
Element 7 – Negotiated expense allocation with production-based component	▶ 50% equal share, 50% production-based expense allocation (or other percentages)
Element 8 – Modified cost accounting expense (shared and based on utilization)	▶ Modified cost accounting of expenses (with combined sharing and utilization-based expense allocation) ▶ Allocation of expenses into three to four "buckets" consisting of direct (physician-specific) expenses, fixed (equal share) expenses, variable (utilization-based) expenses
Element 9 – Strict cost accounting expense allocation based on utilization	▶ Strict cost accounting of expenses based on utilization to maximum extent possible ▶ Use of multiple (e.g., 5 to 10) methods to allocate discrete expense types (e.g., CME and nursing staff on direct, per-physician basis; medical records costs based on chart pulls; rent based on square footage and exam room schedules, etc.). Typically involves high levels of granularity in expense allocation among practice physicians

EXHIBIT 5.5

Example of Matrix Middle Ground Element

Element 5 – Graduated or negotiated revenue/ expense allocation method	▶ Graduated percentage of revenues or net collections (e.g., 60% of first $400,000; 40% of next $200,000; etc.)
	▶ Graduated dollars per WRVU based on production (e.g., $28 per WRVU for first 5,000; $30 per work RVU for next 2,000; etc.)
	▶ Market-based expense allocation (e.g., uniform expense allocation on first $300,000 of revenues; specialty-specific overhead "tax" (based on practice specialty) applied to remaining revenues)
	▶ Graduated overhead assessment based on production (60% of first $400,000 of net collections; 50% of next $200,000; etc.)

© 2006 Johnson & Walker Keegan

be available that could help promote these goals, although all such models would move to the right on the array in Exhibit 5.6 to plans that are more individualistic in nature.

As illustrated in the array of architectures shown in Exhibit 5.6, some of the plan architectures tend to have a more "team-oriented" perspective, while others tend to be more individualistic. Architectures that involve only revenue elements (without an express allocation of expenses in the plan methodology) will be the most heavily "team-oriented."

Conversely, those that combine revenue and expense elements from the matrix will be more individualistic in nature. A plan architecture that combines Revenue Element 4 – pure productivity-based revenue allocation – with Expense Element 9 – pure cost accounting of expenses – constitutes the most individualistic of all architectures. This is the most individualistic model from a cultural perspective given that it focuses almost exclusively on the performance of the individual physician in *both* revenue and expense treatment.

In compensation plan development, one or more of the 18 overall architectures will typically be selected as a "preferred" architecture that will be considered for use in the medical practice. By this we mean that the practice and its physicians will typically determine that they prefer architectures that are more team-oriented, more individualistic, or more in the "middle."

Once one or more preferred architectures is selected, the architecture(s) will then be more fully defined and detailed as part of the plan development process. This additional definition and detailing will involve making plan-specific decisions within the

EXHIBIT 5.6

Array of Compensation Plan Architectures

Architecture	A	B	C	D	E	F	G	H	I	J	K	L	M	N	O	P	Q	R
Revenue Element	1	2	3	4	5	2	3	2	3	2	3	2	3	4	4	4	4	4
Expense Element						6	6	7	7	8	8	9	9	5	6	7	8	9
	TEAM					MIDDLE GROUND								INDIVIDUALISTIC				

basic architectural framework. For example, under a largely team-oriented Architecture C that uses Revenue Element 3 involving a combined equal share and production-based allocation of revenues or income, the practice will address questions such as:

► What portion of total revenues should be allocated on an equal share basis, and what portion should be based on production?

► What measure (or combination of measures) should be used to allocate the production portion (e.g., gross charges from professional services, net collections from professional services, WRVUs, or a combination of one or more of these)?

► At what level or levels should the architecture be applied (e.g., across the practice as a whole, at individual division/specialty, or practice site level)?

When fully detailed, any single compensation plan that is built by a medical practice based upon one of these basic architectures will be further distinguished from other plans by a high degree of variability as to the "science" of the plan – the system of measurements, methods, targets, and other plan characteristics and features. The basic architectures can also be supplemented through the use of additional methods and measures, such as those focusing on quality, efficiency, use of technology, or the like. In all instances, however, the basic foundational elements for virtually any new compensation plan can be described by reference to the elements on the compensation plan matrix, and those elements can be used to describe the basic plan architecture.

The major compensation plan architectures that are commonly developed and used based on the nine elements in the compensation plan matrix are described in detail in the next chapter, along with a brief review of the advantages and disadvantages of each. However, before moving to that review, some additional information and discussion is needed regarding the range of options available for the treatment of practice revenue and expenses.

REVENUE TREATMENT

Two important areas to consider when determining revenue allocation are: (1) the "funds flow" model; and (2) the precise revenue allocation method to be used in the mathematical formula of the compensation plan.

► FUNDS FLOW MODELS

Funds flow models address the treatment of revenues that are used for physician compensation purposes. In simplistic terms, the funds flow model addresses several questions:

- ► What are the various sources of revenues or funds that "come into" the practice?
- ► How are "assessments" or "taxes" determined and applied to these funds?
- ► How is each of the fund sources utilized for compensation purposes?

Given the importance of funds flow issues, detailed discussions during the compensation plan development process will commonly occur relative to different types or sources of practice revenues, including:

- ► Revenue from professional services (e.g., ambulatory encounters, hospital encounters, procedures, and surgeries);
- ► Revenue from risk contracts (e.g., P4P funds, managed care risk-pool refunds and awards, etc.);
- ► Revenue from ancillary services (e.g., technical components of diagnostic services);
- ► Revenue generated by nonphysician providers (e.g., nurse practitioners, physician assistants); and
- ► External income (e.g., expert witness fees, independent medical examinations, medical director stipends, research funds, etc.).

Each medical practice will typically consider and address the treatment of these and potentially other revenue sources available to its physicians. Importantly, however, the funds flow models that are used in academic and nonacademic practice settings will commonly differ, as described below.

Funds Flow Models in Nonacademic Practices

The funds flow model in a nonacademic or private practice is generally straightforward. The typical private practice generally has relatively limited sources of revenue. The largest source of revenue for most medical practices is that generated through professional services. However, the medical practice may also have ancillary services income as well as revenue associated with hospital medical director services, expert witness fees, honoraria, and other similar sources.

In a private practice, these different sources of practice revenues may be addressed separately for compensation plan purposes. For example, a typical nonacademic (e.g., private) medical practice may address two revenue sources: (1) professional fee earnings; and (2) ancillary services revenue. The compensation plan may treat each of these sources in different ways due to political, legal, regulatory, and potentially other issues (further discussed in Chapter 9, "The Legal Element"). As another example, medical practices may elect to apply a uniform rule that all revenues and income derived from services requiring medical licensure will be brought into the practice and used for compensation plan purposes, or it could take the position that some revenue sources (e.g., medical director income) need not "come into" the practice, but instead may be paid directly to the physician.

However, as a general matter, the funds flow and treatment of different revenue sources in a nonacademic or private practice will generally not create *major* problems or concerns, because most of the practice's activities and therefore its income will still be derived from "traditional" professional services fee-generating activities.

Funds Flow Models in Academic Practices

For good or for bad, issues of funds flow tend to be more extensively addressed in faculty practice plans. This is primarily due to the fact that, in such a setting, there are multiple, highly diverse funding sources that may be used to determine and pay faculty compensation. These may include support between and among the health system, the school of medicine, the practice plan, and the faculty-generated revenue associated with clinical activity, research, and outside professional activities. The funds flow model is typically designed in such a way as to create incentives to achieve performance outcomes that are consistent with strategic and tactical plans in support of the academic mission, including clinical, teaching, research, and service activities.

In the academic setting, therefore, in addition to addressing many of the same issues addressed in private practice settings, the funds flow model *also* addresses tithing mechanisms, such as the dean's tax and the departmental tax, and clarifies which revenue sources are to be counted and used for faculty compensation purposes.

As an example, academic institutions often differ with regard to the handling of expert witness fees. Some institutions require that this income be reported to (and deposited with) the university and essentially treat this income as they would professional fee revenue generated from professional services. Others may require that the money be deposited to the university; however, the taxation or tithing of these types of funds may be handled in a fashion that differs from that of professional fee earnings. Still other academic institutions may permit physicians to earn expert witness fees outside of the faculty practice plan but may impose limits on the number of days or hours physicians can devote to these types of outside professional activities. Furthermore, they may require mandatory reporting of all such activities. See Chapter 15, "Compensation Plans in Academic Practices," for a further discussion of funds flow models in academic practices.

Regardless of the type of medical practice, the funds flow model, as part of the compensation plan development process, should be defined clearly so that each physician understands the sources and uses of funds for compensation plan purposes.

► REVENUE DISTRIBUTION METHODS

Medical practice revenues are, of course, essential to the ability to pay compensation to physicians. Many methods are used to measure and allocate revenue to physicians in the context of a compensation plan. The basic indices used to measure productivity and allocate practice revenues for compensation plan purposes include the following:

► Net collections from physician professional services;

► Gross professional fee charges;

► Adjusted or net professional fee charges;

► WRVUs;

► Number of encounters (ambulatory, hospital, surgical, or in combination);

► Other unit-based measures (e.g., practice-defined "hybrid" work units, such as time measures);

► Per capita or equal share (commonly adjusted for clinical full-time equivalency [CFTE]);

► Negotiated basis (e.g., direct revenue allocation for capitation income combined with individual physician professional services net collections as a percent to total net collections for fee-for-service income; or based on a combination of one or more of these basic measures, such as a portion allocated based on individual physician WRVUs as a percent to total WRVUs, and the remaining percentage based on individual physician net collections as a percent to total net collections from professional services); and

► A combination of some or all of the above elements.

As with compensation plans more generally, there is no one "right" method to measure and distribute revenue or income for compensation plan purposes.

The revenue allocation method that is selected may also be linked to the funds flow model of the medical practice. For example, a surgeon may be paid a portion of his or her personally generated professional services revenue for nontrauma call activity, with trauma call income paid via a different distribution method. Trauma call income could, for example, be paid pursuant to a contract between the hospital and the physician practice and distributed using any number of methods, such as on an equal share basis, percentage of production basis, or based on a point scale (e.g., assigning one point per weeknight call and three points per weekend call).

EXPENSE TREATMENT

Just as there is no one "perfect" compensation plan, the myriad of ways to allocate practice expenses will impact physicians differentially based on their production, practice modality, specialty, practice setting (e.g., hospital employment, group practice, or otherwise), and many other factors.

Expenses can be allocated in any number of ways, although the basic mathematical options involve the following allocation methods:

► Based on utilization of the expense item – either actual or estimated;

► Based on production (e.g., some or all expenses are allocated on a percentage of production basis, with the physicians having the highest production bearing the highest portion of the expense, or graduated production methods involving allocation on a percentage of production basis up to a specific threshold, with a reduction in expense allocation as productivity increases);

► Explicit equal share allocation of practice expenses; or

► Using a negotiated expense allocation arrangement (e.g., 50 percent equal share combined with 50 percent based on estimated utilization or production).

To demonstrate the complexity of expenditure treatment – and the misunderstandings that often occur when nomenclature is applied to specific plan methods – Exhibit 5.7 outlines two methods to allocate practice expenses. Both are generally termed "equal share" allocation models; however, as demonstrated by these examples, each of these results in different compensation paid to the physician.

In Example A – a team-based "equal expense" plan – each physician is assessed the same *percentage* of his or her net collections to be used to pay practice expenses. In this example, each physician is assessed 50 percent of his or her net collections from professional services as overhead or practice expense, with the balance available for physician compensation purposes. For example, Physician A's net collections from professional services are $500,000, and 50 percent of this amount, or $250,000, is used for practice expenses, with $250,000 available for compensation purposes. On the other hand, Physician B, with net collections from professional services of $400,000, is assessed $200,000 for practice expenses, leaving $200,000 available for compensation.

In Example B – an individualistic "equal expense" plan – each physician pays the same *dollar level* of practice expenses. In this example, each of the physicians is assessed $230,000 for practice expenses, with the balance available to the physicians for compensation purposes. In this example, Physician A now has $270,000 available for compensation (rather than $250,000, as in Example A), and Physician B now has only $170,000 available for compensation (rather than the $200,000 he had in Example A).

As demonstrated by these examples, the nomenclature used to describe a compensation plan must be expanded to a more detailed level to truly explain the implications of the model on physician compensation.

EXHIBIT 5.7

Example of Expense Treatment

Physician	A	B	C	D	E	Total
Net Collections from Professional Services	$500,000	$400,000	$300,000	$500,000	$600,000	$2,300,000
Physician % to Total Production	22%	17%	13%	22%	26%	100%
Total Operating Expense (overhead)						$1,150,000

Example A.
"Team-Based" Plan: Total Operating Expense Is Distributed Based on an Equal Percentage of Production

	A	B	C	D	E	Total
Net Collections from Professional Services	$500,000	$400,000	$300,000	$500,000	$600,000	$2,300,000
Equal Share of Expense (equal percentage of net collections)	50%	50%	50%	50%	50%	
Dollar Amount Paid by Each Physician (50% × net collections)	$250,000	$200,000	$150,000	$250,000	$300,000	$1,150,000
Amount Available for Physician Compensation	$250,000	$200,000	$150,000	$250,000	$300,000	$1,150,000

Example B.
Individualistic Plan: Total Operating Expense Is Distributed Based on an Equal Dollar Level

	A	B	C	D	E	Total
Net Collections from Professional Services	$500,000	$400,000	$300,000	$500,000	$600,000	$2,300,000
Equal Share of Expense (equal dollar level overhead paid by each physician)	$230,000	$230,000	$230,000	$230,000	$230,000	$1,150,000
Amount Available for Physician Compensation	$270,000	$170,000	$70,000	$270,000	$370,000	$1,150,000
Percent of Net Collections Paid as Overhead	46%	58%	77%	46%	38%	

For some medical practices, cost of practice is easily handled – they simply use a team-oriented compensation plan and pay practice expenses as in Example A above, then distribute the rest as physician compensation. Under this approach, all physicians share practice expenses before they are paid, and each physician gives up an equal percentage of clinical practice revenues to pay practice overhead. Others use approaches more like Example B by allocating an equal portion of practice overhead costs across all physicians such that each physician effectively "pays" the same amount or portion of practice overhead costs, but each will then have different overhead percentages.

Of course, many practices ask whether any such "equal" distribution of practice expenses is appropriate. What about the physician who has two nurses to support his or her practice when his or her colleague has only one? What about the physician who insists on a specific costly supply item that only he or she uses? When physicians take issue with a largely equal cost distribution model, more detailed expenditure treatment models are commonly pursued to attempt to allocate the cost of practice to the physician or group of physicians who actually incur the cost (those using utilization-based expense allocation methods), or based on a percentage of production (with those producing more incurring a larger portion of expenses, as demonstrated in Example A above), or more sophisticated strategies involving tiered or graduated approaches based on production levels.

GAINING PERSPECTIVE ON CURRENT AND POTENTIAL FUTURE PLANS

As noted above, the combination of elements from our compensation plan matrix can be arrayed to reflect different types of plan architectures, as illustrated in Exhibit 5.6. The relative position of a particular plan architecture on the array is important. By understanding a medical practice's current compensation plan by reference to the matrix and by understanding the plan's position on our array of compensation plan architectures, we gain perspective regarding the practice's current culture and approach to finances, as well as on the types of plan alternatives that may be available to the practice.

Of course, a core objective of developing a new compensation plan is to develop one that better fits the particular culture of the medical practice as it exists today or, in some cases, to use the plan to help move a practice's culture in a particular direction (e.g., make the plan more individualistic to promote higher work levels). Thus, the array of compensation plan architectures set forth in Exhibit 5.6 can be used to assess where the practice's current compensation plan is today (e.g., whether it is at one end or another, or whether it is in the middle ground). Moreover, the matrix can be used to examine the range of basic options that may be available for a new compensation plan – where the practice might go with its plan in the future.

For example, a practice that currently uses a plan architecture at the most individualistic end of the array of architectures (e.g., an individualistic model that combines Revenue Element 4 [pure production] with Expense Element 9 [strict cost accounting of expenses]) will find it difficult to create a plan that is even more individualistic in nature. We say this because the current plan is already at the far end of the array of plan architectures. As a result, a practice already using such a highly individualistic architecture would generally have two basic options:

1. It might seek to refine the measures of revenue and expense allocation (to make the plan within this highly individualistic architecture even more individualistic by tracking individual variables to a greater or "more precise" degree); or

2. The practice might consider the need to promote more of a team orientation in its practice culture and financial management (e.g., as a means to help reduce competition within the practice for patients, minimize disputes over cost allocation, or resolve other issues that the practice might be facing in light of the heavily individualistic focus).

On this point, it is important to keep in mind the compensation plan evolution and change process discussed in Chapter 3. That is, since there is no perfect plan, and because perceptions of a plan's adequacy (or inadequacy) change based on a variety of factors, it is almost inevitable that today's plan will be rejected in favor of a plan that is viewed to be more desirable (tomorrow's plan). Furthermore, tomorrow's plan will likely "evolve" over time from an acceptable plan that meets practice and individual physician goals to one that is viewed to be unacceptable (for one reason or another) and therefore in need of change. That evolutionary process may take a long time (e.g., 10 or more years) or a short time (e.g., three to five years), and the speed of evolution may be hastened or slowed by internal and/or external developments. In many respects, however, the change process is inevitable.

In the next chapter, we describe and evaluate the major compensation plan architectures that serve as the basis for the methodological design of compensation plans.

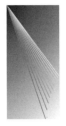

SIX

Compensation Plan Architectures

As discussed in Chapter 5, when different elements of the compensation plan matrix are combined, a number of discrete compensation plan "architectures" emerge. By "architectures," we refer to the basic approach or framework that is used in a plan methodology. That framework effectively considers and addresses the cultural and financial dimensions of compensation. Each architecture can be classified on an array ranging from highly team-oriented to largely individualistic compensation plans.

The nine basic elements in the compensation plan matrix can be combined to identify 18 basic architectures. Those architectures are arrayed from the most team-oriented to the most individualistic, as repeated in Exhibit 6.1. In the compensation plan development process, typically one or more of these architectures is initially selected as a "preferred" framework for the practice. One or more architectures is then more fully "tested" and defined, and the practice defines details of revenue and expense treatment within that architecture in any number of ways. For example, revenue can be distributed based on gross charges from professional services, net collections from professional services, work relative value units (WRVUs), or some other measure. Expenses can be distributed based on production, utilization, negotiation, or some other method. As a result, when a particular practice's compensation plan is fully detailed, it differs from those used elsewhere due to the variability of measurement systems, methods, targets, and other design characteristics.

EXHIBIT 6.1 Array of Compensation Plan Architectures

Architecture	A	B	C	D	E	F	G	H	I	J	K	L	M	N	O	P	Q	R
Revenue Element	1	2	3	4	5	2	3	2	3	2	3	2	3	4	4	4	4	4
Expense Element						6	6	7	7	8	8	9	9	5	6	7	8	9
	TEAM					MIDDLE GROUND								INDIVIDUALISTIC				

In this chapter, we review the major plan architectures as summarized on the array in Exhibit 6.1 and assess their general advantages and disadvantages. We examine these basic architectures by reference to whether each promotes a largely team-oriented, individualistic, or "middle ground" culture, as well as by their approach to the financial dimensions of compensation.

Because of the large number of potentially discrete architectures, we will not review all 18 architectures that can be developed based on different combinations of elements in our matrix. Rather, our primary focus is on the team and individualistic ends of the array. We will couple this with a more general discussion of the architectures in the larger "middle ground" that are derived from different combinations of the nine elements in the compensation plan matrix.

TEAM-ORIENTED ARCHITECTURES

Recall that team-oriented plans generally involve the allocation of practice revenues or income using an agreed upon methodology in order to determine physician compensation. Team-oriented plans pay practice expenses "off the top" out of available practice revenues to create a compensation pool that is then allocated among practice physicians. The compensation plan focuses on distributing the compensation pool rather than focusing direct attention on how practice expenses are allocated. In this regard, team-oriented plans tend to treat the practice as a single economic unit and involve some level of "sharing" rather than functioning as a collection of separate individual physician profit-and-loss centers.

The basic mathematical formula for team-oriented plans is as follows:

$$\begin{array}{r} \text{Practice Revenues} \\ - \ \underline{\text{Practice Expenditures}} \\ \text{Compensation Pool} \end{array}$$

The compensation plan then defines how this compensation pool is allocated among the physicians. The purely team-oriented architectures consist of Architectures A through E. They are reported in Exhibit 6.2 and are reviewed below.

▶ ARCHITECTURE A — UNIT-BASED PLANS
Revenue Element 1

Unit-based architectures use Revenue Element 1, which is situated in the bottom left quadrant of the compensation plan matrix, by using a pure "unit-based" mechanism to determine and pay physician compensation. Architectures that involve this single element are distinguished by their high team orientation in that physicians are paid per unit of service, and the primary focus is on revenue allocation, without regard to expense allocation as part of the plan methodology.

EXHIBIT 6.2 Team-Oriented Architectures A–E

Architecture	Revenue Dimension	Expense Dimension	Examples
A	Element 1 – Unit-based share of revenues or income	No express expense treatment	► Straight salary ► 100% equal share ► Compensation per unit of work (with work measured by professional services gross or net charges, or net collections, WRVUs, or other measures) ► Hourly rates
B	Element 2 – Guaranteed share of revenues or income (e.g., base plus incentive) plus other incentive measures	No express expense treatment	► Base salary plus incentive ► Market-based salary plus incentive ► Nonclinical production-based incentive based on qualitative, patient satisfaction, or other measures
C	Element 3 – Combined equal share and production-based allocation of revenues or income	No express expense treatment	► 70% equal share of net income with 30% production-based incentive (or other percentage combinations)
D	Element 4 – Pure production-based allocation of revenues or income	No express expense treatment	► Total net income allocated 100% based on % of total production (with production measured by professional services gross or net charges, or net collections, WRVUs, or other measures)
E	Element 5 – Graduated or negotiated revenue/expense allocation method	Expenses considered directly or indirectly	► Graduated percentage of net revenues/collections (e.g., 60% of first $400,000; 40% of next $200,000; etc.) ► Graduated dollars per WRVU based on production (e.g., $28 per WRVU for first 5,000; $30 per WRVU for next 2,000; etc.) ► Market-based overhead assessment with floor ► Graduated overhead assessment based on production (e.g., 60% of first $400,000 of net collections; 50% of next $200,000; etc.)

© 2006 Johnson & Walker Keegan

Examples of unit-based architectures include:

► Straight salary;

► 100 percent equal share;

► Compensation per unit of work; and

► Hourly rates.

Unit-based plan architectures may define the "unit" that serves as the basis for the architecture in any number of ways, such as based on time (e.g., per hour or a salary representing compensation per year), or per unit of work (e.g., fixed compensation per WRVU or defined percentage of net collections). Pure unit-based architectures do not include an explicit consideration of practice expenses as part of the plan methodology but instead pay compensation from the net revenue available after payment of practice expenses.

Advantages

► Plan administration is relatively easy;

► Compensation paid to physicians is generally stable;

► Unit-based plans can include a production orientation for setting the level of unit-based compensation (e.g., by considering historic production in setting a fixed salary or by paying a set dollar amount per WRVU or other unit); and

► Practices with straight salary arrangements are often able to more readily form a "care team" approach involving multiple specialties attending to an individual patient's needs, since individual productivity and individual income generation are not emphasized.

Disadvantages

► Questions of fairness of equal share plans may arise if physicians perform at different production or work levels within the practice;

► With equal distribution and salary plans, there are no direct incentives for productivity, cost of practice, or other performance outcomes (and these areas may therefore not receive appropriate attention and focus by practice physicians);

► A straight salary arrangement may undermine a group practice orientation, because it enables individual physicians to focus on their own "local" issues related to patient panels, support staff, facility arrangements, and other areas of concern; and

► Cost of practice may not receive appropriate focus, since physician compensation is not directly tied to expenditure levels.

➤ ARCHITECTURE B – GUARANTEED SHARE PLANS (BASE PLUS INCENTIVE)
Revenue Element 2

Plan architectures that are slightly less team-oriented are those involving different forms of base plus incentive arrangements. These architectures typically provide for a set base salary level that is largely "guaranteed," along with opportunities to earn additional incentive compensation. Examples of team-oriented plans using this architecture include:

- ➤ A fixed base salary plus production-based incentive;

- ➤ Market-based salary plus production-based incentive; and

- ➤ Market-based salary combined with an incentive based on quality, patient satisfaction, or other measures that are determined at the individual physician, specialty, location, or other levels.

The base salary may also be tied to specific performance expectations such that the otherwise "guaranteed" base salary portion of compensation may be modified (typically reduced) for failure to meet the basic (minimum) performance levels.

In base plus incentive plans, the incentive portion of compensation is typically variable and consists of defined performance measures in a number of categories, including clinical productivity, clinical performance and quality, patient access, patient satisfaction, citizenship, etc.

Advantages

- ➤ Base plus incentive plans tend to support a group practice orientation;

- ➤ The base salary can provide for income stability, while the incentive can provide an opportunity for additional compensation based on individual production or other performance measures; and

- ➤ Base plus incentive plans can include multiple performance measures in their incentive component as a means to support diverse practice-related goals (e.g., quality, profitability, patient satisfaction, or other goals at different levels within the practice).

Disadvantages

- ➤ The level of compensation that is determined to be "at risk" in a base plus incentive plan may not be a sufficient motivator of behavioral change;

- ➤ Incentive measures linked to clinical productivity tend to be most easily addressed, while those dealing with more qualitative aspects of performance tend to be more subjective in nature; and

► Because base plus incentive plans typically involve multiple measures, the medical practice's administrative infrastructure and information systems need to be at levels consistent with data requirements.

► ARCHITECTURE C – PERCENT-SHARED, PERCENT-PRODUCTION PLANS
Revenue Element 3

Medical practices using a combination of percent-shared and percent-production plans, as in this team-oriented architecture, focus on revenue treatment without express attention being given to expense allocation as part of the mathematical model. Examples of this type of architecture are plans that pay all practice expenses, then allocate practice income (net of expense) among practice physicians on an agreed upon basis. The agreed upon basis to allocate practice income might include, for example:

► 70 percent on an equal share basis; 30 percent based on individual physician net collections from professional services as a percentage of total net collections from professional services;

► 50 percent on an equal share basis; 25 percent based on individual physician WRVUs as a percentage of total WRVUs; 25 percent based on individual physician net collections from professional services as a percentage of total net collections from professional services; and

► 50 percent on an equal share basis; 50 percent based on subspecialty net collections from professional services as a percentage of total net collections (e.g., cardiovascular surgery, vascular surgery, etc.); then on an equal share basis to physicians within each subspecialty (e.g., equal share within cardiovascular surgery, equal share within vascular surgery, etc.).

As with other models, a variety of measures and combinations of measures can be used, but an essential element of the pure team-oriented version of this architecture is that there is no direct allocation of expenses. Instead, net income is allocated on an agreed upon basis, with a portion shared and a portion allocated based on production. As noted above, the measure of production can also vary and/or involve multiple measures, such as:

► Percent to total gross charges from professional services, percent to total net collections from professional services, or percent to total WRVUs; and

► Combination measures (e.g., 50 percent based on a percent to total gross charges from professional services, and 50 percent based on a percent to total WRVUs).

Advantages

► An equal share portion of compensation can promote teamwork and group practice orientation;

- There is no direct attention to costs, thus avoiding an area of potential conflict or dispute; and

- Plans using this architecture can combine different measures and approaches to create different levels of sharing (e.g., through equal share), different treatments of revenue generation (e.g., measured through net collections from professional services), and different recognitions of physician work (e.g., measured through gross charges from professional services or WRVUs).

Disadvantages

- There is no direct attention to practice operating costs; and

- The level of sharing among group physicians may be difficult to determine and must be negotiated to a level that is viewed to be reasonably "fair" by the majority of physicians.

▶ ARCHITECTURE D – PURE PRODUCTION-BASED PLANS (NO EXPENSE ALLOCATION)
Revenue Element 4

Architecture D describes production-based plans that involve measuring and rewarding the work effort of individual physicians in the practice with no direct revenue sharing. Pure team-oriented, production-based plans focus on revenue or income allocation methods without express expenditure treatment.

Different measures of production or work can be used for plans using this basic architecture, including:

- Net collections from professional services;

- Gross or net charges from professional services;

- WRVUs;

- Panel size or unique patient volume;

- Encounters (ambulatory, hospital, surgical; in combination); and

- Combination measures, such as direct allocation of capitation revenues and percentage to total of individual net collections for fee-for-service professional activity.

Advantages

- With pure production-based plans, physicians typically perceive control over their work levels and income; and

- Since physicians are directly encouraged and rewarded to be highly productive, practices with production-based plans are, indeed, among the most productive.

Disadvantages

► Depending on the measures used in the plan (e.g., net collections from professional services), inequity may arise between revenue and physician work effort due to payer mix variations; and

► Physicians may become focused on production at the expense of other important areas, such as cost of practice, outreach, committee participation, etc.

► ARCHITECTURE E – GRADUATED REVENUE ALLOCATION PLANS
Element 5, with Focus on Revenues or Income

The last team-oriented architecture, Architecture E, uses a graduated methodology to allocate practice revenues or net income to determine physician compensation. Because Element 5 of the compensation plan matrix is directly in the middle of the matrix, this element may use either revenue or expenditure treatment in the compensation plan methodology. The more team-oriented plans that are based on this architecture focus on revenue or income distribution, with only an indirect (or hidden) treatment of practice expenditures, while the more individualistic plans embracing this architecture implement express treatment of expenses (as further described in Architecture N below). Examples of plans using this type of architecture include:

► Graduated percentage of gross charges or net collections from professional services (e.g., 40 percent of the first $400,000; 60 percent of next $200,000, etc.); and

► Graduated dollars per WRVU based on production (e.g., $28 per WRVU for the first 5,000; $30 per WRVU for the next 2,000, etc.).

Advantages

► This architecture allows for a production focus with indirect or "negotiated" overhead assessment;

► Payment of differing levels of compensation based on production or other measures is often used because it is consistent with the financial realities of the medical practice (and any business);

► Surrogate expense treatment may be used but without expense micromanagement and disputes; and

► Physicians desiring a defined income level can understand what they need to produce at a defined minimum level to achieve that level of compensation.

Disadvantages

► The use of surrogate measures for expenditures may be inconsistent with physician perceptions of "fairness" related to practice operating costs;

▶ Depending on the methodology used, this architecture may not reflect revenue variations within the practice consistent with payer mix (e.g., in a graduated dollars per WRVU system, a physician who sees all indigent or Medicaid patients may receive the same compensation as a physician who has a superior payer mix); and

▶ Plans using this architecture may encourage too heavy a production orientation to the detriment of other activities or goals of the practice (e.g., outreach, committee participation, or others).

The architectures described above represent the major team-oriented plan architectures. Of course, different aspects of one or more architectures may be combined to create additional plan variations that still promote a largely team orientation. For example, a practice may elect to combine a base salary mechanism (Revenue Element 2) with an incentive mechanism that uses a graduated payment per WRVU or a graduated percentage of professional services net collections or gross charges in the incentive component (Element 5). This type of plan would then provide a level of income stability via the base salary that is coupled with variable income through a graduated production component. Other incentive measures, such as those directed at quality, patient satisfaction, resource utilization, practice efficiency, information technology utilization, citizenship, and others, can also be incorporated into or used to augment any of these plan architectures.

The elements of the compensation plan matrix that deal with revenue or income treatment may also be combined with those addressing practice-related expenditures or "overhead" in the form of more individualistic architectures that combine revenue *and* expenditure treatment. The architectures that use the most purely individualistic approaches are described below.

INDIVIDUALISTIC ARCHITECTURES

While team-oriented architectures sit on one extreme of the array of plan architectures, those at the opposite end are more individualistic in nature. Such individualistic architectures combine both revenue treatment and expense allocation elements and, as such, use the following financial model or mathematical calculation:

$$
\begin{array}{r}
\text{Allocated Revenues} \\
- \ \underline{\text{Allocated Expenses}} \\
\text{Physician Compensation}
\end{array}
$$

The architectures that are the most individualistic tend to focus on each individual physician's production, coupled with an agreed upon approach to the allocation of practice expenditures. Thus, the most extreme "individualistic" model is that which combines pure production-based revenue allocation (Revenue Element 4) with strict cost accounting of expenditures (Expense Element 9).

Our review of individualistic architectures will begin with this architecture (on the far right end of the array depicted in Exhibit 6.1) and work inward toward architectures that are still largely individualistic but that include more of a team orientation nonetheless. Importantly, however, the "team orientation" found in these individualistic models is through the sharing of *expenses* rather than revenues.

There is no clear trend among medical practices for allocating key expenditures in the medical practice. Expenditure treatment is a difficult decision for a compensation planning committee, as perceptions of fairness may not be uniform among physicians on this issue. Unfortunately, some medical practices tend to self-destruct when grappling with this issue, with the conversation quickly shifting from defining appropriate responsibility for practice costs to a focus on cost shifting. Thus, the actual methodology used to allocate expenditures in a compensation plan will likely occupy considerable debate in the compensation planning process.

The basic individualistic architectures are summarized in Exhibit 6.3 and are further described below.

► ARCHITECTURE R – PURE PRODUCTION-BASED, COMBINED WITH STRICT COST ACCOUNTING PLANS
Revenue Element 4 and Expense Element 9

The most individualistic of all plan architectures is the one that combines Revenue Element 4 (pure production revenue treatment) with Expense Element 9 (strict cost accounting expense treatment). Compensation plans utilizing this architecture concentrate both on revenue and expenditure allocation methods, with the objective being to allocate these financial elements as directly as possible to the individual physician responsible for their generation (in the case of revenues) or utilization (in the case of expenses).

Plans that use strict cost accounting allocate each expense, no matter how small or how large, to the level of an individual physician as directly as possible. Some expenditures might be allocated among a number of the physicians in the practice; for example, the cost of a large equipment purchase might be divided equally among the physicians who will be using the equipment based on utilization. Essentially, however, with strict cost accounting, each expense is specifically allocated to an individual physician.

Physician-specific direct expense allocation is a subset of strict cost accounting. Typically, physician-specific direct costs include professional liability insurance, as well as discretionary items, such as continuing medical education (CME), automobile allowances, cellular telephones, and other similar expenditures that are easily linked to a specific physician in the practice. Often, the cost of the nonphysician provider is directly expensed to an individual physician or a small group of physicians in the medical practice whom this individual supports.

EXHIBIT 6.3 Individualistic Architectures R–N

Architecture	Revenue Dimension	Expense Dimension	Examples
R	Element 4 – Pure production-based allocation of revenues or income	Element 9 – Strict cost accounting expense allocation based on utilization	► Revenues allocated based on personal production, combined with strict cost accounting of expenses based on utilization to maximum extent possible
Q	Element 4 – Pure production-based allocation of revenues or income	Element 8 – Modified cost accounting expense allocation (shared and based on utilization)	► Revenues allocated based on percent of production, combined with modified cost accounting of expenses (with combined shared and utilization-based expense allocation)
P	Element 4 – Pure production-based allocation of revenues or income	Element 7 – Negotiated expense allocation with production-based component	► Revenues allocated based on production, combined with 50% equal share and 50% production-based expense allocation
O	Element 4 – Pure production-based allocation of revenues or income	Element 6 – Equal share expense allocation	► Net income allocated based on personal production; expenses allocated on pure equal share basis
N	Element 4 – Pure production-based allocation of revenues or income	Element 5 – Negotiated or graduated expense allocation	► Revenues allocated based on pure production with market-based overhead assessment with floor ► Graduated overhead assessment based on production (e.g., 60% of first $400,000 of net collections; 50% of next $200,000; etc.)

Strict cost accounting extends this physician-specific direct cost allocation approach to all practice expenditures, allocating costs and expenses as precisely as possible, including to ancillary services. It is only occasionally observed in practice in its "pure" form, however, due to two issues: (1) the cost of the infrastructure to support this level of plan implementation is often determined to not be worth the effort; and (2) this allocation method can potentially create conflict. Most medical practices that desire to allocate a significant portion of the practice's expenditures to an individual physician level adopt what can more pragmatically be referred to as "modified" cost accounting methodologies (as used in Expense Element 8).

Advantages

- ► Physicians are held directly responsible for their own production and expenses;
- ► Physicians are held directly accountable for the cost of practice; and
- ► Plans based on this architecture tend to be financially viable, since all expenditures are allocated before compensation is paid to physicians.

Disadvantages

- ► An extensive administrative infrastructure may be required for strict cost accounting systems;
- ► Conflict over specific expenditure types may be significant, involving recurrent discussion and renegotiation; and
- ► Strict cost accounting may lead to an inappropriate "illusion of precision" regarding practice costs.

► ARCHITECTURE Q – PURE PRODUCTION-BASED, COMBINED WITH MODIFIED COST ACCOUNTING OF EXPENSES (SHARED AND BASED ON UTILIZATION) PLANS
Revenue Element 4 and Expense Element 8

The second most individualistic of all plan architectures combines Revenue Element 4 (pure production revenue treatment), with Expense Element 8 (modified cost accounting). This architecture concentrates both on revenue and expenditure allocation methods, with the objective being to allocate revenues as directly as possible to the individual physician responsible for their generation, while also reasonably defining an expense treatment based on estimated utilization.

By "modified" cost accounting, we mean that expenditures in the medical practice are treated differently depending upon their broad type of expenditure category. Typically, in modified cost accounting, while some expenditures are allocated to individual physicians on a direct allocation basis and some on a variable basis based on physician utilization, the majority are allocated on a fixed (equal physician or equal physician full-time equivalency [FTE]) basis.

Physician-specific direct expenses, such as CME, automobile allowances, cellular telephones, professional liability insurance, and other similar expenditures, are typically allocated directly at the individual physician level in modified cost accounting plans. In these plans, a medical practice may also allocate clinical support staff costs to an individual physician and other physician-specific expenditures, such as equipment or special supplies. However, under this plan architecture, the majority of the expenditures in the medical practice are allocated on a largely equal share basis and generally represent the "fixed" cost of the medical practice, with the variable costs of a medical practice allocated based on utilization (e.g., patient visit volume).

Advantages

► Physician compensation is directly linked to the cost of practice;

► Plans utilizing this architecture require less complex administrative infrastructure than strict cost accounting plans; and

► These types of plans tend to be fiscally sound, because individual physicians are encouraged to be highly productive as well as to exercise cost control.

Disadvantages

► Cost allocation methodologies receive considerable attention and debate; and

► Physicians may perceive that they are being held accountable for expenditures for which they have limited control.

► ARCHITECTURE P – PURE PRODUCTION-BASED, COMBINED WITH NEGOTIATED EXPENSE ALLOCATION (WITH PRODUCTION-BASED COMPONENT) PLANS
Revenue Element 4 and Expense Element 7

The third most individualistic of the plan architectures is the one that combines Revenue Element 4 (pure production revenue treatment) with Expense Element 7 (negotiated expense allocation with a portion based on production). Compensation plans utilizing this architecture concentrate both on revenue and expense allocation methods. In these plans, revenues are allocated directly to the physician producing them (e.g., as a percentage of net collections from professional services or some other measure). However, unlike Architectures R or Q (discussed above), these plans use an acknowledged negotiated expense allocation method, along with some portion of expenses allocated based on production.

The expense treatment in these plans may incorporate aspects of the methods used in modified cost accounting allocation methods, but because a portion of expenses are allocated based on production, physicians who have the lowest level of production "pay" the least amount, and those who have the highest "pay" the most amount. Examples of plans that use Element 7 for expenditure treatment include:

► Production-based revenue allocation treatments with expenses allocated on a 50 percent equal share basis, and 50 percent on a percent to total production basis (e.g., measured by net collections from professional services); and

► Production-based revenue allocation treatments with expenses allocated on a 50 percent fixed (equal share per physician) basis, 15 percent equal share per division (then reallocated in each division), and 35 percent based on individual physician production as a percentage of total production (e.g., with production measured by WRVUs).

Advantages

► Physician compensation is generally linked to physician work effort and cost of practice, but without the level of detail and potential micromanagement that may occur in strict or modified cost accounting methods, because the expenses are viewed and understood to be negotiated;

► When used in multispecialty groups, this architecture allows primary care physicians to be supplemented somewhat by specialists with higher revenue-generating potential;

► Plans utilizing this architecture are relatively simple and easy to understand; and

► The plans may be viewed as fair (or socialistic) based on the perception that those who generate more should be willing to "pay" a larger share of practice operating costs.

Disadvantages

► Cost allocation percentages and methodologies must still be negotiated;

► Production-oriented cost allocation may not be consistent with actual resource utilization (e.g., physicians who are in the hospital more may also have the highest levels of production, but they will be paying a higher portion of the practice clinic costs than others who are in the clinic more frequently);

► Highly productive and/or specialist physicians may protest subsidization of physicians in primary care and/or those with lower levels of production; and

► Physicians may perceive that they pay for expenditures for which they have limited control.

► ARCHITECTURE O – PURE PRODUCTION-BASED, COMBINED WITH EQUAL SHARE EXPENSE ALLOCATION PLANS
Revenue Element 4 and Expense Element 6

Moving toward the center of the array of compensation plan architectures, but still within the individualistic plan architectures, is the architecture that combines Element 4 (pure production revenue treatment) with Expense Element 6 (equal share expense allocation).

Compensation plans utilizing this architecture concentrate both on revenue and expense allocation methods, but they use a clear allocation of expenses on an equal share basis as opposed to allocating expenses based on utilization, production, or some other negotiated basis.

The pure equal share expense treatment in these plans allows for a clear understanding of the mathematical model used to determine compensation. The portion of expenses that is allocated equally may vary somewhat from one practice to another. For example, the following expenditure treatment methods might be used within Expense Element 6 on the matrix:

- ► 100 percent of all expenses are allocated equal share "per physician" (without regard to clinical FTE level);

- ► Physician-specific direct expenses (e.g., CME, personal expenses, and others) are allocated directly to each physician; all remaining expenses are allocated 100 percent equal share "per physician"; and

- ► 100 percent of all expenses are allocated on an equal share basis, but each equal share is adjusted based upon clinical FTE in the practice (e.g., 1.0 clinical full-time equivalency [CFTE] receives a full equal share; .75 CFTE [based on days worked or otherwise] receives 75 percent of an equal share of expenses, etc.).

Advantages

- ► These plans involve simple plan administration, requiring no specific cost allocation methods;

- ► This architecture recognizes that most practice expenses (e.g., 60 to 85 percent of total operating expenses in many practices) are largely "fixed" in that they must be paid regardless of utilization or production levels by individual physicians;

- ► Some level of teamwork is promoted through expense allocation, combined with individual production based on work levels, thus encouraging high levels of production; and

- ► This architecture does not require the level of detail and potential micromanagement found in other expense allocation methods.

Disadvantages

- ► This architecture arguably does not address the fact that a portion of expenses is variable in nature (meaning that it can result in lower producers arguably supplementing those with higher levels of production);

- ► Production orientation may lead to inappropriate behaviors; and

- ► Physicians may feel that since they will share equally in expenses, they should be free to spend as they wish (without appropriate attention to cost control).

► ARCHITECTURE N – PURE PRODUCTION-BASED, COMBINED WITH GRADUATED EXPENSE ALLOCATION PLANS
Revenue Element 4 and Element 5, with Focus on Expenses Only

As with all plans that use Element 5, this architecture is close to a middle ground model. Like team-oriented Architecture E, this plan uses a graduated methodology, but this individualistic version focuses on expenses as opposed to revenue allocation. This plan also combines this graduated expense allocation method with a pure production orientation to revenues.

Plans based on this architecture directly link physician productivity and expense allocation based on graduated thresholds of production. Examples of plans using this approach to expense allocation include the following:

► Pure production-based revenue allocation with graduated overhead assessment based on production (60 percent assessed on the first $400,000 of net collections from professional services; 50 percent assessed on the next $200,000, etc.);

► Pure production-based revenue allocation with market-based overhead assessment with a floor (e.g., all physicians, regardless of specialty, are assessed 60 percent of overhead on the first $200,000 of net collections based on professional services, then are assessed a market-based overhead on all remaining amounts based on the practice specialty);

► Pure production-based revenue allocation with tiered expense allocation models using defined assessment up to a certain level (e.g., 50 percent assessed on the first $400,000 of net collections from professional services; 40 percent assessed on the next $300,000; then 50 percent assessed on the remaining amounts); and

► Pure production-based revenue allocation with market-based overhead with a floor, coupled with variations based on production (e.g., all physicians pay 60 percent on the first $200,000 of net collections from professional services; 50 percent of the next $200,000; then a variable level based on the market and on their production by reference to market levels of production [with those having the lowest production by specialty paying a higher percentage, and those with the highest production by specialty paying the lowest percentage]).

To illustrate this fourth example, a physician who performs at the median level of WRVUs for his or her specialty could also be assessed the median overhead (defined as total operating cost as a percentage of total medical revenue) for this particular level of activity. Above the median level, the dollars per WRVU allocated to the physician may decline, and the cost of practice allocated to the physician (in the form of a defined percentage) may increase at specific intervals.

Advantages

► Plans utilizing this architecture directly reward production;

► This architecture provides some linkage to costs but without potential for micromanagement;

► Production is encouraged through both revenue and expense allocation methods (by allowing those with the highest levels of production to "pay their fair share" but also to benefit from the additional production beyond a defined level);

- ► Plans can incorporate market-based overhead based on practice specialty; and

- ► Plans can be modified to discourage "excessive" production.

Disadvantages

- ► This architecture may lead to frequent renegotiation and assessment of "fairness";

- ► The success of this plan may depend on the particular mix of specialties in the practice;

- ► The linkage to market data may be both helpful (as an objective external reference point) or potentially problematic (on the grounds that the market data are not "representative of my practice"); and

- ► Depending on actual plan methodological design, physicians may perceive that they are inequitably rewarded at the extremes (either high producers or low producers).

ARCHITECTURES IN THE VAST "MIDDLE GROUND"

The architectures described above constitute the most individualistic plan architectures. As with our discussion of team-oriented architectures, different elements on the compensation plan matrix may be combined to create additional architectures that are in a vast "middle ground." These architectures combine different aspects of team-oriented and individualistic plans.

For example, a practice may elect to combine a revenue allocation methodology that allocates practice net collections from professional services on a 10 percent equal share basis, 90 percent based on individual physician production as a percentage of total production for professional services (Revenue Element 3 basis), with a modified cost accounting expense allocation system (Expense Element 8). This type of plan would combine some limited "sharing" of practice revenues with an expenditure treatment methodology that still focuses, to a degree, on individual cost responsibility and accountability. This and other models that use combinations of revenue and expense allocation elements fall in the "middle." Although this particular combination of elements may sit in the middle ground, it is closer to the individualistic rather than the team-oriented end of our array of plan architectures.

Likewise, architectures that allocate practice revenues based on a percentage of production (Revenue Element 4) and that also allocate practice expenses based on a combined equal share and production basis (Expense Element 7) might also be viewed as middle ground models. However, this architecture tends to fall more toward the team-oriented end of the array of plan architectures.

There are eight basic middle ground architectures. Descriptions and examples of these plan architectures are summarized in Exhibit 6.4. Note that although different combinations are possible, these combinations tend to have varying frequencies of application in medical practices.

EXHIBIT 6.4 Middle Ground Architectures F–M

Architecture	Revenue Dimension	Expense Dimension	Examples
F	Element 2 – Guaranteed share of revenues or income (base plus incentive) plus other incentive measures	Element 6 – Pure equal share of expenses	► Base salary plus incentive based on allocated revenues minus expense, with expenses allocated on a pure equal share basis
G	Element 3 – Combined equal share and production-based allocation of revenues or income	Element 6 – Pure equal share of expenses	► Base salary plus incentive based on allocated revenues minus expense, with expenses allocated on a negotiated basis (with some shared, some based on percentage of production)
H	Element 2 – Guaranteed share of revenues or income (base plus incentive) plus other incentive measures	Element 7 – Negotiated expense allocation with production-based component	► Market-based salary, coupled with incentive based on graduated share of revenues over target (e.g., 40% of revenues in excess of $600,000)
I	Element 3 – Combined equal share and production-based allocation of revenues or income	Element 7 – Negotiated expense allocation with production-based component	► Defined equal share in revenue allocation with graduated expense allocation (e.g., 10% equal share of revenues combined with overhead assessed 60% on first $400,000, 40% on next $200,000, etc.)
J	Element 2 – Guaranteed share of revenues or income (base plus incentive) plus other incentive measures	Element 8 – Modified cost accounting expense allocation with utilization-based component	► Base salary plus incentive based on allocated revenues minus expense, with expenses allocated based on modified cost accounting (with some portion based on utilization)
K	Element 3 – Combined equal share and production-based allocation of revenues or income	Element 8 – Modified cost accounting expense allocation with utilization-based component	► Revenues allocated 70% equal share and 30% based on production, coupled with expenses allocated 60% equal share with 40% based on percentage of production (or other percentage combinations)
L	Element 2 – Guaranteed share of revenues or income (base plus incentive) plus other incentive measures	Element 9 – Strict cost accounting expense allocation based on utilization	► Base salary based on specialty, plus production-based percentage of revenues with strict cost accounting of practice expenses
M	Element 3 – Combined equal share and production-based allocation of revenues or income	Element 9 – Strict cost accounting expense allocation based on utilization	► Revenues allocated 70% equal share and 30% based on production (or other percentage combination), coupled with explicit equal share expense allocation

© 2006 Johnson & Walker Keegan

Once the compensation planning committee has discussed and agreed upon one or more broad architectures for the compensation plan, it is now ready to develop the details of the compensation plan's methodology. In the next chapter, we take a closer look at the basic alternatives and methods available to measure physician work and effort.

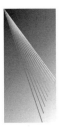

SEVEN

Measuring Physician Work and Effort

Clinical productivity, whether measured by gross charges or net collections from professional services, work relative value units (WRVUs), or some other index, is currently the most prevalent focus for physician compensation plans. Yet, it is important to recognize that not all physicians find themselves in medical practices where they can be equally productive and efficient. Thus, the impacts to physician productivity and practice efficiency need to be recognized – with proactive steps taken to minimize or mitigate these factors – if a medical practice's goal is to encourage and reward physician clinical work and effort.

In this chapter, we review some of the external and internal influences that impact clinical productivity of the physician. We also review the broad types of productivity measures used by medical practices for compensation purposes and describe their advantages and disadvantages. The chapter concludes with an analysis and demonstration of benchmarking physician compensation and production for use in compensation plan design.

THE CONTEXT FOR PHYSICIAN PRODUCTIVITY

Peter Drucker has coined the term "knowledge workers" to describe individuals whose work is based on intellectual capital. Health care is a knowledge-based business, and physicians represent a significant cohort of knowledge workers. In terms of physician compensation planning, *how* to measure and reward knowledge work is the fundamental challenge. The compensation plan in health care organizations represents a basic element of the formal management coordination systems that are used by leaders to align health system and knowledge worker (i.e., physician) goals. The compensation plan effectively outlines what is expected of physicians who belong in the practice so that they can "self-manage," and, as such, it is an essential element for practice success. Of course, if a compensation plan is too complex, then the attention of physicians may be diverted to business and financial issues at the expense of patient care.

Yet, in today's environment, production in the form of clinical service and other revenue-generating activities is essential to the success of the health care organization in which a physician practices, and to that physician's compensation. Medical practices, hospitals, and other organizations generally only receive reimbursement that can be used to pay compensation and costs when they actually provide services. This is clearly the case in the context of fee-for-service or similar reimbursement systems (which reimburse practices based on service volume and intensity), but it is equally true in capitated, pay-for-performance (P4P), and similar reimbursement environments (which reimburse practices for patient care management, practice efficiency, utilization of information technology, and other similar measures).

In one way or another, physicians get paid for what they do; therefore, compensation plans may encourage or discourage the "productive" activities of physicians in furtherance of medical practice–related goals. Physician productivity and work effort are central to these issues, but any evaluation of physician productivity and work effort must also recognize the significant challenges inherent in examining physician productivity.

Questions are plentiful. For example:

- ▶ Is productivity simply an examination of inputs and outputs?
- ▶ Is productivity a measure of the efficiency of the physician?
- ▶ Should productivity measures also take quality of care or patient care outcomes into account?
- ▶ Can individual physician productivity be examined exclusive of the medical practice or parent organization and its policies and processes?

These questions are important and occupy considerable debate. As noted above, however, the issues of incentives, bonuses, revenue streams, and return-on-investment analyses are necessary to health care delivery in our current environment. And to that end, it's fair to say that compensation plans are generally designed to articulate what is expected of physicians in a financially viable framework so that they can continue to be in business to meet the health care needs of their communities.

Because of these realities, most medical practices measure physician productivity and use this measurement in some capacity to help determine physician compensation.

INFLUENCES ON PHYSICIAN PRODUCTIVITY

An extensive body of empirical research exists related to physician productivity and compensation. However, there are distinct methodological challenges to any attempt to examine such issues due, in part, to the significant variation in the medical practice environments in which practicing physicians reside. Numerous other factors and variables may also influence and impact production and compensation studies, such as external reimbursement systems and changing technology. Because of the dramatic changes that have occurred in health care generally and in medical practices in particular over the past 10 to 15 years, much of the research that was conducted in years past may have limited relevance today.

What we do know is that some physicians are more clinically productive than others. This is due to a host of factors, including those listed below (and presented in Exhibit 7.1):

► External environmental variables, such as geographic setting, payer reimbursement mechanisms, and physician-population density;

► Technological variables, such as equipment, electronic health records, and data retrieval and analysis;

► Practice variables, such as specialty, services offered, staffing deployment models, practice facilities, scope of practice (e.g., specialty mix), practice size (e.g., increasing the potential for "shirking" behavior as practice size increases); and

► Individual physician variables, such as experience, practice style, and degrees of professional and personal work/life balance.

Not surprisingly, these factors are likely to impact both productivity and physician compensation levels. Hence, we often find practices working on enhancing their internal medical practice operations at the same time they are redesigning their physician compensation plans.

The focus on productivity itself, however, is not surprising, given the trend of changes in compensation and production for both primary care and specialty care practices. Benchmark data tend to support physicians' perceptions that they are generally "working harder" for less money. For most medical practices, the percent change in physician production has outpaced the percent change in compensation.

EXHIBIT 7.1 Impacts on Physician Productivity

► External Environment
 – Geography
 – Reimbursement mechanisms
 – Health care market

► Medical Practice Factors
 – Practice size and economies of scale
 – Group type – single vs. multispecialty
 – Group culture

► Individual Physician Factors
 – Physician-specific variables
 – Unintended consequences – shirking and moral hazard

PRODUCTIVITY'S NEGATIVE EFFECTS

We have learned that an emphasis on productivity in a physician compensation plan, without balance, can be detrimental to the health of a medical practice. In a compensation plan that emphasizes individual production, it is possible for physicians to "game the plan," since there is no perfect plan out there.

For example, a physician can increase his or her production levels via: (1) churning, which is scheduling patients for multiple visits when perhaps a single visit or, at most, two visits, would clinically suffice; or (2) cherry-picking, which is selecting patients based on payer status or health status that may provide an advantage over colleagues related to production measures. This is not to suggest that all physicians will "game" a plan that relies heavily on productivity factors. In fact, in our experience, only a small minority of physicians may engage in these actions. We draw attention to them, however, so that practices can be alerted and can develop appropriate monitoring methods if they are required.

Another negative effect of a production-focused compensation plan is that physicians in a group practice may tend to run separate, individual physician practices with minimal team-oriented behaviors. Unhealthy internal competition can result, and opportunities to develop a "true" group practice may be thwarted.

Lastly, in productivity-focused compensation plans, a medical practice may experience difficulty engaging physicians in other practice activities beyond clinical work. For example, some practices have had difficulty obtaining participation in committee work, community outreach, hospital directorship assignments, and even executive board membership, due to the impact that these activities have on an individual physician's productivity or professional and personal work/life balance.

MEASURES OF PHYSICIAN WORK AND EFFORT

Measures of physician work and effort typically involve a number of categories that are used either singly or in combination in physician compensation plans. Five measurement categories (see Exhibit 7.2) are typically employed to measure physician work and effort (note: a discussion of measures beyond clinical productivity is presented in Chapters 8 and 10). These include: (1) gross charges from professional services; (2) net collections from professional services; (3) WRVUs; (4) patient encounters; and (5) panel size. Combination measures, such as revenue and expense per WRVU, may also be employed, as may other measures, such as time devoted to clinical pursuits.

As a measure of physician work and effort, each of the five major categories has both strengths and weaknesses, as further described below.

1. GROSS CHARGES FROM PROFESSIONAL SERVICES

Gross charges from professional services are a function of the practice's fee schedule and its service utilization. When used in physician compensation, professional services

EXHIBIT 7.2 Measuring Physician Work and Effort

Gross Charges

Professional services charges at practice's fee schedule, excluding technical component and nonphysician providers.

> Pro: Available from every practice
> Con: Subject to variation and year-to-year changes in fees

Net Collections

Collections from professional services, excluding technical component and nonphysician providers.

> Pro: Represents "real" money
> Con: Subject to payer mix variations and may result in "cherry-picking"

WRVUs – Medicare RBRVS

One-to-one relationship to professional CPT® code billed.

> Pro: Standardized – "apples-to-apples" comparison of work and effort without regard to payer mix
> Con: May impact physician work preferences

Encounters

Total encounters, ambulatory encounters, hospital encounters, procedures.

> Pro: Available from every practice
> Con: Does not relate well to actual work levels

Panel Size or Panel Size Equivalencies

> Pro: Measures actual number of patient "lives" managed
> Con: Some physicians may have "sicker" panels

© 2006 Johnson & Walker Keegan

gross charges typically exclude the technical component, nonphysician provider gross charges, and other nonphysician-specific charge activity. See Chapter 9, "The Legal Element," for a discussion of "incident to" and ancillary services activity.

The advantage of using gross charges is that these data are readily available from every practice. The downside is that a practice's fee schedule is subject to variation from year to year, and it varies from practice to practice, making benchmarking problematic. Moreover, unless a practice uses a standard approach to the establishment of its fee schedule (e.g., establishing the fee schedule using a standard percentage of the Medicare allowed fee), there will even be within-practice variation in fees. In addition, gross charges may not relate well to actual revenue or collections for professional services.

A medical practice that elects to use gross charges to measure physician work and effort (e.g., by paying physicians a defined percentage of charges) needs to perform financial modeling to ensure sufficient revenue levels for income distribution or otherwise link gross charges to actual revenue. For example, an individual physician's percentage of gross charges to total gross charges can be applied to allocate available revenues or profits. A medical practice may also want to combine gross charges with other measures for benchmarking purposes, for example, gross charges per WRVU in determining how a physician's production compares to his or her peers.

2. NET COLLECTIONS FROM PROFESSIONAL SERVICES

Measuring physician work and effort by employing actual revenue or net collections from professional services is a frequently used strategy in physician compensation plans, because it relates to "real" money received by the practice. Net collections are frequently defined as revenue received in the practice less any refunds. The difficulty in using net collections from professional services as a measure of physician work, however, is that it is subject to payer mix variations among the practice's physicians. For example, if one physician has a larger share of Medicaid patients than his or her colleagues, this would most likely have a negative impact on the physician's collection performance. However, when payer mix is relatively consistent across physicians within a single specialty practice, using net collections from professional services to measure physician work and effort is frequently employed.

3. WORK RELATIVE VALUE UNITS (WRVUs)

WRVUs are one of three elements outlined in Medicare's RBRVS strategy to recognize work and cost issues in a medical practice (the other two being the expense of practice component and the malpractice expense component). WRVUs are assigned to the Current Procedural Terminology (CPT®) codes consistent with the physician work effort associated with the particular professional service that is billed.

The advantage of using WRVUs to measure physician work effort is that the measure is standardized. This effectively provides an "apples-to-apples" comparison of work and effort, without regard to payer mix, type of specialty, interpractice fee variation, and other factors. However, if physicians in a medical practice do not code their services at appropriate levels consistent with the work they perform (and document), WRVUs may not be an accurate reflection of their work level. The importance of coding accuracy – for a number of other reasons beyond physician compensation (not the least of which is legal compliance) – should mitigate the downside of using WRVUs to measure physician work and effort.

4. ENCOUNTERS

Some medical practices measure physician work and effort using encounters, either ambulatory, hospital, surgical, or in combination. Encounter data are typically available for each practice, since most practice management systems readily capture the volume of services by CPT code and by place of service. Like WRVUs, encounters provide for standard measures without regard to payment levels. However, the disadvantage of using encounters such as patient visits is that this measure does not relate well to actual work levels. For example, a physician in the practice may have "sicker" patients or may have more advanced seniors in his or her patient mix, thus reducing ambulatory encounters. Or, alternatively, a physician could "grow" ambulatory encounters by instituting routine follow-up visits for patients at levels beyond those required based on clinically accepted standards and protocols.

5. PANEL SIZE

Some medical practices have transitioned to panel size as a measure of physician work and effort. In medical practices with a high percentage of capitated patients, the panel size for individual physicians is often readily available. For other medical practices, a recognized proxy for panel size is comprised of unique patient volume for the past 12- to 18-month period. This means, for example, that a patient who sees his or her physician on three different occasions during the year is counted as "one" unique patient for this physician's panel.

The difficulty in using panel size to measure production is that many patients could be counted more than once if the physicians practice in a group practice mode that involves "sharing" of patients. For example, an obstetrics and gynecology (OB/GYN) practice might rotate obstetrical patient prenatal visits among each of the physicians in the medical practice. In this OB/GYN practice, it would be important to ensure that clearly defined criteria have been used so that the patient is only counted once (e.g., at the first prenatal visit). If new patients are assigned to physicians through a rotational basis (and assuming that the practice does not have a significant patient drop-out rate), the first prenatal visit may represent an acceptable proxy for each physician's obstetrical panel size.

Sophisticated methods of analyzing panel size may also be used for compensation plan purposes. For example, panel size may be adjusted based on gender or age of the patient, or the panel size may be adjusted based on severity of illness or other risk factors.

Note that the above five measures of physician work and effort do not include technical components, supplies, equipment, injections, immunizations, and other similar categories of ancillary services. The exclusion of these services from measurements of production is generally required by benchmark sources and, in some cases, by the legal element of physician compensation (discussed in Chapter 9, "The Legal Element").

MEASURING AND REWARDING QUALITY

The above measures permit an examination of the *quantity* of work (e.g., gross charges, encounters, panel size) and general *intensity* of that work (e.g., WRVUs), that is, for the most part, consistent with the predominant method of reimbursement from health plans that pay based on volume and complexity. We are now seeing, however, P4P reimbursement, with health plans paying contingent reimbursement based on clinical and practice efficiency measures. Directly translating this health plan reimbursement methodology (money from the health plan to the practice) to a medical practice's compensation plan (money from the practice to the physician) is discussed in Chapter 8, "Pay-for-Performance (P4P) and Physician Compensation."

BENCHMARKING PHYSICIAN PRODUCTIVITY FOR COMPENSATION PLAN DEVELOPMENT

Benchmarking is the systematic comparison of key financial, productivity, and other indicators for one physician or practice to those of other "representative" similar physicians or practices. Benchmarking allows for an objective assessment of key performance indicators at two discrete levels: (1) at the individual physician level; and (2) at the practice or organization-wide level. It permits identification of variation, physician "outliers," and opportunities for improvement, and it informs areas in need of further investigation. It also encourages a proactive search by medical practices for new methods and improvements in performance. A description of the benefits of benchmarking for compensation planning purposes is provided in Exhibit 7.3.

Benchmarking physician productivity involves more than simply counting the number of patient encounters, adding up the gross charges, or totaling the revenue that was generated by a physician. Through benchmarking, a comparison with other physicians and with other medical practices can be made to inform the compensation plan development process, and to inform physicians of their relative productivity and performance vis-à-vis their colleagues and peers. As noted previously, this type of education and assessment is typically essential to understanding what is, or what may be, "fair" related to a compensation plan.

EXHIBIT 7.3

Benchmarking for Compensation

► Systematic comparison of key clinical and financial indicators to "similar" practices

► Allows for objective assessment of key performance indicators at various levels:
  – Practice or department
  – Individual physician

► Identifies variation, "outliers," and opportunities

► Informs areas in need of further investigation

► Encourages proactive search for new methods

➤ PURPOSES AND USES OF BENCHMARKING

Benchmarking permits a medical practice to compare its compensation and productivity levels, as well as the practice's financial performance, to other similarly situated physicians or like practices. This is an important step in the compensation development process for several reasons, including: (1) it ensures that appropriate business and operational issues are evaluated as part of the process; and (2) it provides an understanding of legal compliance associated with physician compensation plans. Each of these uses is further described below.

Business and Operational Uses

One of the key business uses for benchmarking in the context of compensation is to create realistic expectations among physicians regarding their salary levels. For example, if the physicians are paid compensation that is above the 90th percentile, yet their production is at the 25th percentile, opportunities to realign compensation may be in order.

Benchmarking also permits a medical practice to evaluate its financial performance in comparison to other practices so that a plan is developed that is consistent with the financial realities of the practice. By illustration, if a practice's current overhead rate is significantly higher than benchmark norms, fewer dollars are likely to be available for physician compensation purposes. Similarly, if net collections from professional services are disproportionately lower in a particular medical practice in comparison to other practices, less revenue is available to cover both cost of practice and physician compensation. Thus, benchmarking for business and operational purposes is commonly performed to assess business issues such as operating costs (e.g., overhead incurred by an organization to support a particular practice) and to provide information regarding compensation and production levels at the individual physician level.

From a business and operations perspective, information derived from the benchmarking process is commonly used to answer a number of key questions, such as:

- ➤ Are the overhead costs, staffing ratios, supply expenses, etc. of a particular clinic or practice at, below, or above the typical costs and levels for practices in the same specialty?

- ➤ What areas of practice operations might a practice focus on in order to reduce costs and/or provide additional resources that will enhance physician efficiency?

- ➤ How well (or poorly) is a particular physician paid in relation to his or her peers?

- ➤ How does the work level of particular physicians compare to the work levels of peers in the same specialty?

- ➤ How well (or poorly) does a particular physician get paid for the work that he or she performs?

The questions outlined above (and others) can be used to provide perspective regarding a particular physician's practice, identify opportunities for improvement, help understand areas in which performance is at expected or better than expected levels, provide a realistic expectation regarding compensation levels, and provide other useful information to understand how a particular practice compares to others in operational terms.

Legal Compliance Uses

Benchmarking is also commonly used in the context of legal compliance efforts. Numerous laws impose requirements related to the payment of compensation to physicians, including laws and rules governing tax-exempt organizations, and the Stark and anti-kickback laws. The overall objective of assessing compensation and production from a legal compliance perspective is to ensure that the level of compensation is reasonable and, in some circumstances, that it is consistent with fair market value (FMV).

As a general matter, compensation is deemed to be reasonable when it is within the range of compensation paid to individuals in the same specialties, in the same geographic region. These issues are further discussed in Chapter 9, "The Legal Element," and Chapter 16, "The Special World of Hospitals and Academic Practices – Assessing Reasonableness and Promoting Compliance."

► AVAILABILITY, UTILITY, AND VALIDITY OF BENCHMARKING RESOURCES

Benchmarking is generally conducted both internally and externally. Internal benchmarking involves comparing one physician in the practice to his or her colleagues who work in the same practice. External benchmarking involves comparing a physician to his or her colleagues in like practices; for example, physicians in the same specialty, the same geographic location, the same practice size, and other similar comparative measures. Both internal and external benchmarking involve measurement and comparison.

The benchmarking source that is selected might be a single survey or a blend of multiple surveys. In addition, based on the subsets of data, the benchmark itself may be a single value or a blend of multiple values. For example, "all respondents" benchmarks indicate values from the entire survey of respondents; however, various subsets of the data typically are also reported, such as by size of group practice, geographic location, type of practice ownership, and many others.

Some physicians will make the case that the benchmarking data are not meaningful to them, citing that their patients are "sicker" or their practice is "different." As we noted previously, it is important that the benchmarking data not be used as an arbitrary goal, but rather to identify the current state of the medical practice (e.g., operating expenses, physician compensation, productivity, etc.) and the extent of opportunity that the medical practice may have as it works toward a new compensation plan design. The benchmarking analysis often leads to useful projects that have direct relevance for physician compensation, such as analyzing the cost of practice differences or discovering the reasons for wide variations among a practice's physicians in terms of compensation or production.

Typically, a medical practice seeks to identify benchmark survey sources that appear to include medical practices of similar type and/or size (e.g., academic vs. private practice and/or small vs. large practices). In Chapter 16, "The Special World of Hospital and Academic Practices – Assessing Reasonableness and Promoting Compliance," we further discuss data issues associated with benchmark surveys. In the Additional Resources section at the end of this book, we list some of the common benchmark surveys currently in use. In all instances, none of the sources is perfect, nor can any be said to be perfectly valid, primarily because each benchmarking source represents only a subset of the universe of physicians and practices generally. As discussed in Chapter 16, however, the currently available benchmark surveys represent the sources of information that exist today, and, as such, can (and indeed are) used in conjunction with the exercise of reasonable judgment.

▶ BENCHMARKING STEPS

Benchmarking is used to provide a "snapshot" assessment of compensation, production, and financial position at a moment in time. Thus, the benchmarking process requires a medical practice to continually benchmark compensation and productivity over time. The basic steps involved in benchmarking include:

Step 1. Identify benchmark source(s) and understand data definitions;

Step 2. Obtain practice data consistent with data definitions;

Step 3. Compare practice data to benchmark source(s);

Step 4. Perform a "gap" analysis to identify areas of opportunity; and

Step 5. Repeat these steps at systematic intervals.

The benchmarking process typically involves evaluation across multiple data elements. For example, the physician's WRVUs and compensation can be benchmarked to industry norms, but equally important is the *interaction* of these two data elements. In this example, this would be measured by calculating compensation per WRVU (e.g., the physician's annual compensation divided by the physician's annual WRVUs). As another example, the physician's compensation level can be benchmarked to industry norms, and his or her net collections from professional services activities can be benchmarked to industry norms. In this example, however, it would also be important to benchmark the *interaction* of the physician's compensation to revenue (e.g., calculation of a compensation-to-revenue ratio defined as the physician's annual compensation divided by the physician's annual net collections from professional services). This ratio reflects how much of the revenue is distributed to physicians as compensation vs. how much is retained in the practice for operating expenses and other uses.

► PHYSICIAN-SPECIFIC FACTORS AND BENCHMARKING

When physician productivity is benchmarked, four individual, physician-specific factors are typically taken into account. These include:

1. Time;

2. Efficiency;

3. Volume; and

4. Quality (or appropriateness) of care.

The following examples demonstrate benchmarking comparison involving these factors. Compensation plans may be designed to support or promote behavior relative to one or more of these areas.

1. Time

Physician time devoted to clinical activities will impact the production level that he or she achieves, regardless of the specific measure of physician work and effort that is employed. Exhibit 7.4 demonstrates the importance of understanding time devoted to clinical activities by the physicians in a medical practice. In this example, a physician who elects to work four days per week and 46 weeks per year is at 80 percent time (.80 FTE), compared to the 100 percent (or 1.00 FTE) physician working a full five days per week over the same 46 weeks per year.

EXHIBIT 7.4 Impact of Time on Physician Productivity

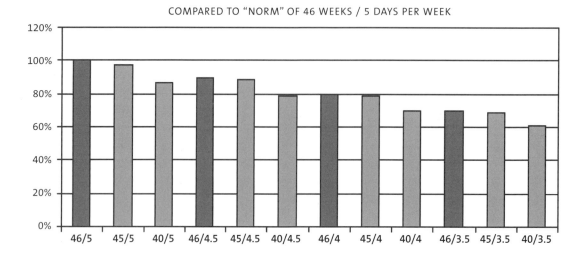

© 2006 Johnson & Walker Keegan

It is important to understand physician time devoted to clinical activity in order to accurately benchmark that physician's clinical production. A physician who works four days a week in a community where the "normal" schedule is five days a week will have production on one measure – time in practice – that is 80 percent of that of his or her peers. That difference can, and generally will, have implications for the physician's production and therefore for the physician's compensation.

2. Efficiency

Efficiency also influences physician productivity. In the context of compensation and benchmarking, the question of efficiency essentially asks: "How much does the physician produce during the time he or she is working?"

Exhibits 7.5 and 7.6 provide examples of internal benchmarking in which physicians' performance during a particular time period is compared. In Exhibit 7.5, the revenue generated by each physician during a half-day session in clinic is graphed. In this example, the question could be raised as to why Dr. C is able to generate more revenue in a defined session of time. Potential explanations include physician subspecialty, payer mix fluctuations among physicians, severity or risk of the patient panel, higher volumes of new patients vs. return patients, or other similar factors.

EXHIBIT 7.5 Measuring Efficiency per Unit of Time – Revenue

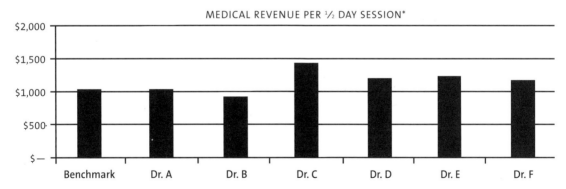

MEDICAL REVENUE PER ½ DAY SESSION*

* Assumes average revenue of $484,523 per physician, 45 weeks of service, 9 sessions per week (405 sessions total)

© 2006 Johnson & Walker Keegan

In Exhibit 7.6, each physician is internally compared to other practice physicians in the same specialty based on WRVUs generated in a clinic session. In this example, we again see that Dr. C reports higher WRVUs than his colleagues. Assuming that coding is accurate, this physician may be performing procedures, may be providing greater service levels, perhaps has a different staffing support model, potentially has a different appoint-

EXHIBIT 7.6 Measuring Efficiency per Unit of Time – Work RVU (WRVU)

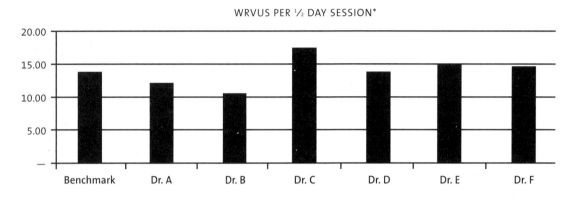

WRVUS PER ½ DAY SESSION*

* Assumes average of 5,700 WRVUs per physician, 45 weeks of service, 9 sessions per week (405 sessions total)

© 2006 Johnson & Walker Keegan

ment scheduling methodology, or other factors that impact the physician's efficiency. As these two examples demonstrate, both practice and physician-specific factors influence the efficiency with which physicians practice. This has obvious implications for physician compensation levels, particularly in productivity-based compensation plans.

3. Volume

Understanding volume is relatively straightforward, at least on the surface. This involves counting the number of procedures, the number of ambulatory encounters, the number of hospital encounters, the gross charges, and other similar measures of work or production performed by a physician for a defined denominator. This type of comparison can be performed for each of the physicians in a practice to provide internal benchmarking comparison, as well as external comparison involving published benchmark data. If the statement is true that "my patients are sicker," then we may expect some volume differences between the work produced by physicians within the same specialty. In addition, recent trends toward "super-specialization" will also impact measures of work volume in a medical practice.

Exhibit 7.7 reflects a comparison of one physician's work volume to CMS-reported volume as measured by CPT code frequency. In Exhibit 7.8, we have reflected a comparison of a physician's activity with that reported by CMS, but we have also reflected the impact on that physician's WRVU levels if the physician's activity had, in fact, resembled CMS-reported data. This type of analysis should not be used to dictate changes to coding; however, it may lead to coding reviews and education to ensure that physicians are, in fact, coding appropriately for services performed and documented.

EXHIBIT 7.7 Measuring Volume

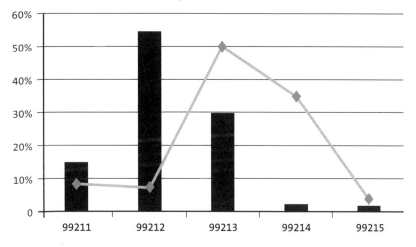

OFFICE/OUTPATIENT ACTIVITY VS. CMS PART B CLAIMS PAID

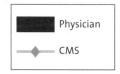

© 2006 Johnson & Walker Keegan

EXHIBIT 7.8 Measuring Volume and Intensity

OFFICE/OUTPATIENT ACTIVITY VS. CMS PART B CLAIMS PAID

Question: What if the physician's coding reflected CMS data?

	Actual Physician Codes	Actual Physician Percentage	WRVU per Code	Actual Total WRVUs	CMS Percentage	Expected Physician Codes	WRVU per Code	Expected Total WRVUs
99211	105	14%	0.17	17.85	9%	66	0.17	11.22
99212	384	52%	0.45	172.80	8%	59	0.45	26.55
99213	224	30%	0.67	150.08	49%	362	0.67	242.54
99214	15	2%	1.10	16.50	31%	228	1.10	250.80
99215	9	1%	1.77	15.93	3%	22	1.77	38.94
	737	**100%**		**373.16**	**100%**	**737**		**570.05**

Note: For illustrative purposes only. Actual coding frequency would depend on medical necessity, documentation, and related factors. Nothing presented here is intended to encourage inappropriate coding, the provision of services not medically indicated, or otherwise in a noncompliant manner.

© 2006 Johnson & Walker Keegan

Beyond physicians' variation in their practice styles, physicians who are working in medical practices that have not been able to streamline their patient flow processes, leverage technology appropriately, and provide the infrastructure and support for physician productivity and efficiency will exhibit volume discrepancies with their colleagues. These will impact a physician's productivity measures and will also likely impact his or her compensation levels.

4. Quality (or Appropriateness) of Care

Measures of physician quality or the appropriateness of care he or she provides are probably the most difficult to benchmark. The key question being asked in this factor is, "What is right for the patient and the patient's condition?" As we previously discussed, many practices are performing internal benchmarking of key quality indicators, and many health plans are essentially conducting external benchmarking of these same indicators to differentiate reimbursement levels to medical practices. As P4P strategies grow, and as electronic health records improve the ability to capture clinical performance data, these measures will likely increase in importance as a benchmarking tool and as distinct performance measures for physician compensation plan purposes.

EXAMPLES OF BENCHMARKING FOR COMPENSATION PLAN PURPOSES

The benchmarking process for physician compensation plan development is typically comprehensive to a high degree of specificity. In this context, benchmarking is used to identify the current state of physician productivity and compensation in comparison to others, but, perhaps more important, to understand the current linkages between productivity and compensation.

The four examples shown at the end of this section in Exhibits 7.9 to 7.12 demonstrate how to benchmark physician compensation and production for compensation plan development. The administrative infrastructure of the medical practice, coupled with requirements imposed by medical practice leaders and physicians, dictates the level to which benchmarking is employed in compensation plan development.

➤ EXAMPLE 1: PHYSICIAN COMPENSATION AND KEY PRODUCTION MEASURES

Exhibit 7.9 demonstrates a simple benchmarking analysis involving compensation levels and three key production measures – gross charges from professional services, net collections from professional services, and WRVUs. In this exhibit, we see that Dr. A, a family practitioner, receives a current compensation level that is 102.56 percent of benchmark medians. However, his production as measured by all three indices – gross charges, net collections, and WRVUs – is lower, at 88.39 percent, 77.27 percent, and 81.16 percent of benchmark medians, respectively.

As we further discuss in Chapter 16, we typically start the benchmarking process by reference to the benchmark median. The question needs to be asked as to whether a medical practice indeed wishes to "look like" the median or like something else (e.g., 90th percentile of practice peers). A comparison of physician compensation levels and physician productivity levels using benchmark medians presents a useful starting point for compensation plan purposes. By examining this type of data, a medical practice can determine if current compensation levels are realistic in relation to physician production levels, or whether there is opportunity to better link compensation to production (assuming that this is an intended goal for the plan).

➤ EXAMPLE 2: COMPENSATION-TO-PRODUCTION RATIOS

An example of benchmarking that demonstrates the interaction between two measures is depicted in Exhibit 7.10. By calculating ratios, we can see the relationship between compensation levels and various production levels of the physician, then compare these ratios to benchmark sources. In Exhibit 7.10, we calculate three separate ratios for the medical practice: (1) compensation-to-gross charges from professional services; (2) compensation-to-net collections from professional services; and (3) compensation per WRVU. We then compare the ratios for the practice to benchmark medians.

As this example demonstrates, the compensation-to-production ratios for Dr. A are higher than median levels in all three production measures employed. Of particular interest is that Dr. A is paid $50.00 per WRVU performed, compared to the benchmark median of $39.13. If the goal of this practice is to align compensation with the work effort and intensity of physicians, then an opportunity exists to refine the compensation plan. In this example, six of the twelve physicians are receiving compensation per WRVU that is higher than median levels, with the other six receiving compensation per WRVU that is lower than benchmark norms. However, only one physician reports a compensation-to-net-collections ratio that is less than the benchmark norm. This suggests that, while this practice may be paying physicians at higher levels on a WRVU basis, the net collections may also be higher due to a more favorable payer mix or for other reasons.

Perhaps more relevant to Exhibit 7.10 is to question why certain physicians receive significantly higher levels of compensation per WRVU as compared to benchmarks, while others are below (in some cases, significantly below) benchmark levels. In this example, it may be particularly important to note that Drs. C and F have the highest WRVU levels within their particular specialties (family practice [FP] and internal medicine [IM], respectively), but both receive compensation per WRVU that is below the median level. The precise reasons for these variations cannot be learned simply from the data, but assessing the benchmarking results can lead to probing questions about physician work levels, reimbursement, the allocation of overhead costs, and others – all of which will be relevant to understanding and providing perspective regarding the current compensation plan and potential alternative plans.

In the case of Exhibit 7.10, for example, the assessment may indicate that the practice's approach to overhead allocation tends to benefit physicians with lower levels of work and production as compared to physicians with higher production levels. If the practice has determined that one of the goals underlying any new compensation plan is to promote additional production and reward hard work, then changes to the expense allocation methodology may be in order. Keep in mind that the purpose of benchmarking is to provide perspective – not definitive answers. However, the perspective that is gained can provide useful information in evaluating the current compensation plan or refining or designing a new plan for a medical practice.

► EXAMPLE 3: COMPENSATION IN THE CONTEXT OF THE PRACTICE'S FINANCIAL POSITION

This third benchmarking example examines the cost of the medical practice in relation to its revenue, assisting in identifying the financial realities associated with any changes to physician compensation levels. In Exhibit 7.11, we can see that this practice has more staff support costs as a percentage of total medical revenue than the median, at 36 percent compared to 31.32 percent, while general operating costs generally approximate median levels. This suggests that it may be possible to "rightsize" staffing in the medical practice – for example, review its staffing levels, skill mix, staffing deployment models, etc. to potentially reduce staffing costs, or alternatively, redeploy the staff to enhance physician productivity and revenue generation. In this example, however, we also see that physicians are receiving compensation and benefits at levels that are higher than the benchmark median as a percentage of total medical revenue. Thus, if the goal is to "pay physicians more dollars," this medical practice will need to find ways to improve its revenue position and/or alter its operating expenses.

► EXAMPLE 4: ACADEMIC PRACTICE AND CLINICAL FULL-TIME EQUIVALENCY (CFTE) ANALYSIS

In Exhibit 7.12, we benchmark an academic department of OB/GYN that consists of 5.00 FTE faculty with a CFTE level of 3.75. CFTE is a subset of the full-time equivalent (FTE) level and signifies the portion of the faculty member's FTE that is devoted to clinical patient care. In this example, we calculate CFTEs for the actual work performed by faculty, using gross charges from professional services and WRVU levels.

In Exhibit 7.12, we can see that, overall, the faculty in this department are paid at 80.40 percent of private practice medians and at 102.06 percent of academic practice medians. The 3.75 CFTE faculty generate gross charges equivalent to 5.01 CFTE for academic practice physicians and 3.68 CFTE for private practice physicians, suggesting a potential opportunity to enhance productivity. By comparing the *intensity* of the work by using WRVUs, we see that there does appear to be the opportunity suggested by the gross charges finding. In this example, the 3.75 CFTE faculty generate WRVUs equivalent to 4.35 CFTE for academic practice physicians and 3.63 CFTE for private practice physicians. This analysis can also be performed at the level of individual faculty members.

Thus, as a department, the data suggest that the faculty are paid at levels that are greater than those for the academic median, although they are paid at levels that are lower than those for private practice physicians. Their production, as measured by WRVUs, is above what we would expect of 3.75 CFTE academic faculty, but below what we would expect of their private practice counterparts. This may be due to many factors (e.g., the CFTE determination method, impacts to practice efficiency, etc.), but it still provides a useful point of reference for the discussion of physician compensation levels for planning purposes, in particular given that academic practice physicians are increasingly expected to have clinical service work levels that are comparable to their private practice counterparts during the time in which they are engaged in delivering patient care services.

EXHIBIT 7.9 Benchmarking Example 1 – Physician Compensation and Key Production Measures

		Total	Dr. A FP w/o OB	Dr. B FP w/o OB	Dr. C FP w/OB	Dr. D IM
	Physician FTE Levels	12.00	1.00	1.00	1.00	1.00
Step 1	**Benchmark compensation levels.**					
	Actual Compensation Levels		$160,000	$165,000	$155,000	$165,000
	Benchmark Medians		$156,011	$156,011	$165,124	$166,420
	Percent of Median		102.56%	105.76%	93.87%	99.15%
Step 2	**Benchmark production levels.**					
	Actual Gross Charges from Professional Services		$400,000	$375,000	$425,000	$500,000
	Benchmark Median		$452,560	$452,560	$484,056	$472,284
	Percent of Median		88.39%	82.86%	87.80%	105.87%
	Actual Net Collections from Professional Services		$240,000	$225,000	$255,000	$300,000
	Benchmark Median		$310,613	$310,613	$363,161	$320,745
	Percent of Median		77.27%	72.44%	70.22%	93.53%
	Actual WRVUs		3,200	3,500	4,500	4,000
	Benchmark Median		3,943	3,943	4,236	3,894
	Percent of Median		81.16%	88.76%	106.23%	102.72%

Note: Benchmark medians provided for example purposes only; source benchmarks selected should be linked as closely as possible to medical practice; for example, by specialty, by geographic area, and by practice type.

Key:
Card Inv = Cardiology: Invasive
Card Non-Inv = Cardiology: Noninvasive
FP w/OB = Family Practice with Obstetrics
FP w/o OB = Family Practice without Obstetrics
IM = Internal Medicine
Pulm = Pulmonary Medicine
Rheum = Rheumatology

Dr. E IM	Dr. F IM	Dr. G IM	Dr. H IM	Dr. I Rheum	Dr. J Card Inv	Dr. K Card Non-Inv	Dr. L Pulm
1.00	1.00	1.00	1.00	1.00	1.00	1.00	1.00
$170,000	$162,000	$175,000	$180,000	$180,000	$350,000	$375,000	$250,000
$166,420	$166,420	$166,420	$166,420	$198,839	$398,133	$351,637	$230,688
102.15%	97.34%	105.16%	108.16%	90.53%	87.91%	106.64%	108.37%
$475,000	$485,000	$450,000	$500,000	$600,000	$1,000,000	$1,200,000	$800,000
$472,284	$472,284	$472,284	$472,284	$538,398	$1,561,296	$1,249,403	$715,328
100.58%	102.69%	95.28%	105.87%	111.44%	64.05%	96.05%	111.84%
$285,000	$291,000	$270,000	$300,000	$360,000	$600,000	$500,000	$350,000
$320,745	$320,745	$320,745	$320,745	$358,070	$670,483	$510,356	$380,165
88.86%	90.73%	84.18%	93.53%	100.54%	89.49%	97.97%	92.07%
3,800	4,000	3,700	3,850	4,500	6,800	6,000	5,800
3,894	3,894	3,894	3,894	4,009	8,310	6,564	5,589
97.59%	102.72%	95.02%	98.87%	112.25%	81.83%	91.41%	103.78%

EXHIBIT
7.10

Benchmarking Example 2 – Compensation-to-Production Ratios

		Total	Dr. A FP w/o OB	Dr. B FP w/o OB	Dr. C FP w/OB	Dr. D IM
	Physician FTE Levels	12.00	1.00	1.00	1.00	1.00
Step 1	**Determine current compensation levels.**					
	Compensation Levels		$160,000	$165,000	$155,000	$165,000
Step 2	**Determine current production levels.**					
	Gross Charges from Professional Services		$400,000	$375,000	$425,000	$500,000
	Net Collections from Professional Services		$240,000	$225,000	$255,000	$300,000
	WRVUs		3,200	3,500	4,500	4,000
Step 3	**Calculate compensation-to-production ratios and compare to benchmark sources.**					
	Compensation-to-Gross Charges Ratio		0.400	0.440	0.365	0.330
	Benchmark Median		0.339	0.339	0.357	0.345
	Compensation-to-Net Collections Ratio		0.667	0.733	0.608	0.550
	Benchmark Median		0.499	0.499	0.474	0.520
	Compensation per WRVU		$50.00	$47.14	$34.44	$41.25
	Benchmark Median		$39.13	$39.13	$41.31	$42.12

Note: Benchmark medians provided for example purposes only; source benchmarks selected should be linked as closely as possible to medical practice; for example, by specialty, by geographic area, and by practice type.

Key:
Card Inv = Cardiology: Invasive
Card Non-Inv = Cardiology: Noninvasive
FP w/OB = Family Practice with Obstetrics
FP w/o OB = Family Practice without Obstetrics
IM = Internal Medicine
Pulm = Pulmonary Medicine
Rheum = Rheumatology

	Dr. E IM	Dr. F IM	Dr. G IM	Dr. H IM	Dr. I Rheum	Dr. J Card Inv	Dr. K Card Non-Inv	Dr. L Pulm
	1.00	1.00	1.00	1.00	1.00	1.00	1.00	1.00
	$170,000	$162,000	$175,000	$180,000	$180,000	$350,000	$375,000	$250,000
	$475,000	$485,000	$450,000	$500,000	$600,000	$1,000,000	$1,200,000	$800,000
	$285,000	$291,000	$270,000	$300,000	$360,000	$600,000	$500,000	$350,000
	3,800	4,000	3,700	3,850	4,500	6,800	6,000	5,800
	0.358	0.334	0.389	0.360	0.300	0.350	0.313	0.313
	0.345	0.345	0.345	0.345	0.394	0.257	0.283	0.324
	0.596	0.557	0.648	0.600	0.500	0.583	0.750	0.714
	0.520	0.520	0.520	0.520	0.573	0.580	0.579	0.569
	$44.74	$40.50	$47.30	$46.75	$40.00	$51.47	$62.50	$43.10
	$42.12	$42.12	$42.12	$42.12	$49.64	$51.86	$49.80	$43.38

EXHIBIT 7.11

Benchmarking Example 3 –
Compensation in the Context of the Practice's Financial Position

		Total	Per FTE Physician	Benchmark Median	Cost as % of Total Medical Revenue	Benchmark Median
	Physician FTE Levels	5.00				
	Total Medical Revenue	$2,500,000				
Step 1	**Determine practice operating expenses.**					
	Staff Support Costs	$900,000	$180,000	$163,751	36.00%	31.32%
	General Operating Costs	$625,000	$125,000	$123,984	25.00%	25.77%
	Total Operating Costs	$1,525,000	$305,000	$300,040	61.00%	57.60%
	Physician Compensation Costs					
	Compensation	$852,000	$170,400	$180,386	34.08%	33.82%
	Benefits	$153,360	$30,672	$28,124	6.13%	4.79%
	Total Physician Compensation Costs	$1,005,360	$201,072	$200,962	40.21%	41.64%
	Total Practice Costs	$2,530,360	$506,072	$505,951	101.21%	100.46%

Note: Benchmark medians provided for example purposes only; source benchmarks selected should be linked as closely as possible to medical practice; for example, by specialty, by geographic area, and by practice type.

EXHIBIT 7.12 Benchmarking Example 4 – Academic Practice CFTE Analysis

	Total	Faculty A Obstetrics/ Gynecology	Faculty B Obstetrics/ Gynecology	Faculty C Obstetrics/ Gynecology	Faculty D Maternal-Fetal	Faculty E Maternal-Fetal
Physician FTE Levels	5.00	1.00	1.00	1.00	1.00	1.00
Physician CFTE Levels	3.75	0.70	0.75	0.80	0.75	0.75
Step 1 — Benchmark current compensation.						
Compensation	$1,055,000	$180,000	$195,000	$200,000	$230,000	$250,000
Academic Practice Benchmark Median	$1,033,740	$191,082	$191,082	$191,082	$230,247	$230,247
Percent Current to Academic Median	102.06%	94.20%	102.05%	104.67%	99.89%	108.58%
Private Practice Benchmark Median	$1,312,171	$237,191	$237,191	$237,191	$300,299	$300,299
Percent Current to Private Practice Median	80.40%	75.89%	82.21%	84.32%	76.59%	83.25%
Step 2 — Report current clinical activity.						
Gross Charges from Professional Services		$600,000	$750,000	$950,000	$1,200,000	$1,500,000
WRVU Levels		4,500	5,000	6,000	6,500	8,000
Step 3 — Report academic practice benchmarks.						
Gross Charges Median		$872,045	$872,045	$872,045	$1,138,677	$1,138,677
WRVU Median		6,273	6,273	6,273	7,709	7,709
Step 4 — Report private practice benchmarks.						
Gross Charges Median		$1,052,879	$1,052,879	$1,052,879	$1,802,540	$1,802,540
WRVU Median		7,204	7,204	7,204	9,825	9,825
Step 5 — Calculate CFTE based on academic benchmarks.	Total					
CFTE Gross Charges (academic)	5.01	0.69	0.86	1.09	1.05	1.32
CFTE WRVU (academic)	4.35	0.72	0.80	0.96	0.84	1.04
Step 6 — Calculate CFTE based on private benchmarks.						
CFTE Gross Charges (private)	3.68	0.57	0.71	0.90	0.67	0.83
CFTE WRVU (private)	3.63	0.62	0.69	0.83	0.66	0.81

Note: Benchmark medians provided for example purposes only; source benchmarks selected should be linked as closely as possible to medical practice; for example, by specialty, by geographic area, and by practice type.

With physician productivity in the spotlight as a key measure for physician compensation, the question "how should a practice measure physician productivity and physician work levels for compensation purposes?" is an important one for medical practices to address. Moreover, the compensation plan development process is informed through benchmarking of current physician compensation and production levels. This influence is largely in the form of providing useful perspective regarding key issues such as:

► How good (or bad) current compensation levels are in relation to peers;

► How good (or bad) physician work levels are in relation to peers; and

► How good (or bad) practice operating costs are by reference to similar practices.

Because of the perspective it can provide, benchmarking is therefore an essential element of the process needed to develop an effective compensation plan.

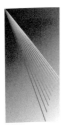

EIGHT

Pay-for-Performance (P4P) and Physician Compensation

While fee-for-service continues to be the most widely used mechanism to reimburse physicians for professional services, a contingent reimbursement strategy termed "pay-for-performance," also known as "P4P," is emerging as a popular methodology for payers who are seeking a way to foster high quality, low cost health care services. P4P programs differentially reimburse physicians based on their achievement of specific clinical and practice efficiency measures. These programs seek to focus physician attention and performance on effective care management and clinical outcomes through the use of discrete measures and incentives. A number of medical practices have extended this reimbursement strategy (payments from health plan to medical practice) to physician compensation plans or incentive plans (payments from medical practice to physician), effectively aligning the reimbursement mechanism that generates revenue to the practice with the payment mechanism that pays physicians for their services.

BACKGROUND

Historically, medical practices have generally thrown up their hands when the issue of differentiating performance or quality has been raised. Many believed that it was simply too difficult to control for the many idiosyncratic factors that impact quality of patient care – specifically, the patient-specific variables of genetics, age, risk factors, comorbidities, socioeconomic status, compliance with treatment plans, and other similar factors. Medical practices that sought to differentially reward physicians based on quality thus tended to focus on "proxies" of quality that involved more easily measured issues of medical record documentation (e.g., timeliness and completeness), patient perceptions of service delivery (e.g., derived from patient satisfaction surveys or patient complaint tracking), and patient access (e.g., access to third available appointment and wait time upon presentation for a scheduled appointment).

Today, however, electronic health records and other sophisticated information technologies have facilitated capture, reporting, and analysis of clinical data by medical practices and payers. Many practices have now negotiated terms in their health plan contracts that permit differential reimbursement based on clinical or quality measures.

In the past, the measures that were selected for contingent reimbursement tended to focus on those that were readily available to the health plan – data submitted on a billing claim form. Increasingly, however, health plans are requiring additional data to be submitted by medical groups that involve data mining of medical records, self-reports of technological readiness, patient access data, and other similar indices.

THE P4P DEBATE

There are strong proponents and strong detractors of P4P as a reimbursement strategy. Proponents argue that contingent reimbursement will help to more quickly transition the health care industry to a focus on prevention and wellness (which is expected to reduce the cost of care), encourage medical practices to institute electronic health records, and permit consumers (employers, health plans, and patients) to differentiate performance of medical practices (and physicians) based on clinical and practice efficiency measures. P4P reimbursement mechanisms are relatively new, and proponents include employers concerned about rising health care costs, health plans seeking to differentiate high quality, low cost physicians, and patients who are seeking a high return on investment as they pay rising out-of-pocket expenses for health care services. Proponents tend to view P4P as an alignment strategy (long overdue), aligning the interests of employers, health plans, medical practices, and patients on high quality, low cost care.

Those opposing P4P programs tend to not oppose the underlying *concepts* of P4P arrangements; rather, they question whether the measures that are selected for contingent reimbursement truly define "quality." These individuals are asking questions related to the long-term impact of linking payment to the measures that heretofore have been selected. For example, what is the impact on physicians and medical groups who treat very ill patients? What is the impact on physicians and medical groups that have a large noncompliant patient base? What is the impact on small practices that do not have the administrative infrastructure to compete for these additional funds? What is the impact on the overall revenue stream for a medical practice as more and more of the dollars are paid in this type of contingent fashion? In general, opponents of P4P are highly skeptical and are concerned that P4P may lead to further declines in reimbursement for professional services, encourage undue competition, and/or may not result in the high quality, low cost outcomes that are anticipated from these programs.

In the future, if P4P comes to represent a large portion of the reimbursement dollar, concerns regarding differential access for specific types of patients and the financial and other impacts on medical practices will need to be addressed. The impact this will have on physician perceptions of clinical autonomy, revenue performance, measures of physician work and effort, and the alignment within internal compensation strategies remains to be seen.

ALIGNING COMPENSATION WITH REIMBURSEMENT

As we have indicated, it is important for a compensation plan to be aligned with the reimbursement mechanism of the medical practice to not only ensure fiscal responsibility but also to optimize revenue performance. For example, if a medical practice has 75 percent of its revenue paid via capitation contracts, a physician compensation plan that rewards physicians based on professional services gross charges or patient visits alone is likely nonsensical. Similarly, if a medical practice generates 75 percent of its revenue via fee-for-service contracts, a compensation plan that only addresses panel size may be misaligned with revenue-generating opportunity. With P4P reimbursement, a similar situation holds. That is, if a significant percentage of the revenue of a medical practice is derived through P4P strategies that predicate reimbursement on specific clinical, patient safety, or practice efficiency measures, a compensation plan based solely on professional services net collections or work relative value units (WRVUs) is likely not aligned with the financial reality that revenue is contingent on measures that extend beyond clinical production.

There does not necessarily need to be a one-to-one relationship between the reimbursement mechanism and the physician compensation mechanism. Some practices, for example, still pay physicians on straight salary arrangements while receiving their revenue via discounted fee-for-service strategies. For our purposes, the importance of P4P in physician compensation relates to one of *alignment*. As reimbursement levels from these arrangements increase to represent a significant portion of a practice's revenue, practices will likely attempt to align their internal physician compensation plans in order to ensure heightened focus on these performance criteria to optimize revenue to the medical practice.

P4P METHODS AND MEASURES

▶ P4P COMPENSATION STRATEGIES

A number of different compensation strategies are used to recognize and reward physicians for P4P measures. Similarly, a number of different contracting strategies are used to generate P4P dollars. We now turn to a discussion of the P4P methods and measures currently adopted by medical practices.

P4P strategies used in the context of physician compensation take one of three forms: (1) direct; (2) indirect; or (3) integrative treatment of these funds for physician compensation purposes.

1. Direct Treatment

In a direct treatment of P4P dollars, a medical practice adopts a direct "pass-through" approach of these dollars to the physicians who "earned" them consistent with the P4P contracted measures. In this direct treatment, this payment is above and beyond what the physician receives due to the physician compensation plan that the practice has adopted. In some cases, the practice may retain an administrative fee related to managing the infrastructure to monitor and document performance and/or to contract, manage, and disburse the funds. Otherwise, all P4P dollars are paid directly to the earning physicians.

The advantage of this direct approach to P4P dollars is that physicians who are directly responsible for earning this contingent payment individually benefit from their work – and they also recognize the magnitude of that benefit.

The disadvantages of a direct approach to administering P4P are twofold: (1) the P4P component of compensation may be wholly inconsistent with the internal physician compensation plan, leading to conflicts regarding priorities and focus; and (2) as the amount of revenue grows from P4P in comparison to "traditional" fee-for-service reimbursement, this direct treatment may be inconsistent with the goals of compensating physicians in the practice. In essence, this represents an individualistic, performance-based compensation plan, with the same advantages and disadvantages of these plans, including a lack of team orientation and focus on cost of practice issues.

2. Indirect Treatment

In an indirect treatment of P4P dollars, a medical practice generally elects one of three options: (1) to treat P4P dollars as simply another revenue source in the funds flow model that is available for physician compensation purposes, with the overall compensation plan generally silent as to the P4P measures; (2) to create a separate incentive pool for these dollars that may be "earned" by the physicians (including those physicians who did not generate the P4P dollars); or (3) to use the P4P dollars for discretionary purposes.

In the first indirect treatment method, the current internal physician compensation plan is not impacted in a material way; however, the method used to credit physicians for their productivity is extended to these funds as well. So, for example, if a practice credits physicians for net collections from professional services by using a percentage of net collections to total net collections basis, then this same percentage is applied to the P4P dollars received by the practice, with each physician receiving his or her portion consistent with the revenue treatment method identified for professional services.

In the second indirect treatment method involving a separate incentive pool for P4P funds, the money is awarded to physicians based on criteria established by the practice that may or may not have a direct linkage to the measures used to generate the P4P dollars.

When an indirect treatment of these funds is employed, any number of methods may be used to distribute this revenue to physicians, including:

► Per physician (equal share);

► Per physician full-time equivalency (FTE) (equal share adjusted for FTE);

► Based on individual physician professional services net collections as a percentage of total net collections;

► Based on individual WRVUs as a percentage of total WRVUs; or

► Others.

In the third indirect treatment method, in some cases, the medical practice may elect a discretionary use of these funds consistent with practice needs. For example, it applies these dollars to practice operating expense, thereby reducing overall expenditures specifically allocated to physicians; or it uses the funds to support new program development, to support physician leadership or administrative stipends, or for other purposes in the practice.

The advantage of the indirect treatment of P4P includes the recognition that a group or team orientation (rather than simply individual physician effort) is needed to ensure high quality, low cost care for patients (which is what the P4P dollars typically represent). Thus, all of the physicians in the practice have an opportunity to "earn" P4P dollars through additional revenue credit and/or through a new incentive pool option, or the practice as a whole benefits from the additional revenue that has been generated.

The disadvantage of the indirect treatment is the general lack of focus and accountability for performance relative to the P4P measures and its promised revenue potential. Since physicians do not perceive a direct reward for generating the funds, there may be less focus on the measures and outcomes. Of course, this disadvantage can be overcome if the P4P dollars are sufficiently great to warrant collective attention to the performance measures and/or if the practice builds in performance expectations related to program participation.

3. Integrative Treatment

The third strategy involves an "integrative" approach to P4P allocation. In these practices, a larger program of clinical engagement or integration[1] is adopted, with that program funded via the P4P dollars. In this strategy, an overall program to recognize physicians for their high quality, low cost outcomes is developed and typically involves multiple measures of performance (often beyond those identified in the contracts with the health plans for these dollars), and typically also applies to all patients (beyond those for which the P4P dollars are derived).

The strategy adopted by a medical practice to compensate physicians involving P4P dollars and measures typically depends on the goals of the compensation plan for a particular medical practice, as well as on the amount of revenue available from P4P-contracted dollars that is used to fund physician compensation.

► P4P Revenue Strategies

There are a number of different revenue strategies used in the contractual arrangements for P4P dollars. Some medical practices have been able to secure *additional* dollars from health plans for P4P incentive rewards at an established rate (e.g., X percent of allowable charges). Other medical practices have contracted with health plans for a flat dollar amount per well-managed patient (e.g., diabetic, asthmatic, heart patient) or have entered into tiered arrangements whereby different dollar levels are paid based on performance in relation to peers.

It should be recognized that some practices are increasingly concerned that while many of the initial P4P programs have led to "additional" dollars paid to the practice, the future may not be all that "rosy." They worry that fee-for-service reimbursement levels will be held at a constant level (or even reduced from current levels), with more and more of the revenue used to reimburse medical practices paid on a contingent basis. Thus, some are concerned that P4P may become a new version of the "withhold" or "risk-pool" arrangements of the past, with no overall additional dollars actually made available to the practice.

Regardless of the revenue strategy that is used to contract for these funds, if the portion of the reimbursement dollar awarded via P4P grows, then this type of reimbursement is likely to increasingly impact the way physician work and effort are measured. Moreover, as P4P measures become more entrenched, "full reimbursement" from health plans will be dependent on the demonstration of physician performance in a manner that is consistent with the expectations of the P4P reimbursement system.

► P4P PERFORMANCE MEASURES

The actual measures used in P4P reimbursement strategies are moving beyond those available on billing claim forms to require some additional reporting by medical practices, such as data consistent with the Health Plan Employer Data and Information Set (HEDIS) indicators or self-reports of information technology utilization, such as computerized physician order entry. As electronic health records become more prevalent, the ease of data capture and reporting for P4P reimbursement methods will improve and likely lead to an increase in the popularity of P4P among health plans and employer groups.

The selection of P4P measures used for physician compensation planning purposes will depend on: (1) the measures identified by the medical practice's payers for this differential reimbursement; and (2) whether the medical practice elects to implement a direct, indirect, or integrative P4P program (e.g., building on these measures to create a broader program of clinical engagement). The following types of questions should be explored as part of the planning process for physician compensation:

- ► How much of the revenue is available through P4P mechanisms?

- ► How should P4P or clinical measures be used in the context of the overall compensation plan for the medical practice?

- ► What are the advantages and disadvantages to the practice of adopting a direct approach, an indirect approach, or an integrative treatment of these funds?

- ► What are the specific performance outcomes we are seeking, and by whom?

- ► How should these measures and funds be aligned in the practice – for example, what specific weighting or point system should be used to align this portion of compensation for the practice's physicians?

▶ In what ways might a P4P performance measure be considered "unfair" to a physician? How should this be dealt with in terms of the compensation plan mechanics?

These questions are generated as the compensation planning committee progresses through the 12-step process outlined in Chapter 2, with specific attention paid to Step 2 (establishing compensation plan goals) and to Steps 6 and 7 (determining the compensation plan architecture and its methodology).

If an integrative P4P program is implemented by using the P4P dollars to develop a broader set of measures to evaluate and reward physicians, it is often useful to develop an overall architecture to guide the selection of P4P performance measures to be rewarded. For example, rather than develop a laundry list of 15 to 20 measures, an overall architecture that situates these measures within a formal framework helps to communicate the underlying purpose of the measure and also permits a medical practice to "exchange" measures – for example, add or subtract measures over time while still preserving the balance of measures intended.

An example of a basic P4P architectural framework is depicted in Exhibit 8.1 and includes four separate quadrants: (1) patient-focused care (e.g., patient safety, patient access, patient satisfaction); (2) resource utilization (e.g., cost of care issues, use of appropriate resources); (3) clinical management (e.g., management of chronic diseases such as diabetes, asthma, and congestive heart failure); and (4) leveraging technology (e.g., e-prescribing, e-mailing test results to patients, permitting patients to access the web site for test results reporting, and the use of electronic health records).

EXHIBIT 8.1   **A Basic P4P Architectural Framework**

Patient-Focused Care	Resource Utilization
Measure 1	Measure 1
Measure 2	Measure 2
Measure 3	Measure 3
Clinical Management	Leveraging Technology
Measure 1	Measure 1
Measure 2	Measure 2
Measure 3	Measure 3

The architectural framework then guides the selection and balance of measures to be rewarded.

In the framework depicted in Exhibit 8.2, we expand the overall architecture to include specific measures in each of the four quadrants that might be selected for reward. Note that there are a wide range of measures that can be selected for a particular category. The actual selection of the measures will depend upon those identified by the health plans for contingent reimbursement and/or those that the medical practice determines are particularly relevant for clinical excellence, clinical integration, or other similar purposes.

EXHIBIT 8.2 Specific Measures That Might Be Selected for Reward

PATIENT-FOCUSED CARE

Measure 1: Access to Appointment

Example: Urgent same-day access, routine access within three days

Measure 2: Patient Satisfaction Scores

Example: Overall 4 or better on 1 to 5 Likert scale

Measure 3: Patient Safety

Example: Improvement in preventable or possibly preventable complications or errors over baseline levels

RESOURCE UTILIZATION

Measure 1: Average Length of Stay

Example: Moderately managed or better by diagnostic group

Measure 2: Office Overhead

Example: Operating costs as a percentage of total medical revenue compared to benchmark median for specialty

Measure 3: Generic Prescribing

Example: Target thresholds established by specialty and determined by sampling techniques or evaluation of payer data

CLINICAL MANAGEMENT

Measure 1: Immunizations/Vaccinations

Example: Child and adolescent immunizations, adult and senior flu shots

Measure 2: Diabetic Care Management

Example: HbA1C, LDL, eye exams, foot exams

Measure 3: Congestive Heart Failure Management

Example: Readmission rate, use of ace inhibitors

LEVERAGING TECHNOLOGY

Measure 1: E-prescribing Tools

Example: Utilization levels as a percentage of total patient base

Measure 2: Electronic Health Records at Sophisticated Level

Example: Progress notes, educational tools to patients, trend evaluation, computerized physician order entry (CPOE)

Measure 3: E-communication to Patients

Example: Secured messaging, e-scheduling, e-test results reporting, e-consults

Within such a framework, a medical practice determines the precise operational definitions for each measure, the points to be awarded for each measure (or portion of measure), and the overall weighting of the factors. The actual points and weights may relate to the level and method of P4P reimbursement, or they may be based on a different approach altogether – for example, determined based on the physicians' or medical practice's perceptions of the importance of the measures in facilitating clinical excellence. It is important to recognize that not all measures will apply to all physicians. Thus, in a multispecialty practice, in particular, the measures may be weighted or given point values differentially based on the specialty, or, alternatively, specialty-specific measures may be identified.

➤ PHYSICIAN PROFILES

Similar to other measures of physician work and effort used for purposes of physician compensation plans, physicians should receive regular progress reports (e.g., quarterly or monthly) regarding their performance on the P4P measures. These physician profiles should include the targets that have been selected for the specific performance measures, as well as share that physician's performance in relation to that of his or her peers.

We highly recommend the sharing of "unblinded" data, thereby making the data fully transparent. If the medical practice's culture will not support this level of information dissemination, then "blinded" data (e.g., where the actual physician names are removed) will still permit an individual physician to learn his or her relative position in relation to that of his or her peers. The sharing of targets and relative performances essentially helps to translate "data" to "information" for the physician and tends to enhance physician engagement and behavioral change.

➤ P4P DOCUMENTATION

The measures used in P4P reimbursement and disbursement arrangements tend to have more complex definitional requirements than the financial or productivity measures more typically used to-date for physician compensation – for example, net collections from professional services or WRVUs. The measures themselves need to be carefully defined and well understood by physicians.

We recommend that the program documentation include at least the following elements:

- ➤ Well-defined operational definitions for each performance measure;
- ➤ Eligibility criteria of physicians (e.g., excluding new physicians or physicians who do not actively participate in one or more elements);
- ➤ Stop-loss provisions (e.g., the impact of very ill patients or noncompliant patients on a particular performance measure);
- ➤ Sources of data that will be used for the program and efforts to validate the source data;

- ► The way in which data capture and reporting will occur;

- ► A structured process relative to the development, adoption, refinement, and potential replacement of individual measures; and

- ► The length of time performance needs to be at a certain level to suggest that performance has been modified and the measure has been integrated into standard practices and care.

As with any compensation program, it is important to create formalized policies and mechanisms to respond to physician appeals, questions, or concerns. Equally important is to revisit the program documentation at periodic intervals to determine whether issues are still valid, whether any unintended effects have occurred, or whether additional program requirements and/or clarifications are needed.

EXAMPLES OF P4P PLANS

The use of "nonclinical" production measures is not new; many medical practices have used patient satisfaction, cost containment, citizenship, and other such measures in their physician compensation plans. In the compensation plan examples presented in Chapters 13 through 15, we frequently isolate a component of compensation related to P4P measures, and the reader is encouraged to review these plans for additional plan examples in addition to the two P4P plans showcased below.

► EXAMPLE 1: DIRECT LINK BETWEEN REIMBURSEMENT AND DISBURSEMENT

The compensation plan outlined in Exhibit 8.3 credits each individual physician with his or her net collections from professional services and earned P4P dollars. In this example, the physician's performance is evaluated on each of the P4P measures to which revenue is contingently paid to the practice. In this case, the practice identified a set dollar amount per patient for the effective management of three chronic care conditions: (1) congestive heart failure; (2) diabetes; and (3) asthma. As demonstrated in this example, different specialties are eligible to receive the P4P dollars, with the exact dollar amount credited to each physician based on the method by which the practice is reimbursed – in this case, dollars per well-managed patient based on the P4P criteria.

This approach can be used in multispecialty practices to recognize the different earning power associated with the contingent reimbursement dollar; however, an appropriate administrative infrastructure is necessary to ensure that individual physician performance is appropriately tracked and rewarded. The advantages of this direct method of awarding P4P dollars is that the reward is linked to the number of patients who are well managed by an individual physician. The disadvantage of this approach is that it can lead to unintended effects that may have a detrimental impact on the practice, such as "cherry-picking" of patients or subspecialization of physicians (e.g., developing a heavy diabetic case load), or it may thwart efforts to develop a true "group practice" or "care team" approach to patient care.

▶ EXAMPLE 2: SEPARATE INCENTIVE POOL AND P4P FRAMEWORK

In this second example, depicted in Exhibit 8.4, the money received from P4P contracted dollars is not directly "mapped" and paid to the individual physicians who earned these dollars. Instead, a P4P framework similar to the one outlined in this chapter is used to reward physicians based on the measures via a points and weights system established by the practice.

The advantage of this approach is that the P4P dollars that may be funded by a handful of payers can be used to reward physicians' performances over their entire patient base as determined by criteria established by a medical practice. The performance to be rewarded may be consistent with the specific measures intended by the payers, or it may be expanded to include other measures deemed important to ensuring high quality, low cost care. The disadvantage of this approach includes the administrative infrastructure required to develop, monitor, and implement the program itself due to the number of performance measures involved and the potential confusion related to the multiple-measures approach by the physicians themselves.

EXHIBIT 8.3

P4P Example 1 – Direct Link Between Reimbursement and Disbursement

		Total	Dr. A FP w/o OB	Dr. B FP w/o OB	Dr. C FP	Dr. D IM
Step 1	**Allocate physician professional services net revenues.**					
	Net Collections from Professional Services	$5,014,559	$365,502	$315,387	$411,133	$370,260
Step 2	**Determine physician % to total production.**	100.00%	7.29%	6.29%	8.20%	7.38%
Step 3	**Apply P4P dollar award to physicians based on their performance.**	$20,000				
	1. Congestive Heart Failure Based on readmission rates and use of ace inhibitors	$10,000	Not Eligible	Not Eligible	Not Eligible	$1,000
	2. Diabetic Care Management Based on HbA1C, LDL, eye exams, foot exams	$5,000	$300	$300	$500	$750
	3. Asthma Care Management Based on emergency room utilization and readmission rates	$5,000	$400	$500	$450	$750
Step 4	**Determine total revenue attributed to physician (net collections and P4P Award).**	$5,034,559	$366,202	$316,187	$412,083	$372,760
Step 5	**Determine physician revenue % to total revenue.**	100.00%	7.27%	6.28%	8.19%	7.40%
Step 6	**Assign cost of practice based on physician revenue as a % to total revenue.**	$(2,517,280)	$(183,101)	$(158,093)	$(206,041)	$(186,380)
Step 7	**Determine physician-specific direct expense.**	$(494,058)	$(36,822)	$(37,872)	$(43,292)	$(38,984)
Step 8	**Determine total W-2 compensation (net of physician-specific direct expense).**	$2,033,221	$146,279	$120,221	$162,749	$147,396

Note: For illustrative purposes only; internal system to monitor and track performance on P4P measures required to determine physician award levels.

Key:
Card Inv = Cardiology: Invasive
Card Non-Inv = Cardiology: Noninvasive
FP w/OB = Family Practice with Obstetrics
FP w/o OB = Family Practice without Obstetrics
IM = Internal Medicine
Pulm = Pulmonary Medicine
Rheum = Rheumatology

	Dr. E IM	Dr. F IM	Dr. G IM	Dr. H IM	Dr. I Rheum	Dr. J Card Inv	Dr. K Card Non-Inv	Dr. L Pulm
	$318,255	$365,378	$346,002	$317,171	$354,851	$548,233	$864,741	$437,646
	6.35%	7.29%	6.90%	6.33%	7.08%	10.93%	17.24%	8.73%
	$0	$500	$500	$2,000	Not Eligible	$2,500	$3,500	Not Eligible
	$1,000	$600	$550	$1,000	Not Eligible	Not Eligible	Not Eligible	Not Eligible
	$400	$1,000	$750	$750	Not Eligible	Not Eligible	Not Eligible	Not Eligible
	$319,655	$367,478	$347,802	$320,921	$354,851	$550,733	$868,241	$437,646
	6.35%	7.30%	6.91%	6.37%	7.05%	10.94%	17.25%	8.69%
	$(159,827)	$(183,739)	$(173,901)	$(160,461)	$(177,426)	$(275,367)	$(434,121)	$(218,823)
	$(41,292)	$(40,292)	$(40,312)	$(35,632)	$(41,002)	$(46,523)	$(49,523)	$(42,512)
	$118,535	$143,447	$133,589	$124,829	$136,424	$228,844	$384,598	$176,311

EXHIBIT
8.4

P4P Example 2 – Separate Incentive Pool and P4P Framework

		Total	Dr. A IM	Dr. B IM	Dr. C IM	Dr. D IM	Dr. E IM
	Physician FTE Levels	5.00	1.00	1.00	1.00	1.00	1.00
Step 1	**Allocate physician professional services revenue.**						
	Net Collections from Professional Services	$1,717,066	$370,260	$318,255	$365,378	$346,002	$317,171
Step 2	**Determine physician % to total net collections.**		21.56%	18.53%	21.28%	20.15%	18.47%
Step 3	**Determine P4P pool.**	$25,000					
	1. Diabetic Management Evaluate each patient chart for the following: HbA1C, LDL, eye exams, foot exams.						
	Determine number of well-managed patients per physician.	25	2	6	6	3	8
	Weight per well-managed patient in the P4P category = 2	2	2	2	2	2	2
	Determine physician credit for well-managed diabetic patient (number of well-managed diabetic patients x weight).	50	4	12	12	6	16
	2. Congestive Heart Failure (CHF) Management Evaluate each CHF patient chart for the following: ace inhibitors, reduction in readmision rate within defined time period.						
	Determine number of well-managed patients per physician.	3	0	0	0	2	1
	Weight per well-managed patient in this P4P category = 5	5				5	5
	Determine physician credit for well-managed CHF patient (number of well-managed CHF patients x weight).	15	0	0	0	10	5

	Total	Dr. A IM	Dr. B IM	Dr. C IM	Dr. D IM	Dr. E IM
3. Average Length of Stay (ALOS) Evaluate each inpatient chart for ALOS.						
Calculate each physician's percent of patient equal to or better than defined benchmark.		80%	68%	55%	75%	85%
Assign points for the category as follows: Physician receives 1 point for ≥ to 80% Physician receives .50 point for 70–79%.						
Determine points based on physician results.	2.5	1	0	0	0.5	1
Weight for this P4P category = 3	3	3			3	3
Determine physician credit for ALOS results (points x weight).	7.5	3	0	0	1.5	3

Step 4 — **Calculate total points for each physician and determine each physician's percent of total credits.**

	Total	Dr. A IM	Dr. B IM	Dr. C IM	Dr. D IM	Dr. E IM
Total physician credits for all three P4P measures.	72.5	7	12	12	17.5	24
Physician percent to total credit.		9.66%	16.55%	16.55%	24.14%	33.10%

Step 5 — **Award P4P dollars to physicians based on percent to total credit.**

	Total	Dr. A IM	Dr. B IM	Dr. C IM	Dr. D IM	Dr. E IM
	$25,000	$2,414	$4,138	$4,138	$6,034	$8,276

Step 6 — **Determine total revenue attributed to physician (net collections plus P4P award).**

	Total	Dr. A IM	Dr. B IM	Dr. C IM	Dr. D IM	Dr. E IM
	$1,742,006	$372,674	$322,393	$369,516	$352,036	$325,447

Step 7 — **Determine physician revenue percent to total revenue.**

	Total	Dr. A IM	Dr. B IM	Dr. C IM	Dr. D IM	Dr. E IM
		21.39%	18.51%	21.21%	20.21%	18.68%

Step 8 — **Assign cost of practice based on physician revenue as a % to total revenue.**

	Total	Dr. A IM	Dr. B IM	Dr. C IM	Dr. D IM	Dr. E IM
	$(871,033)	$(186,343)	$(161,202)	$(184,764)	$(176,024)	$(162,729)

Step 9 — **Determine physician-specific direct expenses.**

	Total	Dr. A IM	Dr. B IM	Dr. C IM	Dr. D IM	Dr. E IM
	$(196,512)	$(38,984)	$(41,292)	$(40,292)	$(40,312)	$(35,632)

Step 10 — **Determine total W-2 compensation (net of physician-specific direct expenses).**

	Total	Dr. A IM	Dr. B IM	Dr. C IM	Dr. D IM	Dr. E IM
	$674,461	$147,347	$119,899	$144,460	$135,700	$127,086

Key:
IM = Internal Medicine

If P4P continues its current trajectory to represent a significant portion of the reimbursement dollar, we suspect that physician compensation plans will follow suit and reduce the current focus on quantity of work (as measured through professional services net collections, for example) or intensity of that work (as measured by WRVUs) to a focus on quality, safety, outcomes, and/or practice efficiency measures. Aligning the reimbursement mechanism (health plan to the medical practice) with the distribution mechanism (medical practice to the physician) is a natural response if the dollars paid for health care are provided in this contingent fashion. The future of P4P programs as a reimbursement and disbursement vehicle will likely depend upon the prevalence by which payers (government and private) adopt this type of reimbursement strategy, plus any contingent requirements the payers may make on health care organizations to further distribute this strategy to the level used in physician compensation planning and incentive plan development.

Note

1. Many P4P initiatives are coupled with active programs of "clinical integration," which are designed to promote compliance with antitrust laws. Although a medical practice or other organization may elect to participate in a P4P reimbursement system, that participation may, or may not, be sufficient to constitute the level of clinical integration required by the antitrust laws.

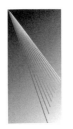

NINE

The Legal Element

P hysician compensation is influenced by a wide variety of federal and state laws and rules that affect both how physician compensation is determined and the amount of compensation that is paid. Entire books have been written on the topic of legal issues and physician compensation, but our focus in this chapter is more practical. Our objectives are to help the reader assess his or her compensation situation, identify the primary legal requirements applicable to that situation, and gain perspective on how a compensation plan might be crafted in light of those requirements.

TWO PRIMARY BODIES OF RELEVANT LAWS

Many laws affect medical practices, but two primary bodies of laws tend to play the most significant roles in physician compensation plans:

1. Laws and rules governing federal health care programs, including the federal "Stark" self-referral law and the federal anti-kickback statute; and

2. Requirements of the Internal Revenue Code (IRC) governing the treatment of compensation in the context of the federal tax code generally, and compensation in the context of tax-exempt organizations more specifically.

The general requirements of each law as applied to physician compensation are summarized below and in Exhibit 9.1.

► LAWS GOVERNING FEDERAL HEALTH CARE PROGRAMS

Laws and rules governing federal health care programs impact compensation in a variety of ways. For example, requirements of the Medicare program certainly influence the reimbursement that is received by a health care organization for physician or other health care services. These rules define both the amount of reimbursement that is received for such services, as well as the underlying requirements to get paid in the first place.

Likewise, certain reimbursement or payment methods, such as managed care and arrangements involving "physician incentive plans" in the context of federal health care programs,[1] and the emerging "pay-for-performance" (P4P) reimbursement systems,

EXHIBIT 9.1 Primary Compensation-Related Legal Issues

Stark Law –
- ► No compensation for referrals of designated health services
- ► Fair market value compensation

Anti-Kickback –
- ► Fair market value compensation
- ► No remuneration for referrals

General Tax –
- ► Reasonable compensation for services
- ► Appropriate treatment as compensation for services or dividend (in some organizations)

Tax-Exempt Organization –
- ► Purpose of compensation arrangement consistent with tax-exempt mission (e.g., charity and promotion of health)
- ► Compensation that is reasonable and consistent with fair market value

© 2006 Johnson

will also impact compensation plans and methods. For the most part, however, these reimbursement systems affect the compensation that is paid from the government to the medical practice, with the practice eventually distributing (and redistributing) that reimbursement (net of expenses) among practice physicians.

The reimbursement systems discussed immediately above have an impact on the underlying compensation methodologies and plans used in the medical practice, but that impact tends to be more indirect than other statutory requirements. The federal physician self-referral or "Stark" law and the anti-kickback statute have a more direct and immediate impact on both the manner in which a practice's compensation plan determines and pays physician compensation, and in some cases, on the amount of compensation that can be paid. Our focus is limited to a review of the general themes and requirements of these important federal statutes.

The Stark Self-Referral Law

The federal physician self-referral or "Stark" law prohibits physicians from making referrals for certain "designated health services" (DHS) to entities with which the physician, or members of the physician's immediate family, have an ownership and/or compensation relationship, *unless* an exception under the law applies.[2] Designated health services include clinical laboratory; radiology and other imaging services; radiation therapy services; physical and occupational therapy; outpatient prescription drugs; inpatient and outpatient hospital services; and certain other services.

The Stark law will commonly be implicated in many relatively typical types of relationships involving physicians, such as:

- ▶ Physician ownership and employment relationships with the physician's medical practice;

- ▶ Physician employment, medical director, and similar relationships with hospitals or other health care organizations; and

- ▶ Direct and indirect contractual service arrangements involving physicians, medical groups, and hospitals.

The Stark law is a "strict liability" law – meaning that where a physician has a financial relationship with any entity that is implicated by the law, the physician is prohibited from making referrals to that entity for DHS, *unless* an exception applies. If a violation of the Stark law's referral prohibition occurs, payment for services furnished in violation of the Stark law is denied, refunds are required for amounts improperly paid, and fines and other penalties – including potential exclusion from participation in the Medicare and Medicaid programs – can be imposed.

Fortunately, physician compensation relationships can commonly be crafted to meet the requirements of an applicable exception to the Stark law, as described in greater detail below.

Anti-Kickback Statute

The federal Medicare anti-kickback statute generally prohibits the offer, solicitation, or payment of any remuneration – essentially, anything of value – in exchange for the referral of patient service opportunities paid for by any federal health care program.[3] The law has potential application to virtually any relationship involving actual or potential referral sources – including physician relationships with medical practices, hospital-physician employment arrangements, and others. The anti-kickback law defines "remuneration" broadly to include anything of "value," including cash payments, but also other items of value, such as below market rent for office space or equipment and other forms of financial or other benefit.

Unlike the "strict liability" Stark law, an improper intent to induce or reward referrals must be demonstrated for an anti-kickback law violation to be found. However, the requisite improper intent can be inferred from the nature of a transaction, such as when the compensation terms in a hospital-physician service arrangement are in excess of fair market value (FMV). Courts have held that the illegal or improper intent may be found where even *one purpose* of the remuneration (e.g., something of value received by a physician) is to influence referrals.

Because the anti-kickback statute can potentially be implicated in many health care provider relationships, anti-kickback "safe harbor" provisions have been promulgated to describe business arrangements that will be deemed to *not* violate the anti-kickback statute. Safe harbors applicable to physician compensation arrangements include those governing bona fide employment arrangements, personal service and management contracts, and others. One of several consistent themes in all safe harbors is a requirement that the level of compensation paid for physician services must generally be consistent with the FMV of the physician's services, without consideration of the physician's referrals.

Business arrangements that meet every requirement of an applicable safe harbor will be deemed to not violate the anti-kickback statute. Those that fail to meet every requirement will not automatically be deemed illegal – nor will they benefit from safe harbor protection. The basic strategy for anti-kickback statute compliance therefore involves taking steps to fit a compensation arrangement squarely into the confines of an applicable safe harbor, or, where that is not possible, ensuring that the arrangement *substantially* complies with a safe harbor or with the requirements of the anti-kickback statute more generally.

▶ INTERNAL REVENUE CODE REQUIREMENTS

The IRC imposes a variety of requirements that impact physician compensation and compensation arrangements. These include basic requirements set forth in provisions of the IRC that impact whether compensation may be properly deducted from taxes as a reasonable and necessary business expense. This core requirement of the tax code is therefore directly related to issues of how practice income is characterized and paid (e.g., as a salary for services, as a dividend, as distribution of income, etc.), and how that income may be treated by taxing authorities at the practice and individual physician levels. Thus, how compensation is paid and how that compensation will be treated for tax purposes will depend on a variety of issues related to the practice's selected legal form and tax treatment, such as:

▶ Whether the practice is organized as a professional corporation that is classified as a business or "C" corporation or as a professional corporation that has elected "subchapter S" designation for tax purposes;

▶ Whether the form of entity used for the practice allows the practice to receive "partnership" tax treatment (e.g., when a professional limited liability company [PLLC], professional limited liability partnership [PLLP], or similar entity) is used; and

▶ Whether the practice is organized and operated as a for-profit (taxable) entity, or whether it is not-for-profit and is "tax-exempt" under section 501(c)(3) of the IRC.

Our focus here is to provide perspective on certain fundamental tax-related issues that will be relevant to compensation depending upon the context – not to provide a treatise on compensation and tax issues. For this reason, we provide a brief review of the IRC's requirements to compensation, along with a discussion of the rules applicable to tax-exempt health care organizations under sections 501(c)(3) and 4958 of the IRC. When a violation of section 501(c)(3) occurs, the organization's tax-exempt status may be revoked, while section 4958 provides for an "intermediate sanction" remedy in the form of an excise tax that can be applied personally to certain persons involved in non–fair market value transactions involving the tax-exempt enterprise.[4]

Other Laws and Rules

Federal laws governing payroll deductions, employee benefits, retirement plans, deferred compensation, and others also affect compensation. Similarly, a patchwork of state laws will also influence compensation. These laws include state-specific provisions that may impose proscriptions that may be largely the same, or, in some jurisdictions, more expansive or significantly different than those imposed by federal law. These include state-specific "mini" Stark statutes and state laws governing charitable organizations, charitable trust doctrines, and others. These and all other applicable laws must be considered and addressed in connection with any physician compensation plan. However, the two primary bodies of law referenced above dealing with federal health care programs (the Stark law and the anti-kickback statute), and provisions of the IRC (governing compensation generally and tax-exempt organizations in particular) will always provide a good place to start.

COMPENSATION AND CONTEXT – APPLYING THE LAWS

The primary laws referenced above impose complex, frequently confusing rules and requirements on physician compensation. Therefore, it is easy to get lost in the legal and compliance minutiae. Our objective is to provide guidance to help the reader assess his or her particular situation in order to identify the primary legal requirements that will typically apply. We also provide perspective on how compensation arrangements might be crafted in light of those requirements.

In furtherance of this practical objective, it is useful to recognize that physician compensation occurs in the context of a relationship between a physician and an organization that is paying for that physician's services. In the context of that compensation relationship, legal issues arise, and the nature of the particular compensation relationship will generally determine what legal issues and rules will apply.

▶ A DIAGNOSTIC MATRIX

Answers to the following four basic questions serve as a diagnostic matrix to help focus on the most important legal issues and rules that will apply to a particular compensation relationship:

1. **Source** – What organization is the source of the compensation being paid?

   ▶ A medical group practice?

   ▶ A hospital?

- ► A health plan?
- ► Another party?

2. **Character** – What is the character of the organization(s) involved?
   - ► A physician-owned medical group?
   - ► A medical group that is owned by a hospital or another party?
   - ► A hospital, academic medical center, or other organization?
   - ► A for-profit corporation, a not-for-profit organization, and/or a tax-exempt enterprise?

3. **Relationship** – What is the nature of the physician compensation relationship?
   - ► An ownership or partnership model in which the physician also owns part of the source organization?
   - ► An employment relationship?
   - ► An independent contractor arrangement?

4. **Payment Structure** – Is the compensation relationship between the source and physician direct or indirect?
   - ► Is the compensation paid directly from the source organization to the physician?
   - ► Or does the payment structure involve an indirect arrangement whereby payment from the source organization goes through another organization before being paid to the physician recipient?

The answers to these questions help to define the laws that will apply to a particular relationship. For example, when the compensation relationship involves a physician and a medical practice in which the physician is also an owner of the practice, then the Stark law will generally be implicated, as will provisions of the IRC dealing with the tax treatment of compensation; however, laws governing tax-exempt organizations generally will not. This is because this type of medical practice – physician-owned – is "privately owned," while a medical practice that is owned by a tax-exempt hospital could be viewed as more "public" in nature by virtue of the hospital's exempt status.

Conversely, when the compensation relationship directly or indirectly involves a tax-exempt hospital that establishes a service arrangement with a physician via an employment or an independent contractor arrangement, the Stark, anti-kickback, and tax-exempt organization laws will all be implicated. The primary laws that tend to be applicable to compensation arrangements involving such "private" (e.g., investor-owned and taxable) or "public" entities (e.g., tax-exempt, including university-owned organizations) are summarized in Exhibit 9.2.

Thus, the source, character, relationship, and payment structure associated with the compensation arrangement will generally define the laws and rules applicable to a particular compensation relationship and plan, as summarized in the diagnostic matrix, reprinted in Exhibit 9.3.

EXHIBIT 9.2 Primary Laws and Contexts

"Private" Settings
- ► "Investor"-owned
- ► Fully taxed/taxable
- ► Medical groups and other organizations

- ► **Primary Laws:**
  - – Stark
  - – Anti-kickback
  - – General tax law
    governing compensation

"Public" Settings
- ► Charitable and university-owned
- ► Tax-exempt [501(c)(3)]
- ► Hospitals and captive medical groups

- ► **Primary Laws**
  - – Stark
  - – Anti-kickback
  - – Tax-exempt organization
    IRC Section [501(c)(3)]
  - – IRC Section 4958
  - – General tax law governing compensation

© 2006 Johnson

EXHIBIT 9.3 Diagnostic Matrix

1. **Source** – What organization is the source of the compensation being paid?
   - ► A medical group practice?
   - ► A hospital?
   - ► A health plan?
   - ► Another party?

2. **Character** – What is the character of the organization(s) involved?
   - ► A physician-owned medical group?
   - ► A medical group that is owned by a hospital or another party?
   - ► A hospital, academic medical center, or other provider organization?
   - ► A for-profit corporation, not-for-profit, and/or tax-exempt enterprise?

3. **Relationship** – What is the nature of the physician compensation relationship?
   - ► An ownership or partnership model in which the physician also owns part of the source organization?
   - ► An employment relationship?
   - ► An independent contractor arrangement?

4. **Payment Structure** – Is the compensation relationship between the source and physician direct or indirect?
   - ► Is the compensation paid directly from the source organization to the physician? Or –
   - ► Does the payment structure involve an indirect arrangement where payment from the source organization goes through another organization before being paid to the physician recipient?

© 2006 Johnson & Walker Keegan

The Stark law is always a good place to start when assessing the legal issues that will impact any compensation arrangement and plan. Whenever a financial and referral relationship exists between a physician and an entity that furnishes DHS, that financial relationship must be permitted by an applicable exception to the Stark law. The context and nature of the relationship will determine what Stark law exception(s) may be used, and the particular exception to be used will determine the specific Stark law requirements that must be applied to the compensation arrangement.

THE PRIMARY LAWS APPLIED IN TWO CONTEXTS

In the remainder of this chapter, we apply our primary laws to compensation arrangements in two distinct contexts:

1. Compensation in bona fide group practices, including:

   ► "Traditional" physician-owned and physician-operated groups; and

   ► "Nontraditional" practices that are owned by a hospital or another organization (including those owned and operated by a tax-exempt enterprise).

2. Compensation in other contexts, including:

   ► Direct hospital-physician employment or independent contractor arrangements; and

   ► Indirect service arrangements between a hospital and physician that involve an intervening medical group or other organization.

Exhibits 9.4 and 9.5 illustrate the basic types of structures and relationships in which these different compensation relationships will commonly occur by reference to whether the compensation arrangement is direct or indirect. Of course, in the complex world of health care delivery, there will be any number of other potential structural models and relationships, although these basic models will generally address the majority of the typical relationships in use today.

► COMPENSATION IN BONA FIDE "GROUP PRACTICES"

Compensation in "Traditional" Physician-Owned and Physician-Operated Group Practices

The Stark Law

Physician-owned "group practices" typically rely on the Stark law's "in-office ancillary services" exception to allow for physician ownership, compensation, and referral relationships with the medical practice. These bona fide group practices may also structure compensation relationships to comply with the Stark law's employment, personal services, or potentially other exceptions – although most "traditional," physician-owned medical groups rely on the in-office ancillary services exception because of the flexibility it provides.

The compensation plans available for physicians in bona fide group practices will generally enjoy the greatest methodological flexibility when compared to those used in other settings due to the application of the Stark law. The Stark law's in-office ancillary services exception may be used solely by medical group practices to allow for DHS referrals within the group practice, while also allowing physicians in the group practice to indirectly share in the income from those referrals. This greater flexibility may be garnered by any medical practice that qualifies as a bona fide "Group Practice" as defined by the law. Medical practices generally rely on the in-office ancillary services exception to furnish laboratory services, radiology services, outpatient prescription drugs, physical and occupational therapy, and other ancillary services through the Group Practice without violating the Stark law.

Note: Because the presence of a bona fide "group practice" under the Stark law is required in connection with many of the concepts discussed in this book, the use of the capitalized term "Group Practice" will be deemed to mean that the relevant group qualifies as a bona fide group practice under the Stark law. Other references to groups and group practices in this chapter will not require that the particular entity qualify as a "Group Practice" as that term is defined and used in the law.

The in-office ancillary services exception has a number of highly technical requirements related to:

1. Who provides and supervises the DHS furnished through the practice;

2. The location in which the DHS are furnished (e.g., in the "same building" in which Group Practice physicians furnish services other than DHS, or in a "centralized building" that is used exclusively by the Group Practice);

3. How the services are billed; and

4. Other requirements specific to the nature of the Group Practice, including how the group operates and the manner in which physicians in the Group Practice are compensated.

Only the last element is addressed in this chapter, as other resources are available to provide guidance on the law's other complex requirements. However, compliance with all elements of the exception is required; a medical practice that complies with the Stark law's compensation test but that fails to comply with other elements will not constitute a bona fide Group Practice and therefore will not comply with the law's highly complex requirements for the in-office ancillary services and other exceptions.

The Stark Law Compensation Test

Any medical group that is a bona fide Group Practice and wishes to qualify for the Stark law's exception for in-office ancillary services must comply with the Stark law's "compensation test."

EXHIBIT 9.4 Direct Compensation Arrangement Examples

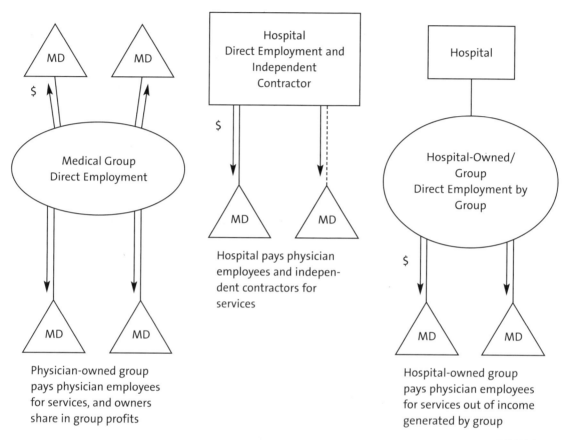

© 2006 Johnson

The compensation test provides that no physician in the medical Group Practice may receive compensation based directly or indirectly on the volume or value of the physician's DHS referrals, *except* through certain indirect compensation methods – defined as "profit shares" or "productivity bonuses." In practical terms, this means that under a Group Practice's compensation plan, there may be no direct correlation between the physician's DHS referrals and his or her compensation. By direct correlation, we mean that physicians cannot be paid for their DHS services based on the volume, gross charges, net revenue, or other direct relationship between referrals and compensation.

EXHIBIT 9.5 Indirect Compensation Arrangement Examples

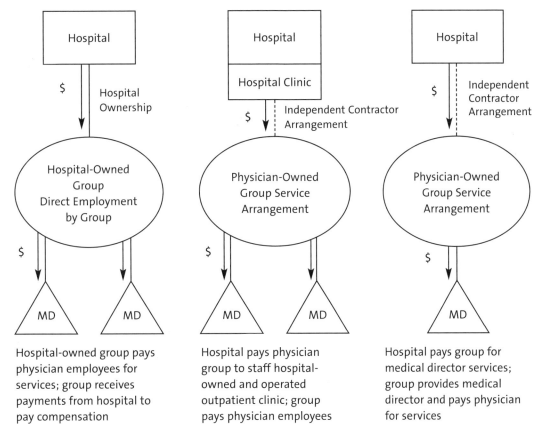

© 2006 Johnson

General Requirements

Before exploring the application of these two indirect methods to compensate physicians for DHS services, two important points are in order.

First, the use of overall profits or productivity bonus methods is only technically required with respect to services defined as DHS that may be paid for by Medicare[5] and, under certain other statutory provision, to Medicaid.[6] Therefore, physicians in Group Practices can be compensated in a different way for non-Medicare services that do not involve DHS referrals (e.g., allowing direct compensation for non-Medicare payable ancillary services). However, most medical groups do not attempt to "carve out"

Medicare DHS from non-Medicare services due to the operational challenges and compliance concerns associated with a Stark law violation.

Second, the compensation test's prohibition on direct compensation for DHS referrals only applies to the DHS the physician refers; it does not apply to compensation paid for DHS or other services that do not involve a referral or that are *"personally performed"* by the physician. This means that, in all instances and in all settings (including outside of medical Group Practices), a physician may be directly compensated for the DHS and other services he or she personally performs. Thus, a physician may always receive "credit" in a compensation plan in the form of gross or net charges, net collections, work relative value units (WRVUs), or otherwise for the *professional* component of an X-ray service or other DHS that the physician truly personally performs.

The Stark law defines "personal performance" strictly to include only those services that a physician performs himself or herself. A physician will not be deemed to have "personally performed" a DHS if anyone else – for example, a nurse, a physical therapist, or any other person working under the physician's supervision – furnishes the services. This means that even services that are properly furnished and paid for by Medicare as "incident to" services will not be "personally performed" by a physician under the Stark law, although, as discussed below, bona fide Group Practices may consider "incident to" services in determining and paying a productivity bonus to a physician in a bona fide Group Practice setting.

Allocating Ancillary Services under the Stark Law

The compensation test for the in-office ancillary services exception allows a Group Practice to distribute revenues, income, or profits from DHS referrals through the use of "overall profit share" or "productivity bonus" methodologies as discussed below.

1. Overall Profit Shares

Overall profit shares compensation methods under the Stark law involve the distribution of a pool of Group Practice revenues or net income (i.e., "overall profits pool"), using an agreed upon methodology. While the term "overall profits pool" is used, this can be interpreted to mean the revenues associated with DHS only, the revenues net of expenses associated with DHS, or the revenues net of expenses associated with DHS plus a portion of the overall general operating expenses of the Group Practice (e.g., overhead). The overall profits pool must consist of at least the revenues or income derived from the practice's furnishing of DHS payable by Medicare or Medicaid. However, the pool may also include a broader subset of practice revenues or profits, including those derived from non-DHS services (i.e., all ancillary services revenues, regardless of payer).

In addition, the overall profits pool may involve all funds from DHS from the practice as a whole, or only DHS revenues or profits derived from subsets of five or more physicians in the Group Practice.[7] This allows practices to create separate overall profits pools for distribution among physicians in a single Group Practice operating division, by site, location, or otherwise, *as long as* the overall profits pool involves the DHS revenues or profits derived from the referrals of at least five or more physicians. The use of separate profits pools generated from the services of five or more physicians is only relevant when the practice wishes to treat subsets of the practice separately for purposes of paying DHS profits; it does not require that the practice must have five or more physicians.

A medical practice can pool and distribute DHS "profits" among practice physicians in the form of compensation, or even in the form of a true profit distribution or return on investment in the form of a dividend on stock or a partnership distribution, based on any methodology that does *not* tie the funds directly to the physician who referred the DHS or generated the revenue.

SAFE HARBOR–TYPE OVERALL PROFITS METHODS

To provide guidance regarding permissible overall profits compensation methods, the Stark law final rule describes three specific methodologies for paying overall profits shares. Medical practices that use one of these three methods will be deemed to be compliant, although practices may also use other reasonable, verifiable methods that pay DHS profits on an indirect basis.[8] These "safe harbor–type" methods involve compensation arrangements in which the Group Practice's overall profits are allocated on a per capita basis, based on the distribution of non-DHS revenues, using any method when the amount of DHS is extremely small, and other ways discussed below.

2. Productivity Bonuses

Unlike "overall profits pool" methods described above, a compensation plan involving a "productivity bonus" as defined in the Stark law does not need to apply solely to a specific pool of revenues or profits from DHS, or any other specific subset of the Group Practice's funds. Indeed, the pool of revenues used to pay productivity bonuses under the Stark law's in-office ancillary services exception can be as large as all Group Practice revenues or profits, or as small as the Group Practice's overall profits pool. As a result, the productivity bonus methods outlined below can also be applied from a methodological standpoint to an "overall profits pool."[9]

The Stark law's use of the term "productivity bonus" may differ from the reader's experience with compensation bonuses. Typically, when medical practices award bonuses, they are "in addition to" the physician's regular compensation. The use of the term "productivity bonus" essentially expands this definition to include the method by which compensation (both bonus and/or non-bonus pay) is determined, depending upon how the productivity bonus is defined. For example, if a Group Practice initiates a productivity bonus approach to compensation involving all of the Group Practice's revenues or profits, then the productivity bonus is used to determine the total compensation of the physician, not simply an "add-on" component or bonus. Alternatively, a productivity bonus can be used solely to determine the incentive portion of compensation as in a base plus incentive system.

A bona fide Group Practice under the Stark law can implement productivity bonuses that are based upon the physician's personally performed services and services that are "incident to" those personally performed services – again, however, without distributing

DHS revenue directly to the physician who generated the DHS referral. However, this ability to receive productivity "credit" for DHS that are furnished on an "incident to" basis is *only* available in the context of bona fide Group Practices that rely on the in-office ancillary services exception. The provision of production credit for DHS that are furnished on an "incident to" basis is not allowed under other commonly used exceptions to the Stark law, such as the employment, personal services, and other exceptions.[10]

PRODUCTION CREDIT FOR "INCIDENT TO" SERVICES

Unfortunately, the availability of production credit for DHS furnished "incident to" a physician's services is also subject to some level of ambiguity under the Stark law. The result is that Group Practices have adopted conservative, moderate, or more aggressive approaches to how such credit for "incident to" services is applied in the context of physician compensation plans. The approach that will be taken to this complex issue in the context of a particular Group Practice's physician compensation plan must be determined in consultation with legal counsel. The basic positions (ranging from most to least conservative) related to the credit for "incident to" services are summarized as follows:

► **Most Conservative Approach**. The conservative approach takes the position that the Stark law and final rule allow for payment of a "productivity bonus based on *services* that [the physician] has personally performed (including *services* 'incident to' those personally performed services [as defined in the incident to rule])."[11] The focus in this conservative interpretation is on *services* (as opposed to "items," as defined under the Medicare program) that are both DHS and that are furnished on an incident to basis. Thus, under this approach, a physician may receive credit for productivity bonus purposes for certain DHS that involve services that are truly furnished incident to the physician's services (e.g., physical therapy services), but the physician may not receive credit for other DHS that do not involve services, such as DHS that are defined by Medicare as "items" (e.g., revenues from outpatient prescription drugs, durable medical equipment [DME] or the like). Therefore, under this conservative approach, a physician would receive productivity credit for physical therapy services that are furnished incident to the physician's services, but the physician would not receive credit in the context of determining a productivity bonus for other items, such as chemotherapy drug profits or revenues.

► **Moderate Approach**. The moderate interpretation generally takes the position that "incident to" credit for purposes of determining a productivity bonus may be provided for anything that is properly furnished and paid for by Medicare on an "incident to" basis. In practical terms, this means that even though drugs are defined as "items" and not as "services" under the Medicare program, outpatient prescription drugs and other items and supplies are still only paid for by Medicare when they are properly furnished "incident to" a physician's services, and when the other requirements of the incident to rule are met.[12] This would mean, for example, that chemotherapy and other drugs that are paid for on an "incident to" basis could be included in determining a physician's production for productivity bonus purposes. It would also mean that physical therapy and other services that are also furnished "incident to" may be included, but other services that are not properly furnished on an incident to basis (e.g., the technical component of an X-ray) may not.

▶ **Least Conservative Approach.** The least conservative approach to "incident to" credit takes the position that any and all services that may be furnished and paid for on an "incident to" basis may be included in determining the productivity bonus. However, this approach also adopts a more aggressive interpretation of what can be furnished and billed on an "incident to" basis. This approach is informed by a series of contradictory statements by the Centers for Medicare & Medicaid Services (CMS) in connection with the original publication and subsequent clarification of the incident to rule.[13] This more aggressive interpretation effectively takes the position that incident to services may include a wide variety of items and services that are paid for under the Medicare program, to potentially include the technical component of radiological and other procedures under certain circumstances, based on a variety of guidance that has been provided throughout the history of the Medicare program.

The presence of interpretations ranging from the most to least conservative with respect to the provision of credit for incident to services in the context of productivity bonuses underscores the importance of sound legal review and guidance in connection with these complex issues. This is particularly true when the most aggressive interpretation is being considered, but it is also critical when even the moderate approach is adopted, given the potential financial implications of an interpretation under the Stark law that is ultimately deemed to be wrong.[14] When it comes to the Stark law, a conservative approach to compliance will have implications for how compensation will be distributed to physicians in a Group Practice.

SAFE HARBOR–TYPE GROUP PRACTICE PRODUCTIVITY BONUS METHODS

The Stark law's final rule provides three specific "safe harbor–type" methods that can be used to pay productivity bonuses, and medical practices that elect to use one of these methods will be deemed to be compliant with the Stark law's compensation test. The methods involve distributing the productivity bonuses based on the physician's total patient encounters or RVUs, based on the allocation of the physician's compensation attributable to services that are not DHS, or based on any method when the amount of DHS is extremely small, or other bases, as discussed below. Productivity bonus methods can also be used to distribute the funds in an overall profits pool.

Distributing Ancillary Services Revenues and Profits

The Stark law requires the use of overall profit shares or productivity bonus methodologies in connection with the distribution of profits or revenues from DHS in a Group Practice. The safe harbor–type methods referenced above constitute permissible methodologies for allocating DHS on an "indirect" basis, although the use of a safe harbor–type method is not mandated.

Indeed, experience shows that many medical Group Practices actually use other methods that are reasonable and verifiable, and that still provide compensation that is only indirectly related to DHS referrals. As a result, Group Practices will sometimes use the following methods for allocating ancillary services in conjunction with an overall profit shares or productivity bonus–based methodology:

1. **Safe Harbor–Type Methods**. This approach involves using safe harbor–type methods for allocating profit shares or productivity bonuses, to include allocating such amounts:

   ► Per capita (e.g., per member of the practice or per physician in the practice); or

   ► Based on the distribution of the Group Practice's revenues attributed to services that are not DHS payable by any federal health care program or private payer; or

   ► Based on the physician's total patient encounters or RVUs; or

   ► Based on the allocation of the physician's compensation attributable to services that are not DHS payable by any federal health care program or private payer; or

   ► On any basis when revenues derived from DHS are less than 5 percent of the Group Practice's total revenues, and the allocated portion of those revenues to each physician in the Group Practice constitutes 5 percent or less of his or her total compensation from the Group Practice.

2. **Payer Treatment**. In this approach, Medicare payable DHS is treated differently from non-Medicare payable DHS for compensation plan purposes.

3. **Overall Profits "Pods"**. This approach involves creating overall profits pools based on physician specialties, locations of practice, or otherwise, while ensuring that each "overall profits pool" is made up of the revenues from DHS referrals from at least five physicians in the Group Practice.

4. **Multiple Profits Pools**. In this approach, a ratio of ancillary services production expressed as a percentage of professional services (e.g., measured by gross charges, WRVUs, or net collections) for each physician in the Group Practice is used to identify different overall profits pools, but without regard to physician specialty, location of practice, or any other factor. Group Practices that use such approaches will commonly develop multiple overall profits pools that are effectively populated by physicians in the Group Practice who have high, moderate, and low levels of ancillary services referrals due to patient mix or practice specialty. This approach is allowed by the Stark law's final rule, which provides that an overall profits pool can consist of the DHS revenues generated from the refer-

rals of at least five or more physicians in the Group Practice. The rule further provides that any means can be used to determine the profits pool or to select the pods of five or more physicians that will comprise the profits pool. Thus, under this approach, where high-, moderate-, and low-utilization profits pools are used, the revenues (or income) from DHS referrals generated by physicians in each respective overall profits pool may be allocated directly to that pool. Each pool, in turn, may indirectly allocate the profits among the physicians in the particular overall profits pool (e.g., equal share, percentage of WRVUs, or the like).

5. **Specialty Treatment**. This approach involves the use of different factors to allocate the profits pool based on physician specialty. Under these approaches, the general differences in ancillary services utilization are indirectly considered in connection with the distribution method. Thus, if the overall profits pool is funded by revenues or income from clinical laboratory and imaging services, physicians in different specialties in the Group Practice might receive different shares of the profits in the overall profits pool based on different factors that are applied on a percent to total basis. Using hypothetical data, this might mean, for example, that a full-time family practice physician might receive a factor of 5; full-time general internal medicine and general pediatrics physicians might have a factor of 4; a full-time orthopedic surgeon might have a factor of 3; a full-time general surgeon might have a factor of 1; and so on. The factors otherwise assigned are further adjusted based on full-time equivalency (FTE), or are based on some measure of relative production (e.g., above or below median benchmark levels using Medical Group Management Association [MGMA] survey data or other data). Under such methods, each physician receives a share of the overall profits pool based on the physician's relative factor, expressed as a percentage of the total factors for all physicians in the Group Practice.

6. **Service Treatment**. This approach involves treating different types of DHS in different ways for compensation plan purposes (e.g., creating an overall profits pool for radiology and other imaging services, another for clinical laboratory services, and another for physical therapy services, etc.) and using different allocation methodologies for each.

7. **Historic Linkages**. In this approach, an overall profits pool is allocated based on historic levels or ratios of ancillary services usage (e.g., a ratio of utilization in year one is used to allocate the ancillary services profits in year two).

8. **Thresholds**. In this approach, individual physicians may participate in the overall profits pool to differing degrees based on the level of their professional service production. For example, a target level of production based on historic production levels (e.g., mean or median professional services production by specialty during the prior one-year period) will be established as the threshold performance level for full participation in the ancillary services profits pool.

Physicians who achieve the threshold level of production will participate fully, while those who do not will participate to a lesser degree (e.g., receiving half of a full equal share rather than a full equal share of ancillary services profits).

These, and potentially other methods, might be considered for use in a Group Practice on the grounds that the Stark law and final rule allow medical Group Practices to use any "reasonable and verifiable methodology" to meet the Stark law's compensation test so long as the compensation that is ultimately determined and paid is not "directly" related to the volume or value of the physician's DHS referrals.

As with the presence of different interpretations relating to the treatment of incident to services as discussed above, these and other creative distribution methods will adopt an approach to compliance that ranges from relatively conservative to aggressive, so sound legal guidance will always be required in connection with these complex issues. And while more aggressive interpretations and approaches may be deemed to be acceptable, remember that when it comes to the Stark law, a conservative approach to compliance will always be the safest approach given the significant financial and other costs that will be associated with a violation.

Anti-Kickback Statute

The federal anti-kickback statute also applies to compensation paid by medical group practices, although in a Group Practice setting, physician compensation arrangements will generally be able to strictly or substantially comply with anti-kickback statute safe harbors relating to investment interests in group practices, bona fide employment arrangements, or personal services arrangements.

These and other safe harbors impose a number of specific requirements, such as compliance with the Stark law's definition of a bona fide "Group Practice" (in the case of the investment interests safe harbor), the presence of a bona fide employment relationship (as defined by the Internal Revenue Service [IRS]), or an independent contractor arrangement that complies with the anti-kickback personal services and management contracts safe harbors. Likewise, these provisions generally impose requirements that are largely similar to those that may be imposed under applicable exceptions to the Stark law, although close attention to the specific requirement of each is always required.

Federal Tax Law – The Internal Revenue Code

In a "traditional" physician-owned medical group, compensation issues generally involve the application of federal tax laws and rules to physician compensation, including the appropriate characterization of that payment as compensation for services or otherwise in light of the form of legal entity and tax treatment of the Group Practice organization. In traditional, physician-owned medical groups, tax-exempt organization concerns will generally not be implicated in the group's internal practice and compensation plan (although these concerns may arise in the context of relationships with third-party organizations, such as hospitals).

General Tax Requirements

The form of legal entity and the tax treatment of the Group Practice will have implications for the tax treatment of physician compensation, as well as for the applicable taxes and withholdings that will be made from amounts earned as compensation. Most medical Group Practices are organized through the use of professional services corporations (commonly referred to as professional corporations, professional associations, or the like), PLLCs, PLLPs, or similar forms. The tax treatment and rules applicable to these organizational forms vary somewhat. Many professional corporations are treated as "C" corporations for income tax treatment, and some professional corporations that have selected "S" corporation designation for income tax treatment are largely treated as partnerships, as are PLLCs and PLLPs.

The specific distinctions between "C" corporation and "S" corporation or partnership tax treatment are beyond the scope of this chapter. As a general matter, the primary distinctions relate to the tax treatment of certain amounts that are distributed to the Group Practice's owners, and the application of certain employment tax and related withholding obligations.

Where the Group Practice is treated as a "C" corporation (as opposed to a partnership) for tax purposes, Section 162 of the IRC will allow the Group Practice to deduct a "reasonable" allowance for salaries or other compensation for personal services actually rendered.[15] Rules in the form of Treasury Regulations require that for compensation to be deducted, it must be paid purely for services and be reasonable in amount.[16]

How compensation is treated for tax purposes is important, because under Section 162, only "reasonable" compensation for services is eligible for deduction as wages, while other amounts earned and paid to the practice's owners should generally be treated as corporate dividends and not as compensation. This compensation vs. dividends distinction is important in the traditional practice context because of the different tax treatment provided to the two different types of payment arrangements.[17]

Conversely, amounts paid in the form of dividends in a practice organized as a corporation that has not elected subchapter "S" designation will be subject to "double taxation" in the form of a tax assessment, first at the corporate level and then at the individual shareholder level. Thus, the IRS is concerned about how the payment is classified, because payments have differing tax implications.

Recent developments have heightened the importance of these distinctions in compensation arrangements. In a 2001 case, *Pediatric Surgical Associates, P.C. v. Comm'r*,[18] a physician-owned medical group that was organized and treated as a "C" corporation for tax purposes was held to have improperly classified dividend payments in the form of salary. The practice's shareholder surgeons received salaries and cash bonuses (distributed from corporate earnings) that included income generated by the practice's nonshareholder physician surgeons. The practice deducted the bonuses paid to the shareholders as officers' compensation, but the IRS disallowed part of the deductions on the grounds that a portion of the compensation was actually a dividend "disguised" in the form of a salary for services; therefore, it was nondeductible. The court concluded that since part of the shareholder bonuses consisted of corporate profit generated by nonshareholder surgeons (and not by the shareholders themselves), the shareholders' compensation exceeded reasonable allowances for their services, and instead constituted a nondeductible dividend.

The standards applicable under Section 162 of the IRC are also applicable to the question of whether compensation paid by a tax-exempt organization is "reasonable," as discussed below. Other factors that have been developed and applied by the IRS (based on the case law) are also considered favorable or unfavorable when determining the reasonableness of compensation. These issues are examined in greater detail below in connection with our discussion of tax-exempt organization concerns.

► COMPENSATION IN "NONTRADITIONAL" (E.G., HOSPITAL-OWNED AND HOSPITAL-OPERATED) GROUP PRACTICES

Most medical groups are physician-owned, but hospitals and other organizations in many states may also own and operate Group Practices. This section provides perspective on the legal requirements applicable to these "nontraditional" (e.g., hospital-owned) Group Practices.

The Stark Law

The Stark law's in-office ancillary services exception can be used in any bona fide Group Practice, to include both physician-owned groups and what we will call "nontraditional" Group Practices. Nontraditional Group Practices are those that are owned by hospitals or another party in which the group consists of a "single legal entity" whose primary function is as a Group Practice that is allowed under applicable state law. This allows a Group Practice to exist even if physicians are not full or partial owners of the enterprise.

Conversely, a bona fide Group Practice for purposes of the Stark law will not include, for example, physicians who are employees of a hospital that are also organized, *for operational purposes only*, into a "group practice" service delivery model. This is because, under such a direct hospital employment relationship, the requisite "single legal entity" formed primarily to function as a Group Practice is lacking.

However, as long as the applicable state allows a hospital or other organization to own and operate a Group Practice,[19] the in-office ancillary services exception is available for use in such nontraditional practice models, and the basic Stark law issues and options related to compensation plans in connection with "traditional" physician-owned medical groups will apply to such nontraditional Group Practices.

Anti-Kickback Statute

The basic anti-kickback statute concerns discussed above with respect to traditional physician-owned groups also generally apply in the context of nontraditional Group Practices (e.g., safe harbor compliance related to ownership interests in the Group Practice, employment, and contractual relationships). However, the very nature of the nontraditional practice structure may raise additional anti-kickback concerns that are generally not present in more traditional physician-owned models.

Nontraditional Group Practice models commonly involve an ownership and/or other financial relationship between a "captive" physician Group Practice and a hospital or another health care provider. Because of this structure, additional anti-kickback concerns may be implicated if a compensation arrangement considers financial or other performance at a level that is outside of the nontraditional Group Practice, such as when a compensation system considers "system-wide" (e.g., hospital and captive nontraditional Group Practice) performance in connection with the determination and payment of physician compensation. Legally appropriate compensation systems can be established that consider system-wide performance, but only with close attention to legal compliance details, including compliance with the Stark law and the anti-kickback statute.

Tax-Exempt Organization Law

Where a nontraditional Group Practice is also tax-exempt, a number of highly complex requirements are imposed on the exempt organization's payment of compensation to Group Practice physicians. These same types of rules and issues will also apply when a tax-exempt organization is involved in another physician compensation relationship. Although these rules are applicable to nontraditional Group Practices, they are most commonly applicable to other compensation arrangements involving tax-exempt hospitals and physicians; therefore, they will be examined in detail in that context below.

► COMPENSATION IN SETTINGS OTHER THAN BONA FIDE "GROUP PRACTICES"

In this section, we briefly address the rules that generally apply to direct and indirect relationships involving organizations that are *not* bona fide "Group Practices" under the Stark law. As a general matter, when the source organization is *other than* a bona fide Group Practice as defined by the Stark law, exceptions other than the Stark law's exception for in-office ancillary services will need to be utilized and complied with. These exceptions, along with applicable safe harbors to the anti-kickback statute and, in many instances, the requirements applicable to tax-exempt organizations, define the legal rules that will apply to the particular compensation plan and relationship.

Direct Compensation Relationships Involving Hospitals and Organizations Other than Group Practices

The Stark Law

In a non–Group Practice setting, physicians will have either direct or indirect relationships with the organization that is the source of their compensation. Common "direct" relationships involve direct employment by a hospital or academic institution, or direct independent contractor arrangements between the source organization and an individual physician for medical director or other similar services. The Stark law's requirements as applied to a particular direct compensation arrangement will vary somewhat depending upon whether the relationship involves an employment or independent contractor arrangement. The common types of direct compensation relationships, including those involving group practices and other organizations such as hospitals, were previously illustrated in Exhibit 9.4.

In the case of direct employment arrangements, the Stark law's employment exception allows for payment of compensation from an employer to a physician or other employee who has a bona fide employment relationship with the employer for the provision of services. Certain additional requirements and conditions must also be met; for example, the amount of compensation under the employment arrangement must be consistent with the FMV of the services. It also must be commercially reasonable. Furthermore, the compensation may not be determined in a manner that takes into account, either directly or indirectly, the volume or value of any referrals of DHS by the referring physician, except that a productivity bonus may be paid based solely on the physician's "personally performed" services (without consideration of DHS referrals).[20]

The Stark law's exception for employment arrangements allows for the payment of a "productivity bonus"; however, in contrast to the law's in-office ancillary services exception, the determination of that bonus amount may *not* include any consideration of DHS that are furnished or performed by any other person, including those that are furnished on an "incident to" basis.

For direct independent contractor service arrangements, the Stark law's "personal services arrangements exception" is commonly used for medical director or other service relationships that exist directly between hospitals and physicians. This exception imposes its own specific requirements including that: The arrangement must be governed by a written agreement that covers the physician's services; and the compensation to be paid over the term must be set in advance, may not exceed FMV for the services, and, generally, may not be determined in a manner that takes into account the volume or value of *any referrals or other business* generated by the physician.

In contrast to the employment exception, the personal services exception to the Stark law imposes even narrower restrictions on the determination and payment of a productivity bonus, because the compensation may not consider the volume or value of DHS referrals "or any other business generated between the parties." This means that any productivity bonus may consider only the services personally performed by the physician, and may not consider, for example, the physician's referrals of designated health services or *any* other services, including those reimbursed by private payers.

The employment and personal services exceptions referenced above are typically relied upon in direct compensation arrangements between physicians and hospitals, academic medical centers, or other health care organizations that furnish DHS. They may also be relied upon in the context of bona fide Group Practices. However, the considerably greater flexibility allowed under the Stark law's in-office ancillary services exception makes it the "exception of choice" when a bona fide Group Practice is involved.

Anti-Kickback Statute

In direct compensation arrangements, such as those referenced above, anti-kickback safe harbors dealing with bona fide employment and personal services and management contracts will also typically be considered in structuring the compensation arrangement. The terms of these safe harbors differ in some respects from the Stark law exceptions with similar names, although the general terms and key themes are similar under both statutes. These include, for example, the presence of bona fide employment arrangements, requirements that compensation may not exceed FMV for services actually provided, and the absence of any consideration of referrals in connection with the compensation arrangement.

Tax-Exempt Organization Concerns

When a compensation relationship is between a physician and a hospital or other organization that is tax-exempt under Section 501(c)(3) of the IRC, the special requirements applicable to tax-exempt enterprises will apply. The basic concerns related to compensation under Section 501(c)(3) and the related provision, Section 4958 of the IRC, are illustrated in Exhibit 9.6. The rules governing tax-exempt organizations are complex, but a close read of the laws and rules suggests that the basic requirements tend to relate to the following basic concerns and themes:

1. The *purpose* of the compensation arrangement and the requirement that the arrangement must promote the organization's tax-exempt purposes;

2. The *process* the tax-exempt organization uses to determine and pay compensation;

3. The *methodology and features* of the compensation plan; and

4. The *amount* of compensation actually paid, with the requirement that the tax-exempt organization pay no more than "reasonable" compensation.

EXHIBIT 9.6 Tax-Exempt Organization Laws and Compensation-Related Concerns

IRC Section 501(c)(3)
- ▶ Level – Reasonable compensation; consistent with market for specialty, region, etc.
- ▶ Method of compensation – Consistent with charitable mission

IRC Section 4958 – Intermediate Sanctions
- ▶ "Excess benefit transactions" – Any "non–fair market value" exchange benefiting a disqualified person
- ▶ Difference between actual and fair market value

We now turn our discussion to the core requirements related to purpose, process, method, and amount.

Purpose: The Compensation Plan's Consistency with Tax-Exempt Status

The compensation plan in a tax-exempt enterprise must be consistent with the mission of the organization. Tax-exempt health care organizations are generally focused on charitable (e.g., delivery of health care) and/or educational purposes; therefore, the compensation plan must not involve characteristics that could undermine the organization's focus and pursuit of these purposes.

This means, for example, that compensation plans that focus physicians on the generation of revenues (e.g., cash) as the *sole* criteria for awarding compensation could be deemed to be inconsistent with tax-exempt status, because such methods might encourage a physician to exercise patient selection in a manner that could reduce the delivery of health care services provided to the indigent. Whether a particular compensation plan is consistent with the organization's tax-exempt status will depend upon a factual analysis.

The requirement that the plan must be consistent with the organization's tax-exempt mission does not, however, eliminate the use of many common physician compensation plan methodologies. For example, departmental productivity-based compensation plans directed at multiple goals, such as increasing individual productivity and lowering costs, while also maintaining quality care, have been approved by the IRS for use in a variety of settings. Such methods have been approved because they are deemed to promote and encourage the accomplishment of an organization's tax-exempt purposes.[22]

On the other hand, compensation arrangements that effectively convert the principal activity of the tax-exempt organization into a joint venture arrangement with physicians will raise concerns. By illustration, arrangements that determine net revenues or income in a particular department or division, and that pay all or substantially all of that net amount to employed physicians in the form of incentive compensation, may be viewed as creating a joint venture–type of relationship that is inconsistent with the organization's mission, because few of the organization's net profits are made available for other tax-exempt objectives.

Process: The Manner in Which the Compensation Arrangement Is Developed, Implemented, and Administered

The IRS has consistently stated that physician compensation arrangements between a tax-exempt hospital or other health care organization and a physician should optimally be developed through arm's-length negotiations and bargaining. In practical terms, this means that the compensation plan methods and the ultimate levels of compensation to be paid to the physician (or any other person providing services to the tax-exempt organization) should be established and/or approved by someone *other than* the physicians benefiting from the compensation. In fact, certain safe harbor requirements of

Section 4958 of the IRC regarding intermediate sanctions provide that an independent committee or independent boards of directors without a conflict of interest should make such compensation decisions.

Of course, a central theme in this book is that the process of compensation plan design (the "art") is just as important as the compensation plan methodology itself (the "science"). This remains true even in a tax-exempt organization. However, in this unique context, the dual requirements of promoting physician understanding and "buy-in" regarding the compensation plan, and the need for independence and absence of conflict of interest in compensation-related decision making, can potentially conflict. Yet, these dual requirements can both be incorporated into an appropriate compensation plan development process in a tax-exempt enterprise by using a process that will generally include:

- ➤ A compensation planning committee comprised of physician and nonphysician (management) representatives to participate in the development of the compensation plan; but

- ➤ Another committee and/or independent board of the tax-exempt organization to have ultimate authority and approval over the plan methods and over the amount of compensation paid, due to the need for independence.

This approach helps ensure the existence of an arm's-length relationship between the organization and the physicians being compensated. It also provides a means to promote the required level of physician input into the process in order to promote physician buy-in of plan goals, methods, and results.

Method: The Compensation Plan's Methodology and Other Features

The two most relevant methodological features applicable to compensation plans involving tax-exempt enterprises relate to: (1) whether the plan considers the tax-exempt organization's net earnings or net income; and (2) whether the plan includes an express limit or "cap" on compensation.

By its terms, IRC Section 501(c)(3) provides that no part of the "net earnings" of the tax-exempt organization may inure to the benefit of any private shareholder or individual. What constitutes the organization's "net earnings" is not black and white, because tax-exempt organizations are allowed, for example, to pay compensation for services required to promote the organization's mission and purposes, so long as that compensation is "reasonable" (discussed below). Yet, when the organization's net earnings revenues or income are considered in the compensation plan methodology, special attention is required.

The IRS has approved a number of compensation arrangements that consider the tax-exempt organization's net earnings, including those that pay incentive compensation based on the actual vs. the budgeted margin of revenues from operations over expenses for a hospital as a whole; performance in relation to an annual "target operating margin" that is coupled with the definition of individual "controllable margins" for individual operating units within the hospital (with "controllable margins" measured based on gross revenues for the unit, minus the unit's controllable expenses); and others.[23]

These and other determinations lead to a number of "rules of thumb" that can be applied to compensation arrangements involving tax-exempt organizations.

► First, if net earnings or net income are used to measure physician productivity and work effort for compensation plan purposes, the arrangement must nevertheless help to promote the tax-exempt organization's charitable purpose, such as keeping actual expenditures within budgeted levels, where expenditures determine the amounts the organization is able to charge for its charitable services.

► Second, where net earnings and similar financial measures are used in the compensation plan, they must also be expressed in a well-defined formula that is also related to, and consistent with, the organization's charitable mission. Thus, methods that promote the achievement of performance in relation to a target (i.e., budgeted operating margins) will generally be preferred to methods that base incentive compensation on the actual "profit margin" in a particular department or division within the organization.

► Third, the total amount of compensation available for payment as incentive should optimally be defined and limited in advance. Such amounts might be expressed as a flat dollar amount (e.g., $10,000 per physician) as a percentage of physician base or guaranteed salaries (e.g., no more than 10 to 20 percent of base salaries), or as a predefined portion of net revenues or profits net of expenses that are derived from the tax-exempt organization's operations.

The IRS also looks favorably on compensation formulas in tax-exempt organizations that include an explicit cap or maximum on the total amount of compensation that can be paid, and/or on the amount of incentive payment that can be directly received by an individual from the tax-exempt enterprise. A cap or absolute limit on the total amount of compensation is not required in all instances, but a cap is strongly preferred as a means to help ensure that the organization does not go beyond the practical requirement (discussed below) that it not pay more than "reasonable" compensation. This preference for a cap imposes a limit that is applicable in the unique context of a tax-exempt organization that is obviously very different from that experienced in a more traditional, physician-owned practice.

A cap on compensation may be expressed in any number of forms, to include, for example, capping the amount of incentive compensation payable to individual physicians to no more than 10 percent of a physician's regular base salary, or that incentive compensation may not exceed a defined portion (e.g., 30 to 50 percent) of the physician's total compensation. Caps or limits on compensation may also be linked to market data (e.g., a cap set at the 75th or 90th percentile benchmark), or set at a defined percentage (e.g., 120 percent) of the median. As discussed in Chapter 16, "The Special

World of Hospital and Academic Practices – Assessing Reasonableness and Promoting Compliance," linking the cap to median values is typically preferred, since the median value is generally subject to lower year-to-year fluctuation. The presence of a cap can help to promote the overall reasonableness of physician compensation levels.

Amount: The Requirement That Compensation Must Be "Reasonable"

Tax-exempt organizations may pay compensation for services as long as the total amount of compensation is "reasonable." For such purposes, "reasonable" compensation is generally defined by the application of IRC Section 162 (discussed previously), or under other applicable rules as "[t]he ... amount that would ordinarily be paid for like services by like enterprises (whether taxable or tax-exempt) under like circumstances."[24] In addition, Section 4958 of the IRC also requires that the compensation paid to certain "disqualified persons" must be consistent with FMV.

Unfortunately, while it is relatively easy to say that compensation must not exceed levels that are reasonable, translating this concept into practice is easier said than done. The IRS will not provide advance rulings regarding the reasonableness of individual compensation levels, and, to date, there is little definitive guidance to assist an organization in determining whether a *specific* amount or level of compensation to be paid to a specific individual is, or is not, reasonable.

In practical terms, determinations regarding the reasonableness of compensation typically consider a variety of different types of evidence as to the comparability of compensation levels, including:

► Compensation levels paid by similar organizations (taxable and tax-exempt), for functionally comparable positions;

► Compensation levels paid for physicians engaged in the same specialty and/or in the same types of administrative activities;

► The availability of similar services within the organization's geographic area;

► Current compensation surveys, such as those published by MGMA, American Medical Group Association (AMGA), and others, that reflect compensation levels for the same physician specialties on a national, regional, and local geographic basis; and

► Actual written offers from similar institutions competing for a specific individual physician's services.

Importantly, the requirement that compensation must be reasonable does not require that physicians who are associated with tax-exempt organizations receive less than their colleagues in the nonexempt world, yet industry standards and the operation of the market are the only real measures of reasonableness. The application of both the standards of "reasonable" compensation and compensation that is consistent with "FMV" is explored in greater detail in Chapter 16.

► INDIRECT COMPENSATION ARRANGEMENTS INVOLVING HOSPITALS AND ORGANIZATIONS OTHER THAN GROUP PRACTICES

An "indirect" compensation relationship or arrangement may generally be defined as one in which an organization stands in-between the organization that is the source of funds used to pay compensation and the physician who receives that compensation. Examples of indirect arrangements were previously illustrated in Exhibit 9.5 and include:

► An emergency room physician staffing company or group that employs or contracts with individual physicians and that also contracts with a hospital to staff a hospital emergency room; and

► A health care delivery system in which a hospital owns and operates ambulatory care clinics, under a contract with a group of physicians (which may or may not qualify as a bona fide Group Practice under the Stark law) to furnish services in the hospital-owned clinic under arrangements in which the hospital bills for and receives reimbursement for the physician's services.

In both of these examples, the hospital is the source of compensation, but that compensation is first paid to the intervening organization (e.g., the separate group or another organization) and is then paid from the intervening organization to individual physicians who are employed or contracted to the organization. Where an indirect compensation arrangement is present, Stark, anti-kickback, and tax-exempt organization issues also generally apply to the arrangement, although the unique nature of the indirect compensation relationship – namely, the presence of an intervening entity – adds an additional twist to the legal issues and considerations.

When an indirect arrangement is present, the Stark law exceptions applicable to direct compensation arrangements (including the in-office ancillary services exception, and exceptions for direct employment and personal services arrangements) will generally not be available. However, other exceptions, including the Stark law's exception for FMV compensation arrangements, and for indirect compensation arrangements, will be available and may be used. The specific requirements of these exceptions are beyond the scope of this chapter. However, as in all other requirements, key themes that are essential for compliance with these exceptions include the presence of FMV compensation for services actually provided, and the absence of any consideration of DHS referrals in the determination of physician compensation levels.

Likewise, the presence of an indirect arrangement will not eliminate the importance of the anti-kickback and tax-exempt organization requirements, although they will make their application more indirect. Here, too, the same issues discussed above, including promoting compliance with applicable anti-kickback safe harbors and paying attention to the purpose, process, method, and amount of compensation when a tax-exempt organization is involved, will be essential to compliance.

THE ROLE OF LEGAL AND ACCOUNTING COUNSEL IN COMPENSATION PLAN DEVELOPMENT

In light of the complexity of the legal and tax environment influencing physician compensation and physician compensation plans, it is not possible for a single chapter to provide extensive application of every rule to physician compensation arrangements. However, readers may use our basic diagnostic matrix involving questions related to:

- ➤ The *source* of compensation (e.g., group practice or other organization);
- ➤ The *character* of the organization(s) involved in the compensation relationship;
- ➤ The *nature* of the relationship (e.g., ownership, employment, or contractual); and
- ➤ The *structure* of the payment arrangement (e.g., direct or indirect).

Using the diagnostic matrix allows readers to focus on the legal rules that will be most pertinent to a particular compensation relationship. Those general rules can be used in connection with the development and consideration of alternative compensation plan methodologies, and to understand the applicable legal requirements and rules.

In every instance, an essential step in the compensation plan development process will involve consideration of the plan methodology by legal and accounting counsel who have expertise in physician compensation arrangements. Such expertise should include knowledge of the Stark and anti-kickback laws, tax-exempt organizations and other legal concerns, and their application to compensation arrangements. The involvement of such counsel should optimally occur at several points in the development process:

- ➤ First, early on in connection with the educational process, legal counsel should provide education regarding the basic rules that will be pertinent to the particular arrangement and should answer questions that may be relevant to potential plan methodologies.

- ➤ Second, counsel should be involved periodically throughout the plan development process, in connection with the development and refinement of plan "details," to ensure that the plan in development does not use methods or involve assumptions that will later be deemed illegal. The objective at this point is to stay "on track" from a legal compliance perspective, although detailed review will generally not be required for a plan that is a "work in progress."

- ➤ Third, once the "final plan" is outlined and defined, legal and accounting counsel should optimally review and approve any plan that is ultimately adopted. The review at this point will be more focused and detailed to include, in many instances, consideration of how particular revenue sources are treated in connection with the compensation methodology, consideration of tax issues, and the like.

Overall, legal, tax, and related issues do influence compensation plans and physician compensation levels. Although these concerns may be viewed as a potentially hazardous minefield, experience demonstrates that close attention to the process of plan development and to compensation plan details can result in compensation plans that promote both the organization's core compensation-related goals and compliance.

Notes

1. 42 C.F.R. § 417.479.

2. Social Security Act § 1877.

3. Social Security Act § 1128B(b).

4. By illustration, if the FMV of services is $100,000 and a disqualified person receives $150,000 for those services, the person can be assessed a personal excise tax ranging from 25 to 200 percent of the value of the excess benefit, or a tax (in this example) on the $50,000 that was in excess of the FMV of the services.

5. DHS are generally defined as items and services within the following broad categories that may be paid for under the Medicare program: clinical laboratory services; physical therapy, occupational therapy, and speech-language pathology services; radiology and certain other imaging services; radiation therapy services and supplies; durable medical equipment and supplies; parenteral and enteral nutrients, equipment, and supplies; prosthetics, orthotics, and prosthetic devices and supplies; home health services; and inpatient and outpatient hospital services. With respect to certain categories of DHS, CMS provides a definitive listing of services that are defined as DHS (and, for example, those diagnostic services that are not included in the list will not be defined as DHS). No such exclusive listing is provided for the other DHS categories. Identification of the particular DHS being ordered or referred by individual physicians is an essential part of developing a legally compliant compensation plan.

6. Although other provisions of federal law effectively apply the law's self-referral prohibition to Medicaid, no formal guidance has yet been published related to such services.

7. 42 C.F.R. § 411.352(i)(2).

8. 42 C.F.R. § 411.352(2)(i)–(iii).

9. Although the Stark law refers to "productivity bonuses," the legal meaning of this term does not always conform with that commonly used in production-based incentive or similar physician compensation arrangements. Thus, many physician compensation plans will be characterized as "productivity-based" plans because they tend to focus and pay compensation based, in one degree or another, on the physician's "production." However, even such production-based plans must ensure that the requirements of the Stark law are met by ensuring that there is no direct payment of compensation for a physician's DHS referrals. To make matters worse, the Stark law refers to the use of "productivity bonuses" in a variety of contexts, and in relation to a number of different Stark law exceptions. For example, under the Stark law, "productivity bonuses" are allowed under the in-office ancillary services exception as described here, but also in the context of the Stark law exceptions for employment arrangements, personal service arrangements, and others. Yet the requirements of what can be included in determining "production" for productivity bonus purposes will vary under different exceptions to the Stark law (e.g., by allowing incident to credit in the context of the in-office ancillary services exception only). It is for this reason that our diagnostic questions

relating to the nature of the organization that is the *source* of compensation, and the nature of the *relationship* between that source and the physician, are of significant importance.

10. The Stark law's exception for "physician services" also requires the presence of a bona fide Group Practice as defined by the Stark law. Because this exception generally has only limited application, it is not discussed here.

11. 42 C.F.R. § 411.352(i).

12. The Medicare program defines specific "incident to" requirements that are set forth at 42 C.F.R. Section 410.26. An examination of these specific requirements is beyond the scope of this chapter.

13. See 66 Fed. Reg. 55267 (Nov. 1, 2001) (initial publication of incident to rule); and 67 Fed. Reg. 79993 (Dec. 31, 2002) (providing clarification of previous publication).

14. For example, because the Stark law effectively imposes a "strict liability" prohibition on payment and requirements of refunds when payments are improper, an "advice of counsel" (e.g., "my lawyer said it was okay") defense may be of limited value in the event of a challenge.

15. IRC § 162(a)(1).

16. Treas. Reg. 1.162-7.

17. The standards under IRC § 162 also have general application in the context of tax-exempt organizations.

18. T.C. Memo. 2001-81.

19. The types of legal proscriptions that may impact the ability of a nonphysician to own and operate a medical practice vary from state to state. For example, some states restrict non-physician ownership of medical practices under arrangements via state medical licensure and other statutes that impose restrictions on the "corporate practice of medicine." Others impose similar restrictions via statutes defining the qualifications to own interests in professional corporations or associations for the practice of medicine, while other states either impose no restrictions on who may own and operate a medical practice, or they specifically allow certain organizations (such as hospitals) to own and operate physician medical practices.

20. 42 C.F.R. § 411.357(c).

21. 42 C.F.R. § 411.357(d).

22. See GCM 35638, and 39674.

23. See GCM 39674, GCM 39674, PLR 8808070, and PLR 9112006.

24. Treasury Reg § 53.4958-4(b)(1)(ii)(A).

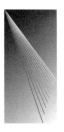

TEN

Special Issues in Physician Compensation

For most medical practices today, their compensation plan architectures will focus to a large degree on the key cultural and financial dimensions discussed in the prior chapters. Some medical practices, however, want to recognize and reward physicians for other activities, such as practice efficiency, resource utilization, patient satisfaction, participation, teamwork, community service, research, teaching, and many others.

In this chapter, we first present a general framework that outlines two distinct methods to treat nonclinical production in physician compensation planning: a direct method and an indirect method. We then discuss eight special issues that may need to be addressed in medical practices as they determine the "best" method to reward physician work and effort. Each of these issues presents a unique challenge in the compensation planning development process and will need to be resolved by the compensation planning committee in its deliberations as it works to revise or craft a new plan for the medical practice.

GENERAL FRAMEWORK FOR REWARDING NONCLINICAL PRODUCTION

Medical practices that wish to reward physicians beyond clinical productivity commonly adopt one of two methods in compensation plan design to encourage and reward these nonclinical production criteria: (1) the direct method; or (2) the indirect method.

The *direct* method involves explicitly defining the specific performance to be rewarded, along with a measurement and reward system consistent with performance levels. The *indirect* method involves building performance requirements into the compensation plan itself; for example, articulating a performance expectation in order to "earn" base salary levels or identifying a minimum set of performance expectations in order to be eligible for incentive.

► DIRECT METHOD – PAYMENT FOR NONCLINICAL PRODUCTION ACTIVITIES

The direct method of rewarding physicians for nonclinical production essentially builds another layer upon any basic plan architecture that might be used. The key steps to employing the direct method for compensation planning purposes are to:

1. Define the desired behavior or outcome;

2. Develop a measurement system that can discriminate rewards based upon the behavior or outcome;

3. Create a pool of funds or otherwise fund the incentive measure; and

4. Allocate dollars to individual physicians consistent with the physician's performance.

Since nonclinical production activities typically involve a more qualitative assessment, actual performance of the physician is typically "translated" to a quantitative score, or the qualitative assessment is assigned a specific dollar value or range of dollar values.

For example, a "low," "medium," or "high" qualitative evaluation of the physician's performance could be made by the medical director in the area of teamwork, with that subjective evaluation translated to a specific dollar amount or dollar range awarded. Likewise, a point system can be used to allocate points for specific work; for example, the number of community outreach programs or administrative activities in which the physician participates. An incentive pool can be identified for this work and allocated on a percentage-to-total basis among the medical practice's physicians.

This direct method of incorporating these types of measures into an incentive or bonus arrangement for physicians is currently not widely employed in private (e.g., physician-owned) practices. Based on the authors' experience, academic practices tend to incorporate these types of approaches into their compensation plan design at higher frequency levels, due to the goal of ensuring a "triple–threat" faculty member, division, or department (e.g., balancing the three academic missions of research, teaching, and clinical service). Likewise, hospital-affiliated practices will more commonly incorporate such approaches through an additional or "additive" incentive measure.

► INDIRECT METHODS – PERFORMANCE EXPECTATIONS AND PHYSICIAN RECOGNITION

Rather than directly rewarding physicians for nonclinical production activities via incentive or bonus arrangements, many medical practices elect an indirect method to acknowledge activities that go beyond clinical production by addressing such activities through the use of performance expectations. Performance expectations represent the minimum expected workload and performance requirements assigned to a physician in order to be part of the practice. The identification of performance expectations effectively links the compensation plan with the performance management process of the practice. For example, performance expectations related to clinical productivity, patient satisfaction, and even interpersonal effectiveness can be articulated, coupled with financial penalties for repeat offenders or potential nonparticipation in the incentive plan if certain base expectations are not met.

By defining performance expectations for all physicians, physician outlier behavior can be addressed by practice leadership. In addition, leverage can be applied to ensure that a physician performs at an acceptable threshold established by the practice. This can take multiple forms, including:

► Reducing base compensation or other arrangements if a physician does not meet minimum acceptable performance standards;

► Initiating steps that have been detailed in the practice's performance management process for evaluating physicians in the practice;

► Determining acceptable levels of performance to serve as a threshold for qualifying for an incentive payment;

EXHIBIT 10.1 Physician Performance Expectations

Category	Measure
1. Clinical Productivity:	► Revenue, WRVUs, Gross Charges, Time, Hours of Availability, Assigned Sessions, On-Call Time
2. Service:	► Administrative Roles, Leadership Roles, Committees, Professional Societies, Community Outreach
3. Fiscal/Financial:	► Cost of Practice, Cost per WRVU, Cost as a Percent of Total Medical Revenue, Billing and Coding Compliance
4. Quality:	► HEDIS Measures, Emergency Department Utilization, Laboratory Utilization, Pharmacy Utilization, Referrals, Medical Records Documentation, Patient Satisfaction
5. Access:	► Next Third Available Appointment, Physician Availability, Wait Times
6. Team-Orientation:	► Interpersonal Effectiveness, Teamwork, Levels of Engagement, Esprit de Corps
7. Teaching (if applicable):	► Hours of Teaching, Assigned Precepting, Resident Supervision, Medical Student Lectures
8. Research (if applicable):	► Extramural Funding, Percent Grants Submitted vs. Rewarded

► Transitioning a physician from "full-time" to "part-time" status due to his or her inability to meet certain performance expectations;

► Removing "partnership status" for physicians who transition from "full-time" status; for example, physicians who request a work slowdown or who begin their retirement countdown (see Chapter 11 for a more detailed discussion of generational issues and physician transition plans); or

► Other similar leverage points.

Performance expectations (also termed codes of conduct, practice doctrines, etc.) describe the expected performance levels of physicians in a number of areas that serve as success factors for the medical practice. Typically, they include consideration of multiple categories and measurements, as outlined in Exhibit 10.1.

A second indirect method to address nonclinical production activity of physicians is through informal rewards and recognition. Activities performed by the medical practice's physicians that go above and beyond the performance of others are often singled out for recognition in appropriate formats and forums, and in other ways. Typically, the medical practice's culture will dictate the extent to which such informal rewards are used (and valued).

SPECIAL ISSUES IN PHYSICIAN COMPENSATION

There are a number of special issues that arise as a medical practice works to revise its current compensation plan or develop a new compensation plan. In this section, we discuss some of the more frequent special issues that are encountered and that often need to be addressed by the compensation planning committee. We present specific methods to manage these issues as part of the compensation plan development process. The special issues discussed in this section include:

1. **Methods to identify base salary levels.** When a base plus incentive plan is adopted by a medical practice, the issue of how to determine the base salary is often raised. We present five different methods for approaching base salary determination.

2. **Compensating physicians for satellite and outreach activities.** Many medical practices have multiple practice sites that need to be staffed by physicians. However, often the services provided at the satellite office are either not at the same volume levels or at the same level of intensity as the services the physicians would be performing if they were assigned to the main practice site. We address the special issue of recognizing the work and effort of physicians assigned to outreach locations to ensure they are not unduly penalized for this work.

3. **Compensating physicians for leadership and administrative services.** Physicians who agree to perform a leadership or administrative role in the practice are frequently not able to maintain the same level of clinical service as com-

pared to their practice colleagues. If the medical practice has focused its compensation plan on clinical production, a method is needed to recognize and reward these physicians for their nonclinical roles. An approach that is often used in these situations involving linking payments to market value for these types of services is presented.

4. **Compensation plans for new physicians.** Rarely are new physicians immediately integrated into the current compensation plan of a medical practice. Instead, new physicians are often recruited with some type of "guaranteed" level of income for a set period of time. Four areas that need to be addressed when determining compensation plans for new physicians are discussed, with examples of methods used by medical practices to address these issues. In addition, we provide comments on considerations and strategies related to the hiring of new physicians and the potential protection of short-term income levels for physicians in the same practice specialty as the new physician.

5. **Compensation plans for nonphysician providers.** This book has focused on compensation plans for physicians; however, as discussed in Chapter 9 regarding "incident to" services, nonphysician providers often play a large role in leveraging the physicians to achieve targeted production and work levels. We have discussed the treatment of expenses associated with nonphysician providers in many of the plan architectures and examples related to strict and modified cost accounting. In this section, we discuss common approaches used to compensate nonphysician providers for their work. The methodology used to compensate nonphysician providers is role-dependent; there is typically a direct linkage between the type of work delegated to nonphysician providers and the compensation method used to recognize and reward that work.

6. **Market differences in subspecialty compensation levels.** In a number of markets, it is difficult to recruit scarce specialists that are needed. How to handle this special issue in the context of compensation planning is discussed so that medical practices are able to recruit and retain these types of physicians, paying them compensation levels that may exceed what they personally can generate in terms of net collections from professional services.

7. **Nonobjective performance criteria in compensation plans.** There are a number of measures that do not currently have objective criteria by which to measure physician performance. Handling this special issue involves turning the "subjective" evaluation into a more "objective" or quantifiable result so that compensation can be rewarded differentially based on individual physician performance.

8. **Compensation plans involving system-wide incentive measures.** Physicians who are members of an integrated delivery system or health system network are often able to participate in a system-wide incentive plan. In this section we dis-

cuss approaches to developing system-wide performance measures that are currently in use.

Each of these eight special issues is discussed below. We first discuss the purpose of addressing this issue for a medical practice. The purpose is then followed by specific methods to measure, monitor, and/or incorporate this issue in the context of compensation planning and development.

▶ ISSUE 1: METHODS TO IDENTIFY BASE SALARY LEVELS

Purpose

When a base portion of compensation is identified in a compensation plan (e.g., base plus incentive plans), its determination will fundamentally impact the other components of compensation. The method selected to identify base salary levels will impact the proportion of total compensation that is attributed to "base" salary. The decision regarding which approach is "best" for a medical practice must involve consideration of what is "fair," along with financial modeling of alternatives as part of the overall compensation plan design process.

Methodology

The five methods that medical practices typically employ in order to determine base salary levels are outlined below.

Method 1: Base Linked to Historical Compensation

In this method, the base salary is set as a percentage of the physician's historical compensation level; for example, at 70 to 80 percent of past total compensation.

Example of Method 1

If the physician received $150,000 in total compensation during the past year, the base salary is set at 70 percent of this amount, or at $105,000.

Method 2: Base Linked to Market Norms

A variety of benchmarking tools are available that outline the market norms for a particular physician practicing in a given specialty. Some of these data sources are highly detailed and include data by gender, by years in practice, by geographic region, by type of medical group, and other factors.

In this second method of establishing base salary levels, the market data are used to determine an appropriate base salary level. The market data that are actually selected for the base salary may be at a specific percentile level (e.g., the 25th percentile), or defined in relation to a percentile (e.g., 80 percent of median). An example of Method 2 is presented in Exhibit 10.2

EXHIBIT 10.2   Example of Base Salary Linked to Market Norms

	25th Percentile	Median	75th Percentile	90th Percentile
Internal Medicine	$132,633	$159,252	$194,984	$245,668
General Surgery	$209,333	$264,375	$350,605	$438,883

Note: Benchmarks in the above table are for example purposes only.   © 2006 Johnson & Walker Keegan

Method 3: Base Linked to Specialty and Production

Adopting this third approach, a medical practice actually links the base salary to both the specialty and the individual physician's productivity level within the specialty. An example for Method 3 is presented in Exhibit 10.3.

EXHIBIT 10.3   Example of Base Salary Linked to Specialty and Production

If: Production Percentile	Then: Percentile of Market Compensation
50th percentile or less	25th percentile for specialty
51st to 65th percentile	50th percentile for specialty
66th to 80th percentile	Midpoint 50th to 75th percentile
81st to 89th percentile	75th percentile for specialty
Above 90th percentile	90th percentile for specialty

© 2006 Johnson & Walker Keegan

Although compensation levels are linked to published benchmarks in Methods 2 and 3, because of the year-to-year variation in benchmark data, linkage of compensation and production levels to median values will commonly be recommended as a means to reduce year-to-year variability. Thus, the basic Method 3 referenced above might be modified, as outlined in Exhibit 10.4.

In all instances, the precise linkages to market would be determined in connection with the modeling process. As a general matter, the two variations of Method 3 link compensation to a market level that would be slightly below the production percentile or percentage of median. This is because the values in benchmark production and compensation tables do not directly correlate. See Chapter 16, "The Special World of Hospital and Academic Practices," for more information.

EXHIBIT 10.4 Example of Base Salary Linked to Specialty and Production – Modified

If: Production Percentile	Then: Percentile of Market Compensation
Less than 80% of median	70% of median for specialty
80% to 100% of median	80% of median for specialty
101% to 120% of median	Median for specialty
121% to 130% of median	110% of median for specialty
Above 130% of median	120% of median for specialty

© 2006 Johnson & Walker Keegan

Method 4: Ranges of Bases

Method 4 involves a range of bases, essentially permitting a physician to advance within an established range. An example of Method 4 is presented in Exhibit 10.5.

EXHIBIT 10.5 Example of Base Salary Including Ranges of Bases

Step	Base Range: $60,000 – $85,000
Step 1	$60,000
Step 2	$66,000
Step 3	$72,000
Step 4	$78,000
Step 5	$85,000

© 2006 Johnson & Walker Keegan

Method 5: Base Tied to Seniority or Academic Rank

The final method used to identify base salary levels is typically found in academic settings. Base salary may be tied to academic rank and involve a stepwise approach consistent with progression through the academic ranks. An example of Method 5 is presented in Exhibit 10.6.

Although seniority continues to be considered as one of several factors in determining and paying compensation in some settings, relatively few practices use seniority (e.g., time with a particular medical practice) as the basis for determining all or part of compensation, and even fewer are considering seniority in a formal sense in connection with new compensation plans.

Steps	Assistant Professor	Associate Professor	Professor
Step 1	$40,000	$55,000	$70,000
Step 2	$43,000	$58,000	$73,000
Step 3	$46,000	$61,000	$76,000
Step 4	$49,000	$64,000	$79,000
Step 5	$52,000	$67,000	$82,000

EXHIBIT 10.6 Example of Base Salary Tied to Seniority or Academic Rank

© 2006 Johnson & Walker Keegan

► ISSUE 2: COMPENSATING PHYSICIANS FOR SATELLITE AND OUTREACH ACTIVITIES

Purpose

Many medical practices engage in extensive outreach services at satellite practice locations. These activities are frequently viewed as essential to the medical practice's business plan, as outreach services are an important means to generate consultations and other services from patients located in more remote locations.

The challenge with outreach activity is the common perception (and frequent reality) that the production and the quality of work life at the outreach location are deficient in comparison to a physician's primary or "home-base" practice location. As a result, not every physician will want to engage in such activities, and some physicians will seek to "cherry-pick" the particular location based on its perceived desirability.

Methodology

While there is no perfect mechanism to both encourage and equitably reward outreach activity, two such methods are provided below: (1) travel time credit; and (2) "efficiency-of-production" calculations.

Method 1: Travel Time Credit

Because travel time to outreach locations involves a lost opportunity for clinical practice production, some limited production travel time "credit" may be provided using a standard, negotiated system. For example, assuming that WRVUs are used in connection with the production component of compensation, additional "travel time" WRVUs can be assigned based on outreach activities.

Three basic factors are commonly used for purposes of assigning travel time WRVUs:

1. An estimate of the time to travel from one primary (or main) clinical practice

location to the outreach location (e.g., from Community X, where the main hospital is located, to different communities);

2. Selection of a "representative" or "typical" evaluation and management (E&M) current procedural terminology (CPT) code (commonly a Level 3 established patient office visit) related to the offsite work; and

3. An estimate of the typical number of units of the representative CPT code (e.g., Level 3 established patient office visit) that can be performed by the typical physician during one hour.

Example

► It takes 1.25 hours to travel from Practice Site X to the "Smithville" outreach location;

► The representative CPT code is a 99213 (Level 3 established patient office visit), which generates .67 WRVUs each; and

► The typical physician can perform three Level 3 services per hour.

The calculation of travel time WRVUs credited to the physician to travel from Practice Site X to the Smithville outreach location would be as follows:

► Travel time WRVUs per hour = 2.01 (.67 x 3)

► Travel time from Practice Site X to Smithville = 1.25 hours

► Travel time WRVUs = 2.251 (one way to Smithville from Practice Site X = 2.01 x 1.25 = 2.251). Total travel time WRVUs for complete outreach (to and from the site) = 5.025.

The result of such calculations can be arrayed on a grid outlining the agreed upon total travel time WRVU credit for outreach locations, which might look something like

EXHIBIT 10.7 Determination of Travel Time WRVUs

Outreach Location	From Practice Site X	From Practice Site Y
Barnstone	13.40	
Milligan	6.70	
Lincoln	6.70	
New Castle	1.34	2.68
Laguna	5.36	
Parkview	2.23	
Pueblo	2.23	

© 2006 Johnson & Walker Keegan

what is presented in Exhibit 10.7 (depending upon the satellite location and the origin of the physician's location as either Practice Site X or Y).

Travel time production credit is then added to other actual production when determining compensation levels. Other measures of clinical production beyond WRVUs (e.g., average gross charges or average net collections from professional services) may also be used in determining travel time production credit. Production credit based on such factors will commonly not make a large difference to the compensation levels, but the provision of some level of production credit will commonly address the political realities associated with the compensation system development process in light of outreach requirements.

Method 2: Efficiency of Production

The second method to reward physicians for outreach activity involves measuring the efficiency of a particular physician at his or her primary practice location and then applying this efficiency measure to the time spent at the satellite site(s). The goal is to not penalize the physician for outreach activity, when he or she could be more productive at the physician's primary clinical service delivery location(s).

An efficiency component is calculated for each physician based on: (1) the physician's performance at his or her primary practice location; and (2) the physician's scheduled time in that location.

Seven steps are used in this approach to rewarding physicians for outreach activity:

Step 1. Allocate Funds to Efficiency Component

Allocate a defined percentage (e.g., 30 percent) of total funds available for payment of physician compensation through the efficiency component to compensation.

Step 2. Determine Physician Time at Various Locations

Use a standard schedule to determine the amount of time each physician is assigned to the physician's primary and outreach locations.

Step 3. Identify Primary Locations

Identify primary hospital and clinic locations (defined as those *other than* outreach locations) for each physician. For example, the primary location might be assigned as follows:

- ▶ Dr. Green – Practice Site X and Community Hospital A;
- ▶ Drs. Jones, Smith, and Johnson – Practice Site Y and Community Hospital B; and
- ▶ Dr. Wilson – Community Hospital C.

Step 4. Measure Physician Production at Primary Location

Measure clinical service production for each physician *solely* at the physician's *primary practice* location(s) for purposes of the efficiency component. Measurement is limited and unique to the scheduled time that the physician is assigned to the primary location(s).

Step 5. Employ Standard Measure for Production at Primary Locations

Employ a standard measure, such as professional services net collections or WRVUs generated by the physician's personal services in his or her *primary location(s) per hour of scheduled time*. For example, using WRVUs as the unit of measurement, this is calculated by dividing the WRVUs generated at the physician's primary location(s) by the scheduled hours at the primary location(s) for each physician. The use of scheduled time allows for a uniform comparison of the relative practice efficiency of physicians with different levels of scheduled time (e.g., the work efficiency of a physician with 1,600 hours of scheduled time at a primary location can be compared to a physician who has only 1,200 hours at his or her primary location).

Step 6. Determine WRVUs for Each Physician in Primary Locations

Calculate the actual WRVUs per scheduled hour in the *primary practice* location for each physician. For example, Dr. A might have 12.0 per hour; Dr. B might have 8.0 per hour; etc.

Step 7. Allocate Efficiency Component of Compensation Pool

Allocate the efficiency component of the compensation pool based on each physician's WRVUs per hour of scheduled time in the primary practice location and on the time assigned to outreach activity, expressed as a percentage of all physicians. Thus, in the example above, for the same time spent in outreach activity, Dr. A would receive a larger share of the efficiency component compensation pool, because Dr. A's WRVU production per scheduled hour is higher than Dr. B's.

► ISSUE 3: COMPENSATING PHYSICIANS FOR LEADERSHIP AND ADMINISTRATIVE SERVICES

Purpose

Many medical practices compensate physicians for their internal and external leadership responsibilities. For example, the president of the medical practice might receive a set compensation in relation to his or her duties. For physicians in the practice who demonstrate external leadership (for example, by serving on hospital boards), many practices find it appropriate to recognize this role via compensation, reduced clinical assignment, or some other method.

In many physician-owned medical practices, physicians who hold leadership roles can and will make more money practicing medicine than they will by assuming a leadership position. Thus, for these physician leaders, some levels of compensation to recognize their "lost" revenue associated with clinical activity is viewed as appropriate, although that level of compensation is rarely, if ever, sufficient to make up for the actual losses in production.

To address this fact, some practices "require" physicians to assume leadership positions, rather than permit personal choice. However, a mandatory leadership requirement in a medical practice can also create a new problem for the medical practice, because all physicians are not equally skilled in the business of medicine issues required for today's complex health care environment.

Methodology

One approach to dealing with the issue of pay for leadership and administrative services involves linking the payment to the market value of these services. It involves: (1) determining the total amount of money that the practice is willing to pay for administrative services using "market" as a starting point; and (2) dividing that aggregate amount among the positions that the practice requires using a standard formula. The specific steps involved in this methodology are outlined below.

Step 1. Define position descriptions for leadership and administrative services that are performed by the practice's physicians.

Step 2. Use market data as the starting point for determining the total amount that should be paid *in the aggregate* for these administrative positions (e.g., such as that found in the MGMA Management Compensation Survey or other agency surveys). That is, based on what the positions are "buying" in terms of services, what would other practices pay for similar services?

Step 3. Use a standard formula or set of criteria to allocate the aggregate amount of compensation designated for the administrative positions. Such a formula might use a combination of several factors to allocate the market level of total pay:

▶ Number of physicians directly "managed" and/or affected through the job;

▶ Relative importance of the position to group success and operations; and

▶ Whether the practice or an outside party pays for this position.

Step 4. Divide the total amount allocated (Step 2 above) among the positions based on the formula (Step 3 above) to determine the compensation to be paid for each position.

Example

Market data are often used to provide a good starting point for determining the aggregate amount to be used to pay for the services. For example, let's assume that, based on benchmarking data, the cost of general and administrative personnel (which include medical directors, administrators, the chief financial officer, and others) on a per FTE physician basis is $10,000 at the 25th percentile level and $12,000 at the median level for general internal medicine practices.

Using the 25th percentile as the starting point, and assuming 8.00 FTE physicians in the medical practice, then $80,000 ($10,000 multiplied by 8.00) might be used to pay for administrative services performed by physicians. That amount would then be allocated among the various administrative positions.

A questionnaire is then submitted to physicians to obtain their feedback on which administrative positions should be reimbursed and at what levels. A sample of such a questionnaire is provided in Exhibit 10.8. It is typically accompanied by specific job descriptions for each of the administrative positions to be considered for the medical practice.

Physicians are asked to rank the "importance" of the positions that have been identified as needed. Importance refers to how critical the position is to the organization and/or its providers and the difficulty and time commitment of the position. In this example, a score of 10 signifies the highest (most critical/difficult/time commitment), and 1 signifies the least (critical/difficult/time commitment).

Through this systematic approach, the medical practice can make decisions on which leadership and administrative positions should be funded. Physician perceptions regarding the importance of each position and its level of difficulty and time commitment inform the decision regarding the portion of the identified funds to be allocated to each position.

► ISSUE 4: COMPENSATION PLANS FOR NEW PHYSICIANS

Purpose

Typically, physicians who are new to a medical practice will be paid via a compensation plan that is different from that of their partners or colleagues who have been in the practice for some time.

EXHIBIT 10.8   Questionnaire for Obtaining Physician Feedback on Leadership Roles and Compensation

Position	Needed? (yes or no) Paid for by whom?	Importance/Difficulty/Time Commitment Circle one number to rank using 1 (as the lowest) and 10 (as the highest)											
Group President		Lowest	1	2	3	4	5	6	7	8	9	10	Highest
Group Secretary		Lowest	1	2	3	4	5	6	7	8	9	10	Highest
Group Treasurer		Lowest	1	2	3	4	5	6	7	8	9	10	Highest
Hospital X Medical Director		Lowest	1	2	3	4	5	6	7	8	9	10	Highest
Hospital Y Medical Director	Hospital	Lowest	1	2	3	4	5	6	7	8	9	10	Highest
Physician Inpatient Unit Director		Lowest	1	2	3	4	5	6	7	8	9	10	Highest
Nursing Home Medical Director	Nursing Home	Lowest	1	2	3	4	5	6	7	8	9	10	Highest
Other (write in)		Lowest	1	2	3	4	5	6	7	8	9	10	Highest

© 2006 Johnson & Walker Keegan

Methodology

Four areas need to be addressed when determining compensation plans for new physicians.

1. **Plan Architecture.** The most common forms of compensation plans for new physicians are straight salary and base plus incentive plans – typically for a one- to two-year period – that provide a competitive level of compensation, while recognizing that the group's current physicians are essentially supporting the physician until his or her practice has been established.

2. **Performance Expectations.** Many practices are recognizing the importance of outlining performance expectations for the first two years of employment so that the new physician recognizes what is expected of his or her performance and productivity. These performance expectations are designed, in large part, to encourage and institute good work patterns and practices based on what would be expected for practice development and growth.

3. **Incentive.** Some medical practices also have elected to provide for an incentive component beyond the negotiated salary once specific productivity or financial thresholds have been met. Such incentives generally provide for a defined share of revenues in excess of a defined threshold, where the threshold is developed with the objective of reasonably covering the salary, benefits, and share of practice overhead incurred by the physician. Thus, a practice may pay a physician a straight base salary (e.g., $200,000) in years one and two, but in year two, it may provide an opportunity for an incentive equal to a percentage of the physician's net collections from professional services in excess of a defined dollar amount (e.g., 30 percent of net collections in excess of $450,000).

4. **Physician Buy-in Policy.** The new physician compensation plan methodology selected by a medical practice will also be impacted by its practice buy-in policy. Some practices elect to negotiate a salary with the new physician for two years and minimize the buy-in obligation. Other groups require a financial buy-in in order to compensate the group for essentially supporting the physician while he or she grows a patient base.

In addition to these areas, many medical practices will plan for and establish criteria related to the hiring of new physicians, to include consideration of how a new physician will impact the compensation levels of physicians already in the medical practice.

Decisions regarding whether to hire a new physician will depend on numerous factors, including the nature of the medical practice (e.g., physician-owned or hospital-affiliated), the work levels of the physicians already in the practice, unmet patient demands and related factors. In most settings, the retention of an additional physician in a particular practice specialty will be undertaken in furtherance of a professional resources staffing plan such that the practice has already identified the number of physicians it wishes to employ in each respective specialty. These plans, however, can be augmented by additional criteria that are considered in connection with hiring and recruitment decisions. For example, many medical practices will establish the criteria that, absent a clear-cut need, the practice will only hire an additional physician when the practice's existing physicians in the relevant specialty have production levels that are well above median or other expected levels. This might mean, for example, that a new physician will be hired when the physicians in the relevant division or specialty have production in excess of 110 (or some other) percentage of median, but that a new physician will not be hired when production levels are below this benchmark. Practices will also consider such factors as expected retirements, physician demographics (ages), and the like in connection with hiring decisions.

By establishing criteria for when a hiring decision can or should be made, these practices help to focus attention on the issues that will impact income levels. This type of focus will also help to ensure that the practice and its other physicians consider all relevant factors when making hiring decisions, as opposed to simply agreeing to a new hire because it helps address other needs (e.g., reducing on-call obligations).

An additional question relates to how the practice intends to treat or potentially "protect" the income levels of the practice's existing physicians when a new physician is hired. This question is typically most prevalent in the context of hospital-affiliated or similar practice settings that are not physician-owned. In these settings, the employer (e.g., hospital) may have a desire to hire additional physicians to meet service delivery goals, without regard to the impact that the new physician may have on the work levels of the preexisting physicians. In these settings, a reasonable, and limited, program of practice and income "protection" may be considered so that the compensation levels of individual physicians are protected for a period of time. Such programs are typically limited in scope (e.g., providing additional production credit within defined parameters or ensuring that established physician compensation levels will not fall below a defined level), and duration (typically for no more than six months to one year). Such programs are typically designed to protect the compensation earned by those physicians who are already meeting or exceeding performance expectations (e.g., those whose production is in excess of median or other benchmark levels), but not others.

► ISSUE 5: COMPENSATION PLANS FOR NONPHYSICIAN PROVIDERS

Purpose

Throughout this book, we have discussed various methods to treat nonphysician provider clinical activity within the physician compensation plan itself. These methods have included:

- ► Identifying a stipend to recognize supervisory roles of physicians;
- ► In some settings, billing of nonphysician provider services as "incident to" the

services of physicians, then assessing the cost of the nonphysician provider as a direct expense to the physicians who benefit from this leverage;

► Including net income from nonphysician providers in the revenue pool that is distributed to physicians (e.g., professional services net collections less expense of the nonphysician providers, with the balance distributed to physicians in the practice);

► "Crediting" physicians with the net collections billed in the nonphysician provider's name and "assessing" those physicians with the cost of the nonphysician providers; and

► Treating nonphysician provider activity as a separate cost center, with any overage generally maintained by the practice as a whole or distributed in some predetermined fashion.

We have not yet, however, addressed the issue of compensation planning for nonphysician providers themselves. By nonphysician provider, we mean individuals who are able to generate revenue – either billed as incident to activity under the physician's name or on their own. Nonphysician providers include nurse practitioners, certified nurse midwives, physician assistants, physical therapists, certified nurse anesthetists, and a host of others. The scope of practice and the level of oversight of these providers vary by state; thus, different expectations of their performance and different levels of supervision are required based on the geographic location of a medical practice.

Methodology

In general, the type of compensation plan that is selected for nonphysician providers in a practice relates to both of the key elements we identified for physician compensation plans – cultural dimensions (individualistic to team-oriented models) and financial treatment (revenue and/or expense treatment) associated with the plan. For nonphysician providers, however, the actual role the nonphysician provider performs in the practice needs to be taken into account.

Role of the Nonphysician Provider

The role of the nonphysician provider in the practice will dictate the type of plan that is developed. The four major roles of nonphysician providers include:

1. **Physician Leverage.** When recruited to "leverage" a physician, the nonphysician provider may be asked to see urgent patient visits, review lab and test results, fill prescription refill requests, manage inbound and outbound telephones, and perform other delegatable duties of the physician.

2. **"Independent" Work Scope.** When the nonphysician provider has an independent scope of work, the nonphysician provider has his or her own assigned

patients and is expected to manage these patients relatively independently (e.g., a certified nurse anesthetist).

3. **Special Skills Need.** Nonphysician providers hired due to their special skills typically augment the physicians and permit expansion of market share or services offered to patients. For example, a female nurse practitioner may be recruited to expand routine gynecology services within an obstetrics and gynecology (OB/GYN) practice that is heavily obstetrics-based. In this role, her special skills permit the practice to expand service offerings to the community. In this role, she may perform an independent work scope (similar to number 2 above); however, the recruitment of this position was consistent with a special skill needed by the medical practice.

4. **Specialty-Specific Role.** Here, the nonphysician provider typically works as a member of the care team for a particular specialty. For example, a physician's assistant in a cardiovascular surgery practice may be assigned to be a surgical assistant. A nurse practitioner or physician's assistant may be assigned to make hospital rounds and assist in admitting and discharging patients.

If a medical practice, for example, views the nonphysician provider as essentially an extension of an individual physician, permitting the physician to see more patients, handle more difficult cases, etc., that provider may be viewed as part of the cost center for the physician. The compensation plan involving the nonphysician provider will likely be linked to that of the physician, or at least be aligned with it, so that the physician and nonphysician provider are not working at cross-purposes.

If, on the other hand, the nonphysician providers have their own work scope (e.g., certified nurse midwives), then they may be treated as a separate unit for compensation plan purposes. The compensation plan involving these providers may be separate and distinct from the physician compensation plan, yet again, the issue of alignment is important to ensure that internal competition for patients is not created or that providers are not otherwise working in divergent ways.

The level by which the nonphysician provider is effectively integrated into the practice also has implications for the compensation plan that is designed. For example, if a practice tends to view the nonphysician providers in a more supportive role, it is likely to take a more traditional approach toward compensation – for example, a straight salary arrangement. If, on the other hand, the practice expects the nonphysician providers to market the practice and views them as key to enhancing the patient base and/or the net revenue, then the practice may choose to provide incentives in order to encourage active attention to increasing market share.

Compensation Plan Architectures for Nonphysician Providers

The basic compensation plan architectures presented in Chapter 13 are available for these types of providers as well; however, we typically see one of three models used in conjunction with compensation plans for nonphysician providers:

1. **Architecture A – Unit-Based Plans.** Consistent with this architecture, non-physician providers receive a straight salary. In these arrangements, performance expectations related to their schedule, patient volumes, revenue generation, and other requirements are typically detailed so that the nonphysician providers know what is expected of their performance while permitting the practice to appropriately budget for their expense (compensation, benefits, and related cost of practice).

2. **Architecture B – Guaranteed Share (Base Plus Incentive) Plans.** In a base plus incentive plan, nonphysician providers typically receive a base salary that is tied to market rates – again, with performance expectations articulated for minimum expectations. Beyond this base salary, nonphysician providers can earn an incentive that is defined in advance. For example, a nurse practitioner who exceeds the base expectations expected of her position may qualify for a specific percentage of professional services net collections over and above that which is generated for her base (e.g., 10 to 25 percent). As another example, a physician assistant who works extra shifts may be eligible for a flat-dollar rate per shift. As a final example, on-call pay can be defined to be in addition to the base salary, with a set dollar amount paid for weekday and weekend call activity.

3. **Architecture D – Pure Production Plans.** In this architecture, a pure production plan is in place. In this plan, the nonphysician providers are treated as a separate cost center and are expected to generate their own revenue and cover their own expense of practice (to include indirect costs as appropriate). They typically take a "draw" each month based on expected total compensation levels, with reconciliation conducted quarterly to address shortfalls in revenue. Any overage at the end of the year is then split between the practice and the nonphysician providers based on predetermined criteria.

Again, however, any of the other plan architectures are also available to be used for nonphysician providers, provided that appropriate legal and regulatory issues are addressed. See Chapter 9, "The Legal Element," for a discussion of "incident to" treatment issues and issues related to compensation in the hospital-owned or hospital-affiliated practice and in tax-exempt organizations.

Due to the demographic changes in the patient population (e.g., the aging of the baby boomers and the increase in chronic care conditions) and in physician availability (subspecialization, geographic maldistribution), we expect to see more nonphysician providers in the medical practice setting. The ability to recruit and retain these providers may require medical practices to revisit the compensation plan strategies they have developed in order to create appropriate recognition and reward systems.

► ISSUE 6: MARKET DIFFERENCES IN SUBSPECIALTY COMPENSATION LEVELS

Purpose

It can be argued that the market and physician work levels ultimately determine physician compensation. However, in some practice specialties that are highly sought after, the demand for physicians arguably exceeds the compensation that can be earned from their production alone. This is found in certain medical and surgical subspecialties and in certain markets. Thus, a method is needed to reallocate dollar amounts in the medical practice to recruit and retain physicians in these subspecialties. Not surprisingly, such a mechanism creates its own political and other issues that must also be considered. From the perspective of a compensation plan, however, the core objective of promoting objectivity via the use of a standard methodology is important to any such approach.

Methodology

While there is no perfect method to recognize and reasonably take into account variations in subspecialty compensation based upon market, two common approaches are employed:

1. **Differential Base Salary Based on Market.** Provides a market-based base salary that is guaranteed and that reflects variations based upon subspecialty; and

2. **Adjusting Production "Credit."** Provides some reasonable subspecialty adjustment within the determination of production "credit" in the context of determining and paying physician compensation. Examples of these two approaches are provided below.

Method 1: Differential Base Salaries Based upon Market

Purpose

This approach reasonably recognizes differences in base compensation levels paid by different medical and surgical subspecialties, while also taking into account actual production for individual physicians.

Step 1. Determine Measures Used to Set the Base-Salary Level

Determine the specific compensation measures that will be used on a consistent basis in setting base salary levels. Given year-to-year variation and variations based upon different measures of market levels (e.g., as reported in survey instruments published by MGMA, AMGA, and others), medical practices will commonly use multiple measures in order to reduce annual variation. As a result, different tables from a single benchmark source and/or multiple benchmark sources may be selected and used (e.g., all physicians, regional median data, and others). Define these benchmark sources, tables, and measures in advance, and apply them on a uniform basis from year to year. Moreover, rather than using or selecting a single value from a single table, consider employing an average of the various medians from multiple tables.

Step 2. Determine Portion of Compensation to Be Considered Base Salary

Determine a defined portion of each physician's total compensation (e.g., 50 to 70 percent) that will be paid as a guaranteed base salary. Link that base salary to market levels of compensation for the physician's particular subspecialty. If wide variations in productivity are present in relation to benchmark norms, additional gradations may be provided based upon relative productivity levels by reference to benchmarks (e.g., below 80 percent of median, 80 percent of median to median, median to 120 percent of median; above 120 percent of median). (An example of this type of approach using gradations in productivity to determine base salary was presented earlier in this chapter, in Issue 1, Methods to Determine Base Salary.) This salary becomes a fixed expense of the practice that is paid on a guaranteed basis.

Step 3. Determine Methodology for Nonbase Compensation

The remaining portions of each physician's compensation are determined based on other methodologies (i.e., incentive based on production or other methods) as outlined in the plan examples in Chapters 13, 14, and 15.

Method 2: Adjusting Production "Credit"

Purpose

This approach uses a quantifiable approach to provide for some limited adjustment to production credit based on market forces related to subspecialties.

Step 1. Identify Compensation Levels for Each Subspecialty Based on Market Data

For example, market data (e.g., MGMA, AMGA, and others) report that different subspecialties are paid at slightly different levels based on the market.

Step 2. Determine the Compensation Differential between Subspecialists

Step 3. Identify WRVUs Generated by Each Physician in the Performance of Each Subspecialty Area

For example, if a cardiologist were to perform services as an invasive cardiologist and as an interventional cardiologist, segregate the WRVUs (based on CPT codes) for each of these areas.

EXHIBIT 10.9 Adjusting Production Credit to Compensate Subspecialists

Example of a Cardiology Practice

Specialty	WRVUs
Electrophysiology (EP)	1.27
Invasive	1.13
Interventional	1.29
Noninvasive	1.00

© 2006 Johnson & Walker Keegan

Step 4. Adjust the WRVUs generated by the physicians based on the compensation differential for each subspecialty.

Example

Market data reflect different compensation levels for cardiologists in each of their four main subspecialties – noninvasive, invasive, interventional, and electrophysiology. In Exhibit 10.9, we have indexed the market data to slightly *adjust the WRVUs* generated for each of these subspecialties *consistent with the fluctuations in compensation levels* reported in the survey instruments.

In Exhibit 10.9, the WRVUs of noninvasive cardiologists were set at 1.00, with each of the other subspecialties indexed off this level based on market compensation differentials. When this approach is employed, the adjustments are applied solely to the procedures (CPT codes) identified for each cardiology subspecialty. Thus, for example, a cardiologist who performs both invasive and interventional services would have his or her WRVUs adjusted differentially; WRVUs attributed to invasive cardiology services would be increased by 13 percent, with interventional cardiology services increased by 29 percent.

Either of these two approaches – differential base salaries based on market or adjustments to production credit – may be used when medical practices are faced with challenges in compensating physicians at required levels for recruitment and retention that may be in excess of what the physician might earn in a pure production compensation plan.

▶ ISSUE 7: NONOBJECTIVE PERFORMANCE CRITERIA IN COMPENSATION PLANS

Purpose

Factors beyond clinical service productivity are important to any effective compensation plan. For this reason, many medical practices and other organizations seek to measure and reward nonclinical production-based factors, including citizenship, program development, leadership, patient satisfaction, and other measures that may involve more qualitative assessment.

While the goal of measuring and rewarding differences in performance related to such factors is common, determining a means to actually measure and reward performance using such nonclinical production-based and "nonobjective" factors is the Achilles heel of many physician compensation plans. Physicians will frequently observe that the idea is great in theory but difficult, if not impossible, in practice due to the inherently subjective nature of such issues. Thus, many of these areas are often addressed in an indirect method via performance expectations for base salary, as opposed to identifying specific incentive payments to reward physicians in these areas.

Any measurement and reward system linked to nonobjective measures will always have to confront the inherent challenges of subjective measures, the potential for favoritism, and other concerns. Nonetheless, many groups have sought to develop systems that provide a reasonably objective and fair method of evaluating citizenship and other factors that are, by their nature, inherently subjective. Essential to such systems is the need to:

► Limit the total portion of compensation that is subject to such nonobjective methods;

► Define, clearly and in advance, the specific performance criteria and expectations that will be evaluated and measured through such a nonobjective component;

► Provide a clear and reasonably transparent system that will be used to perform the evaluations, minimizing the potential for subjective bias (in the form of neither overly negative nor overly positive evaluations);

► Acknowledge that the measures are not perfect, but that it is important to use some imperfect measure as a means to "shine the light" on certain important performance features.

Methodology

While no approach is perfect, the following two methods are directed at these goals:

Method 1: Confidential Peer Rankings

The first method involves a simple, confidential, and reasonably objective method to allow for "peer" rankings of individual physicians and to identify performance outliers.

As we review the methodology, we have used "citizenship" as the performance that the medical practice wants to reward; however, any number of nonobjective performance measures can be rewarded based upon this methodology. We provide a means to reward physicians with above-average citizenship, while not rewarding those with below-average citizenship. In most instances, practice physicians will be judged to be "average" on individual measures, but the methodology allows for the identification of performance outliers who are either above or below the norm in the practice.

Step 1. Define Incentive Pool "Citizenship" Allocation

Define a percentage of the incentive pool (e.g., 10 to 20 percent) that is otherwise available for payment of compensation as the portion that will be subject to allocation for "citizenship."

Step 2. Establish Performance Expectations Regarding Citizenship Behaviors

Step 3. Evaluate Each Individual's Citizenship Behaviors

Conduct this evaluating using a 3-point scale (3 = Above average; 2 = Average; 1 = Below Average) using written and confidential evaluations by committee. For example, a five-person committee could be formed comprised of the following parties:

- ► Two physicians selected from the practice's executive committee;
- ► The medical director;
- ► The chief executive officer; and
- ► One "at-large" physician selected by the physician being evaluated.

Step 4. Select "At-Large" Physician to Evaluate Committee Members

To evaluate physicians on the committee, physicians select one additional "at-large" physician who will stand in for and evaluate each individual physician who also serves on the committee.

Step 5. Remove One High and One Low Value for Each Performance Expectation Evaluated

The average of the remaining values for the particular performance expectation is used to reward physicians for citizenship behaviors. Each physician is expected to score no less than a 2 (average) on each measure (after removal of high and low values).

Step 6. Award the Citizenship Dollars as Follows:

- ► An "average" score on a single performance expectation receives an average share of the amount allocated to this pool. Assuming that there are six performance criteria, and a total of $40,000 per physician is placed into the pool for allocation through this method, the "share" paid for average performance on each of the six criteria would equal $6,666 per physician.
- ► A "below-average" performance on a particular measure results in a reduced (e.g., 50 percent or even 0 percent) "share."
- ► An "above–average" performance results in a full "share," *plus* a pro rata portion of any amount withheld from physicians who scored below average on the particular measure.
- ► If all physicians score "average" or above, then the total amount allocated to the particular performance expectation (all physicians) is distributed on a percent-to-total basis, using each physician's average score for the particular expectation.

Example

The following example provides a hypothetical calculation of this methodology.

Assumptions

- ► Each physician is evaluated using six different performance expectations (columns 1 through 6 in Exhibit 10.10).

- ► Five committee members provide evaluations (rows A through E in Exhibit 10.10).

- ► Exhibit 10.10 shows actual rankings on the five performance expectations (hypothetical data).

- ► Exhibit 10.11 shows rankings and averages after removal of one high and one low ranking.

- ► The nonobjective performance-criteria pool is awarded as follows:

  - – Full share for average ranking (2) on performance criteria;

  - – 0 percent of full share if below average (2) on performance criteria;

  - – Those that are ranked above average (2) to receive the full share plus a pro rata share of the amount not paid to those ranking below average.

Using Exhibits 10.10 and 10.11 as examples, this physician (Dr. X) would receive a reduced portion (e.g., 50 percent or even 0 percent) of a full share on the "relationship with referring physicians" performance criteria, because he or she had a 1.67 (below average) rating. However, this physician would receive more than a full share on the

EXHIBIT 10.10   Peer Rankings to Reward Nonclinical Production Activities

Issue/Factor and Ranking by Evaluator for Dr. X

	Positive Attitude	Relationship with Referring Physicians	Relationship with Staff	Relationship with Hospital	Level of Participation	Peer Interaction
Evaluator						
A	3	3	2	2	3	3
B	3	2	2	3	2	3
C	1	1	2	3	2	1
D	1	1	3	2	2	2
E	2	2	2	1	2	3

EXHIBIT 10.11 Peer Rankings – Averages after Removal of High and Low Values

Issue/Factor and Ranking by Evaluator for Dr. X

Evaluator	Positive Attitude	Relationship with Referring Physicians	Relationship with Staff	Relationship with Hospital	Level of Participation	Peer Interaction
A				2		
B	3	2	2		2	3
C			2	3	2	
D	1	1		2	2	2
E	2	2	2			3
Avg. Rank	2.00	1.67	2.00	2.33	2.00	2.67

fourth and sixth measures ("relationship with hospital" and "peer interaction"), because he or she scored above average on these.

Method 2: Physician Time Commitment

In the second methodology, physicians receive bonus payments for nonobjective performance measures based on their time devoted to these activities. This requires a mechanism to capture (and monitor) the time spent by physicians in these activities. As in the prior methodology, we will use "citizenship" performance as the example to demonstrate this approach; however, other areas can also be evaluated via this fashion (e.g., administrative activity).

Step 1. Determine Nonclinical Production Payment

Determine the dollars to be paid for nonclinical production criteria (e.g., citizenship or behavior) on a per physician basis (note that an incentive pool approach can also be used).

Step 2. Define Performance Areas That Qualify for Reward

Step 3. Maintain Time Records Related to Physician Participation in the Performance Areas

Step 4. Reward Physicians Based on Time Devoted to These Activities

Example

The medical practice has allocated $15,000 per physician to be paid for citizenship behaviors. The following performance areas qualify for this award:

- ▶ Foundation board;
- ▶ Charity or nonprofit board;
- ▶ Government or school board leadership;
- ▶ Local community board leadership;
- ▶ Services that support charitable missions;
- ▶ Preceptorship;
- ▶ Resident training;
- ▶ Leadership in county, state, and national medical organizations; and
- ▶ Leadership roles that benefit the community.

The time devoted by each physician to the above activities is recorded. Each physician may earn a maximum of $15,000 for these activities based on the following allocation formula:

4 hours per month/48 hours per year = 50 percent of individual pool
6 hours per month/72 hours per year = 75 percent of individual pool
8 hours per month/96 hours per year = 100 percent of individual pool

AND

Participation in one major corporate event; and
Attendance at four system physician-at-large meetings

Nonobjective Performance Criteria

Medical practices typically identify a number of categories of performance that they desire to reward but that lack purely objective, quantifiable measures. For each category, specific performance expectations need to be developed by the medical practice in order to apply a methodology, such as presented above, to measure and reward these nonobjective performance areas. Because the measures deal with subjective issues and use subjective measures, the total amount of compensation "at risk" or in play will need to be limited and well managed.

We now provide examples of performance expectations in nine common categories:

1. Professionalism;
2. Teamwork;
3. Collegiality;
4. Integrated delivery system or network development;
5. Research and program development;
6. Medical staff leadership;

7. Compliance;

8. Patient satisfaction; and

9. Use of technology (e.g., electronic health records).

1. Professionalism

► Attends and is appropriately prepared for physician meetings as requested or required (e.g., monthly group meeting, subspecialty conference, journal club, etc.);

► Accepts and adheres to practice policies and procedures with respect to patients and work scheduling;

► Accepts and fulfills responsibilities assigned in a timely and productive manner and implements policies, directives, principles, and organizational values of the medical practice in a conscientious, timely, and productive manner;

► Adheres to all human resources policies prohibiting harassment of any kind; and

► Maintains positive relationships with referring physicians, hospital leaders, practice peers, and practice support staff.

2. Teamwork

► Assists colleagues in providing high quality care to patients, including conducting consults within an agreed upon time frame, working walk-in patients into the schedule, assisting with add-on case volume, and other similar activities;

► Participates in budget, planning, and strategic development activities for the practice as requested;

► Engages in agreed upon outreach activities as defined in the yearly clinical activity plan;

► Participates in reasonable administrative activities (to be defined); and

► Actively and constructively identifies opportunities to enhance medical practice planning and operations.

3. Collegiality

► Acts as an informational resource for staff, satellite locations, and referring physicians, to include answering questions, referring questions to an alternative person appropriately, and conducting grand rounds;

► Maintains excellent communication; maintains positive working relationships with employees, other providers, vendors, and the public; cultivates an attitude of respect, confidence, and pride in the practice; and

► Conducts himself or herself personally in a professional manner; is courteous and pleasant; speaks to other physicians, staff members, and patients in an appropriate, nonabrasive, and nonaggressive manner; does not display rude or arrogant behavior or speech.

4. Integrated Delivery System or Network Development

► Embraces and undertakes outreach assignments as needed;

► Works diligently to build market share at satellite locations; and

► Fosters strong working relationships and loyal alliances at the hospital with the referring physicians and the hospital's leadership at the primary and satellite locations.

5. Research and Program Development

► Researches new developments in subspecialty services, including medical, pharmaceutical, and changes in standards of care and practice;

► Participates in ongoing medical research activities approved by the Institutional Review Board (IRB) by actively recruiting patients for approved research studies;

► Acts as a leader in the development of the practice's research department, assuming the role of principal investigator for studies that are cost-effective and clinically advantageous;

► Acts as a pioneer from a clinical and/or program development standpoint by advancing clinical skills to bring new technology to the practice and building programs and volume to support this technology; and

► Participates in strategic planning and marketing with the medical director, the chief executive officer, and hospital leaders, as requested.

6. Medical Staff Leadership

► Accepts and embraces requests to serve on practice, hospital, and other committees as requested by the medical director, the practice's executive management committee, hospital leaders, and medical staff bylaws;

► Assumes clinical medical directorships as appointed by the medical director; and

► Collaborates with designated medical and administrative directors for specialty and subspecialty services.

7. Compliance

► Complies with infection control standards, procedures, and policies;

► Complies with Health Insurance Portability and Accountability Act (HIPAA) regulations;

► Attends and actively participates in coding and compliance activities as directed during the year (X hours minimum per year);

► Submits inpatient and outpatient charges and completes documentation (e.g., medical records, operative reports, etc.) within defined time periods (which will be no less than malpractice carrier guidelines [e.g., 24 hours of patient encounter for outpatient, 72 hours of patient encounter for inpatient]);

► Achieves acceptable levels of compliance in coding review of inpatient and outpatient activity, and in other documentation assessments, as consistent with the compliance program;

► Complies with programs and directives of the medical practice pertaining to fraud and abuse compliance, including but not limited to billing, write-offs, referral relationships, and relationships with outside vendors; provides complete and clinically accurate documentation of services rendered, including procedural and diagnostic coding;

► Ensures confidentiality of all known legal, financial, and contractual matters at the hospital and medical practice; and

► Respects patient confidentiality in public communications.

8. Patient Satisfaction

► Achieves targeted scores for patient satisfaction (as measured by objective tools);

► Meets established expectations for wait time to third available appointment;

► Meets established expectations for wait time in the reception area;

► Meets established expectations regarding patient complaints; and

► Meets agreed upon citizenship requirements as measured by peers and by an internal performance review process.

9. Use of Technology

► Attends required electronic prescribing training;

► Incorporates electronic health records into normal practice patterns; and

► Uses a personal digital assistant (PDA) or other identified electronic method to document hospital services as a means to optimize charge capture.

► ISSUE 8: COMPENSATION PLANS INVOLVING SYSTEM-WIDE INCENTIVE MEASURES

Purpose

With more medical practices situated in large integrated delivery systems and networks, many hospitals and physician practices will award bonuses that reflect performance related to the achievement of system-wide goals.

Methodology

The typical approach to awarding a system-wide incentive or bonus follows.

Step 1. Determine the Criteria to Permit a Bonus Pool

A system-wide incentive is typically awarded based upon financial or other performance of the hospital and medical practice in relation to agreed upon targets, such as meeting budgetary targets, increasing productivity by a defined percentage during the year, or increasing market share by a defined percentage.

Step 2. Identify a Bonus Pool

In networks and hospital systems, such a bonus component is typically defined in advance at a specific level (e.g., $10,000) per physician, with the total amount placed in a "bonus pool." This means that, in the event the target requirement is met (e.g., division and system-wide margin targets are achieved), the incentive is automatically funded at a defined level. When financial performance is used as the criteria, the incentive funds may be "tiered" based on financial performance up to a defined level (e.g., $5,000 per physician FTE for achievement of a 3 percent system margin; $10,000 per physician FTE for achievement of a 6 percent system margin).

Step 3. Determine the Allocation Methodology

The bonus pool is typically awarded based on group-wide performance on an agreed upon basis. For example, the allocation methodology could be on a flat amount per physician, or it could be on a combined equal share and production basis (e.g., a portion based on the physician's FTE level and a portion based on the physician's percent to total WRVUs). The particular incentive measure will generally influence the allocation methodology.

Step 4. Award Bonus

The bonus is awarded based on performance at the individual, group, or other levels. Importantly, the bonus amounts that are awarded through such system-wide or similar levels are typically limited in amount (e.g., no more than a defined percentage of base salaries or total compensation). This is designed to prevent a windfall benefit and to help ensure that the ultimate level of compensation is still reasonable and consistent with fair market value (FMV) and legal compliance requirements.

Each of the above eight special issues presents challenges in compensation plan design; however, as demonstrated, they are not insurmountable. By approaching these and other similar issues in an objective, systematic fashion, and by identifying the purpose, the methodology, and a stepwise approach, these types of issues can be addressed and integrated into the overall compensation plan design.

ELEVEN

Physician Transition Plans – Physicians in Part-Time, Slowdown, and Similar Status

Physician transition plans permit a practice to proactively plan for nonstandard physician work schedules, whether they are due to generational issues, illness, or simply a desire to alter a physician's work/life balance in a manner that is different from the norm established for the medical practice. They also permit physicians to plan for changes in their work life by articulating up front the impacts to a desire or need to go to part-time status, reduce on-call obligations, and the like. The key from our perspective is for a medical practice to develop a plan now – hopefully before it is needed – so that a precedent-setting decision based on any one individual physician's circumstance is not made that will be detrimental to the other physicians in the practice or to the future health of the medical practice itself.

Some of the physician transition issues can be addressed by a medical practice, in whole or in part, through performance expectations established by the practice (discussed in Chapter 10). Others will require a more formal physician transition plan and strategy that consider how the practice will respond to requests for a transition arrangement, and the impact such an arrangement will have on a physician's compensation, partnership, governance, and other roles in the practice.

PRACTICE "TRANSITION" – WHAT AND WHY

We use the term "transition" to refer to physician work schedules or other arrangements that diverge from what is viewed to be "typical" or "normal" for a particular medical practice. From the perspective of the physician seeking a transition arrangement, the desire for such an arrangement typically revolves around two broad work-related goals:

1. To work on less than a "full-time" basis, including working a reduced or part-time work week, taking more vacation and other time off, or taking advantage of a temporary sabbatical; and

2. To reduce or terminate "on-call" obligations.

► THE GROWTH OF PHYSICIAN TRANSITION PLANS

The need for physician transition arrangements is likely to increase in the future due to changing physician and population demographics, evolving physician preferences, and the changing needs of medical practices themselves.

Generational Issues

Of course, a physician partner at 63 years of age and a physician employee at 37 years of age will tend to view the compensation discussion differently. A physician in his or her more senior years is recognizing near-term retirement and is attempting to understand the impact this will have on many of life's dimensions, including compensation, lifestyle, personal relevance, and other less tangible issues. A physician right out of residency will typically be concerned with applying what he or she has learned, paying off student loans, starting a family, and achieving a balance in his or her personal and professional life.

Generational issues are not new. A medical practice is a highly diverse collective of individuals with different goals, needs, desires, and perceptions. The physicians differ with respect to age, specialty and earning potential, personal situation, personal life experience, and other factors, and they hold varied views regarding what to expect for themselves and what they expect from work and from life.

The generational issues in medical practice tend to revolve around three issues: personal autonomy, lifestyle, and money. Physicians who are full partners in the practice may perceive that they should also have full autonomy to decide their own hours, the number of days they take for vacation, and which patients they will admit to their practice. Unfortunately, when physicians form a group practice, or even when they work as employees in a hospital, academic practice, or other setting, other individuals are impacted by their decisions.

The emergence of generational issues in a medical practice should not come as a surprise. We believe that generational issues should be discussed openly in a medical practice and that the practice's governing documents and rules of the game should include methods by which generational issues and other practice transition issues will be addressed.

We recommend that medical practices outline in advance the response they will take to the following types of questions:

1. What if I want to reduce my hours?

2. What if I want to take less (or no) call?

3. How can I take off more time?

4. When can I "close" my practice to new patients?

5. What if I want to limit my practice to a certain type of patient; for example, gynecology only instead of obstetrics and gynecology?

6. What if I am injured and can only perform a portion of my duties; for example, I can work in the office setting but not in the operating room due to a back injury?

7. What type of "buy-out" can I get if I retire in the next year?

Demographics

It is not just the baby boomers who are aging. Today, physicians are aging as a work force. Just as a large portion of the population in general is middle age or above, physicians as a group tend to be relatively older such that more than half are age 45 or older. In addition, the number of physicians entering the profession has remained fairly constant, while the U.S. population has grown. What this means is that the physician-to-population ratios, which have enjoyed steady increases in the past, are now beginning to stagnate. Combine these realities with the facts that: (1) many physicians – like the general population – are seeking a more manageable work/life balance; (2) there is a maldistribution of physicians in some specialties and in some markets; and (3) the incidence of chronic care conditions is increasing due to the aging of the U.S. population – not only the aging baby boomers, but a greater percentage of the population older than 75 years of age that typically consumes additional medical resources. It is therefore not difficult to anticipate an imbalance between physician supply and patient demand for the foreseeable future, absent fundamental changes to the U.S. health care system. These changing population demographics will influence the number of persons available to become physicians, the number of physicians that will be in practice at any one point in time in the future, as well as the number of individuals seeking medical care.

Changes in medical practices themselves will also influence the need to have more physicians (rather than fewer). As medical costs increase, more physicians are needed to help pay the increased cost of practice operations. As practices consolidate to create larger practices, the likelihood that physicians will desire some form of transitional practice arrangement also increases, for this is one of the reasons practice consolidation takes place. These and other factors are likely to come together to make physician transition issues more prevalent in the years ahead.

In a medical practice setting, the ability of individual physicians to achieve their personal goals depends upon both the physician's personal agenda and on the practice's other physicians. Physicians may desire to move to a transition arrangement by reducing or eliminating on-call obligations or by working a reduced schedule, but their ability to do so depends upon the presence of other physicians to help pick up the on-call duty that has been eliminated, and to otherwise help pick up the slack. When it comes to physician transition arrangements, all physicians are in the "same boat," such that a physician's ability to achieve his or her unique transition goals will depend on the presence and willingness of other physicians to help achieve those goals. That is the way it is today, and that will likely remain the case for the foreseeable future.

Of course, an entire medical practice can "transition" itself to a new model involving more vacation, less on-call, etc. that applies to all physicians in the practice, which in and of itself will lead to its own challenges. However, the intent of this chapter is to discuss transition plans to address the physician "outlier" – that is, the physician who requests a change in status beyond the norm embraced by his or her practice colleagues.

The number of physicians in a medical practice often bears no relationship to economies of scale arguments for practice size. In some practices, the size of the group (or its specialty departments) is simply based on the number of physicians needed for an "acceptable" call group. When medical groups are constituted on this basis, physician transition issues will likely receive heightened scrutiny. A physician who elects to reduce on-call activity will obviously impact his colleagues. A physician transition plan permits the requesting physician and the medical practice's other physicians to respond in an appropriate fashion and in a way that is consistent with established policy, avoiding precedent-setting arrangements that may negatively impact the financial or other health of the medical practice.

DEVELOPING A TRANSITION PLAN

Medical practices approach physician transition arrangements in different ways. Some see a transition as an expected event that they attempt to address in a proactive manner. They view the transition arrangement as a natural part of the change process. These medical practices will typically be able to craft an appropriate transition arrangement entirely through their own efforts, or with some minimal assistance from an external consultant.

Other practices adopt a more reactive approach to transition arrangements. Practice transition in these settings tends to occur in conjunction with a crisis. In this case, crafting a transition arrangement will require a large, almost revolutionary change in the practice's way of doing things. Such practice transition may occur due to disability, illness, or other reasons, but it is generally viewed as a disruptive process that will require focused attention by practice leaders, and frequently by seeking additional help from external consultants and, in some instances, lawyers in the context of an adversarial process.

From our perspective, the most appropriate approach to practice transition involves a planned, proactive approach. Developing a plan in advance will not always guarantee that that plan will work perfectly or that it will not need to be modified. Yet, a transition plan provides a framework and road map from which small deviations can be crafted on an as-needed basis, rather than trying to plan in the midst of a crisis or perhaps in response to a "most favored nation" physician's request to alter his or her practice.

▶ GOALS AND PRINCIPLES OF TRANSITION PLANS

As with other types of plans, a transition arrangement should also be based on goals and principles, rather than it constituting a "special deal." For such purposes, any number of principles or criteria should optimally be used to guide the transition plan development and decision-making process, including the following:

► Develop a common set of rules that can be applied consistently;

► Use objective criteria for decision making to the extent possible;

► Protect the long-term interests of the group;

► Promote recruitment and retention;

► Craft arrangements that would generally be viewed as acceptable if everyone eligible took advantage of them;

► Reasonably honor existing arrangements; and

► Reasonably address the goals and desires of individual physicians.

The development of a physician transition plan typically involves two broad phases: (1) assessment; and (2) development.

▶ THE ASSESSMENT PHASE

Three broad assessment areas need to be considered in connection with transition plan development, and each is examined below:

► Practice demographics;

► Physician and practice preferences and goals; and

► Existing arrangements.

Practice Demographics

Demographics are always important to transition arrangements. To assess the potential need for a transition arrangement, practices can perform a simple analysis to assess the age of the practice's physicians. To do this, group physicians into age groups with five-year increments (e.g., under age 40, from ages 40 through 44, etc.), and count the number of physicians in each age group, both today and in the future (e.g., 5, 10, or more years down the road).

Physician demographics can provide useful perspective regarding the likely or potential preferences that individual physicians might have for transition arrangements. For example:

► Physicians (both male and female) of childbearing age, or whose spouse may be of childbearing age (typically younger than age 40), are more likely to seek part-time schedules to care for children, but they may also be able (perhaps reluctantly) to continue taking a full on-call obligation.

► Physicians who are age 55 or older are likely to engage in a transition arrangement involving reduced on-call obligations or practice slowdown in the form of more time off, sabbaticals, or otherwise.

Understanding the physician demographics, along with the potential and actual preferences of physicians, will help to identify the transition issues that may be relevant for a particular practice. Exhibits 11.1-A, 11.1-B, and 11.1-C provide examples of a hypothetical medical practice's assessment of physician demographics. Assessing the demographic information will give the practice perspective regarding what might be expected in the future. As a general matter, practices that have a large number of physicians who are age "bubble" (e.g., the 45 to 49 age group in Exhibit 11.1-A) will be more likely to have transition challenges than those who have a relatively flat spread of ages within the practice.

Practice Demographics (Today)

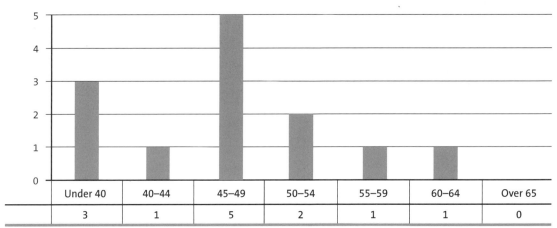

Under 40	40–44	45–49	50–54	55–59	60–64	Over 65
3	1	5	2	1	1	0

© 2006 Johnson & Walker Keegan

EXHIBIT 11.1-B **Practice Demographics (5 Years from Today)**

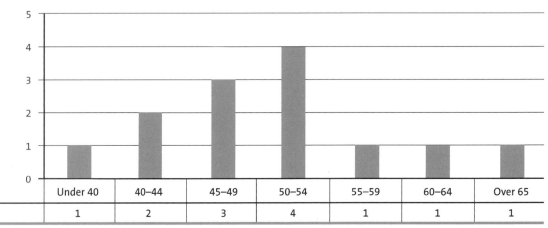

Under 40	40–44	45–49	50–54	55–59	60–64	Over 65
1	2	3	4	1	1	1

© 2006 Johnson & Walker Keegan

EXHIBIT 11.1-C Practice Demographics (10 Years from Today)*

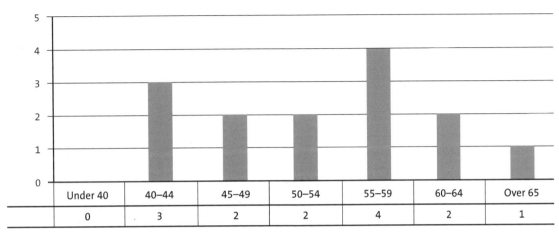

	Under 40	40–44	45–49	50–54	55–59	60–64	Over 65
	0	3	2	2	4	2	1

*Assumes 2 new physicians approx. age 40–42 within 7 years of today

© 2006 Johnson & Walker Keegan

Physician and Practice Preferences and Goals

Physicians will frequently have both stated and unstated goals related to practice transition. Their preferences and goals may be stated and assessed by reference to any number of criteria, including:

▶ Actual statements by physicians related to transition that are made to other practice members;

▶ The occurrence of major changes in the physician's life, such as childbirth, marriage, divorce, health problems, graduation of children, caring for elderly parents; and/or

▶ Changes in clinical production and de facto transition or slowdown strategies.

The practice will also have certain goals and preferences related to physician practice transition. Some practices wish to understand when a transition arrangement might be likely with sufficient advance warning in order to allow the practice to take action (e.g., to recruit a new physician when a senior partner slows down prior to retirement). Others need to develop methods to allow the practice to continue the involvement of as many physicians as possible in order to help ensure the practice's financial solvency. The goals – of both physicians and practices – are important drivers of the development of any physician transition plan and in the mechanics of any plan that is developed.

Every practice must also recognize and understand that the plan and solution that are developed – whatever they may be – will constitute an important precedent that will be viewed as the standard for arrangements that may be considered and/or crafted in the future. Thus, in evaluating any transition arrangement, the practice should consider the arrangement by reference to the core question:

> *What if everyone who could participate in this arrangement actually did elect to participate in this arrangement?*

The transition plan should be developed with the practice's interests – not the interests of one particular physician or one founding member – in mind. If the medical practice is to maintain a viable position in the health care market, it needs to ensure that the plan protects overall medical practice interests. A transition plan that is excessively "rich" or beneficial to the physician in transition will, in all likelihood, not be sustainable, because it will not be able to be used with every physician in the practice.

Existing Arrangements

Medical practices also need to evaluate existing contractual, compensation, and other arrangements that may relate to the physician in transition. Some medical practices already define what is required for a full-time practice format. Some will also determine and define requirements related to on-call obligations. For most medical practices, however, the practice will need to come up with specific approaches to different types of transition arrangements.

▶ THE DEVELOPMENT PHASE

From the medical practice's perspective, a physician's request for practice transition tends to raise three broad issues: (1) lifestyle concerns; (2) power and authority; and (3) money, as further described below.

1. **Lifestyle Concerns.** A change in work schedule or on-call obligations impacts the lifestyle of the requesting physician, as well as the lifestyle of the other physicians in the practice. Beyond actual impact to physicians' work levels and professional and personal work/life balances, lifestyle concerns raised by such requests often include questions regarding the transitioning physician's dedication to the practice and the security of his or her position for the future including ongoing access to health insurance and other benefits during the period of transition and beyond.

2. **Power and Authority.** Issues of power and authority are also raised in these arrangements. Questions regarding the changes to the transitioning physician's status as an owner, partner, or employee in the practice; the physician's role in medical practice governance; and autonomy and control over the physician's practice will need to be addressed. A medical practice must typically determine whether moving to a transition practice arrangement is considered a "right" or a "privilege." The timing of other activities, such as hiring replacement physicians and practice buy-out, also needs to be determined.

3. **Money.** The financial impact of these arrangements is a pragmatic concern for the practice. In addition to the core question of how the physician in transition will be compensated, this also includes questions regarding how that arrangement will impact the compensation earned by the practice's remaining physicians. Furthermore, there will be questions regarding how the transition arrangement may impact practice expenditures and cash flow, and how the practice's transition, employment, compensation, buy or sell, and other arrangements will all work in harmony. These and other money-related issues will generally need to be considered and resolved.

Issues to Address in Physician Transition Plans

Many medical practices choose to not directly address reduced time and transition issues in their physician employment, partnership, compensation, and other arrangements. For these practices, there is no formal transition strategy or plan – only the recognition (or perhaps, more commonly, a lack of recognition) that transition issues can, and will, need to be addressed upon the occurrence of an event, such as a physician's request for more time off, reduced call, or a part-time work schedule. This approach can certainly work, but it is generally not recommended due to the challenges of planning in the midst of a crisis.

When the practice elects to develop a formal transition plan, the following issues are generally addressed in one way or another.

Transition as a Right or a Privilege

Practices may elect to treat transition arrangements as both a right, a privilege, or, in many instances, in both ways.

Transition as a Right

Under the philosophy that transition is a "right," the ability to engage in some form of transition arrangement is left up to the individual physician. Essentially, the medical practice allows each physician to make his or her own choice regarding work levels, and any physician can elect to work as hard or as little as the physician desires. This is commonly accomplished by reference to the minimum requirements for a full-time physician, and by allowing physicians some level of flexibility to manage their own work schedule by reference to these requirements.

Because of the fixed operating costs in any medical practice, this approach tends to work best in practices that have productivity-based compensation plans with express expense allocation, as it essentially requires the physician taking more time off to receive lower compensation due to his or her decreased work levels. Even in these situations, however, more and more practices are recognizing the utility of carefully defining parameters for transitioning physicians in terms of work and expectations – thus, transition as a "right" has become transition as a "right with limits" in order to ensure appropriate resources for doing the work. Thus, these practices may determine that it is

EXHIBIT 11.2 Physician Classification and Time-Off Rules

Physician partner employees shall be classified as Class A, B, or C employees, with each Class having the rights defined below:

Class "A" Partner Employees may take up to thirty (30) days of "Vacation/Leave" per year. Each Class A Partner Employee shall be a voting member in the Partnership.

Class "B" Partner Employees may request and be granted approval to take more than thirty (30) but not more than fifty (50) days of Vacation/Leave per year. Each Class B Partner Employee shall be a voting member in the Partnership during the time in which the Class B Partner Employee is classified as such. A Partner Employee who requests classification as a Class B employee shall request a change to Class B status no later than six (6) months prior to the desired effective date of the Class B status, and may remain in Class B status for a cumulative period not exceeding four (4) years, at the conclusion of which the Partner Employee shall be deemed to have voluntarily terminated his or her employment as a Partner Employee of the Partnership.

Class "C" Partner Employees may request and be granted the right to take more than fifty (50) but not more than eighty (80) days of Vacation/Leave per year, or who has taken, during any twelve (12) month period during the term of employment, more than fifty (50) days of Vacation/ Leave, without regard to whether prior permission for such Vacation/Leave was granted in advance of the leave. Class C Partner Employees shall not be voting members in the Partnership.

A Partner Employee who requests classification as a Class C employee shall submit a request to change to Class C status, no later than twelve (12) months prior to the desired effective date of the Class C status. Each Partner Employee shall be entitled to remain in Class C status for a period not to exceed (1) year, at the conclusion of which the Partner Employee shall be deemed to have voluntarily terminated his or her employment as a Partner Employee.

© 2006 Johnson & Walker Keegan

---

acceptable for a physician to work fewer days or to have more time off (viewing this as a right), but certain other transition preferences – namely, reduction in on-call obligations – are not an absolute right. Exhibit 11.2 illustrates physician classification and time-off rules.

Transition as a Privilege

Other practices view transition arrangements as more of a privilege – one that is earned by longevity and previous commitment to a full-time practice. Under these programs, a physician is allowed to move into transition after X years of service and at the age of Y. This approach to practice transition may include more time off/vacation, reduced (or eliminated) on-call obligations, or a combination of these. Such arrangements are almost always coupled with a reduction in compensation. This type of approach is illustrated in Exhibit 11.3, which defines the rules governing reduced on-call obligations (but at a financial cost, and only for a limited time).

EXHIBIT 11.3 Full-Time Service and On-Call Transition Rules

Full-Time Practice. Each physician employee shall work a full-time schedule, providing services in the Practice Specialty four and one-half (4.5) days per week. In addition, Employee shall share night call and weekend call with the other physician-employees of Employer. Employee may cease providing on-call services only upon the terms and conditions set forth below.

General Requirements and Conditions. Employee may only cease on-call obligations upon satisfaction of, and agreement to, all of the following terms and conditions:

1. Employee may cease on-call obligations upon attaining 62 years of age;

2. No more than ten percent (10%) of the employee physicians in Employee's practice specialty have ceased on-call coverage obligations;

3. Employee's status as a full-time employee of Employer without on-call obligations shall continue for the lesser of three (3) years, or until Employee reaches 65 years of age; and

4. Employee satisfies the Employer's advance-notice requirements; and for each period in which Employee ceases on-call coverage obligations, Employee's "Total Compensation" shall be reduced by 25%.

Advance Notice and Other Requirements. Employee shall be obligated to provide Employer with advance notice of Employee's desire to cease on-call obligations as provided hereunder, along with the date upon which Employee desires to cease on-call obligations, no less than 365 days in advance of the anticipated effective date.

© 2006 Johnson & Walker Keegan

Exhibits 11.2 and 11.3 also illustrate other common requirements imposed in transition arrangements, as discussed below.

Definition of a Full-Time Physician

Medical practices use different standards for defining a typical or expected "full-time" level of practice. Some define it by days per week (typically 4.5 or 5 days per week), and/or a defined number of days per year, plus equal participation in on-call, outreach, and similar obligations. Others define it by the actual work expected of the physician within a defined time period (e.g., day or clinic session). The appropriate approach for a particular practice will typically be based on the practice's historic ways of doing things.

The physician transition plan typically clarifies the definition of a "full-time" physician in the medical practice and what is required of "partnership status" as part of the definition of basic performance expectations for all practice physicians. For example, a medical practice could indicate that full-time physicians engaged in both clinic and surgical practice can be partners, however, physicians engaged in clinic practice only cease to hold partnership status. If the compensation plan includes an equal share component to revenue or income allocation, minimum levels of work and performance are typically imposed.

As a general matter, part-time *partner* status is typically defined in the range of 60 to 75 percent of what is required for a full-time schedule. Physicians can certainly work reduced schedules, but they typically do not retain partnership status for governance purposes.

Governance Implications

The modified status of physicians in transition is typically accompanied by governance changes. Those changes may be immediate (e.g., if a physician drops below a defined level of clinical FTE, that physician can no longer be a partner), or they may be predefined and transitional in nature (e.g., a physician can remain in a particular transition status for no more than a defined time period). Linking these issues to governance is important because of the challenges that can be placed on an organization's long-term viability if a large number of partners are working transitional or reduced schedules. Not only do reduced-time or transitional partners tend to naturally vote in a manner that is consistent with their situation, but the practice also needs to ensure that it meets its patient care obligations, financial commitments, and other similar ongoing concerns.

Time Limits

Regardless of the approach taken, even if a physician is entitled to participate in a transitional practice arrangement, the physician is generally not allowed to continue in such an arrangement indefinitely. Imposing time limits on the transition status is therefore common. With respect to the reduction or termination of on-call arrangements, for example, the time limits will typically range from three to five years, or in some cases up to seven years. At the end of that period, the physician will commonly cease being a partner and/or employee, although the practice will commonly reserve the ability to create a nonowner employment relationship following the termination of the transition period.

Other Limits

All physicians in a medical practice are typically expected to participate in on-call arrangements on an equal basis. However, practices will commonly allow physicians to cease on-call obligations under defined circumstances, with limits, and with a financial cost, provided that the practice has a minimum number of physicians (e.g., five or more) available for call at all times.

Call termination is also commonly subject to eligibility requirements linked to: (1) the date on which call termination is first available; (2) the physician's age; and (3) the years of service with the practice.

Nonpartner Employment and Other Status

Most practices also include, as part of the transition arrangement, the ability of the practice to continue a former owner or partner's employment in a nonpartner capacity. In such circumstances, the former owner or partner will not receive partnership distributions or a partnership vote, but he or she will continue to remain as an employee of the group. Because this is pursuant to a nonowner/partner employment arrangement, however, the relationship continues at the discretion of the practice.

Treatment of Income beyond Professional Fees

If the medical practice maintains a financial interest in a revenue-generating opportunity beyond physician professional fees, a change in the status of a physician may also involve a change in the status relative to this income. For example, a medical practice that has its own ambulatory surgery center (ASC) may decide that the ASC profits are shared among partners on an equal share basis in the context of the practice's compensation plan; however, formal participation in the profits will cease once the physician ceases partner status.

Likewise, physician participation in office-based ancillary services income following termination of the transition arrangement must also be addressed. This is particularly the case given that, in a large number of practices, the income from ancillary services technical components constitutes an increasingly important share of practice income. Consistent with the idea that the practice as a whole needs to be protected in the transition arrangement, many practices elect to not allow physicians who are in a transition arrangement to participate in ancillary services income. For others, however, the activities of a senior physician who maintains an office-based practice that enhances patient access and that may also result in substantial ancillary services usage is also viewed as important to the practice's long-term success. In this case, the practice may provide at least a partial share of ancillary services income to such a physician as a means of aligning incentives to the practice's reimbursement and service mix realities.

Transition Plan Mechanics

Two areas have particular relevance in constructing the transition plan mechanics: (1) ways to handle reduced on-call obligations; and (2) compensation implications involving revenue and expense treatment.

Reduced On-Call Obligations

On-call obligations are typically viewed as the most unpleasant portion of medical practice today. As a result, practices will adopt any number of different approaches to respond to requests for on-call reduction or termination entirely. Some will, for example, provide that every physician in the practice must continue to take on-call or cease working in the practice altogether. More commonly, however, practices will allow physicians to reduce or eliminate on-call upon certain conditions. The reduction might allow, for example, reduction of night on-call but not weekend on-call, or limitation of the number of on-call days. Those that allow for an outright elimination of on-call will typically impose requirements related to the number of physicians in the practice needed for an acceptable on-call schedule, and/or linking the elimination of on-call for a particular physician to a combination of the physician's age and his or her years of service. In almost all instances, however, the reduction or termination of on-call obligations will be linked to a financial "cost" to the physician.

The financial impact of reduced on-call is typically accomplished through one of two general means. Most frequently, negative incentives in the form of an actual reduction in compensation will accompany the reduction of on-call obligations. Such incentives may be in the form of a defined price per day (e.g., reduced compensation of a defined amount, such as $2,000 per day for weekends or holidays, and $1,500 per day for night on-call). In most instances, the price per day of on-call will generally be insufficient in relation to the cost of taking on-call. Reduced on-call obligations generally result in reduced production and disrupt the quality of life of other physicians, but the development and imposition of a price are deemed essential from the perspective of fairness, and as a means to impose at least some "pound of flesh" on the physician who is no longer subject to on-call obligations. Any such price will also commonly consider and incorporate an "escalator" arrangement to ensure that the price of on-call automatically changes with time (e.g., by linking changes in the price to changes in the practice's median income per partner).

For practices that have an equal share compensation plan, a plan with a base salary component, or even a plan with a significant level of revenue sharing, the cost of on-call will be a significant reduction (often 20 to 50 percent) in the share of the total compensation otherwise due to be paid to the physician. Some practices will even base the penalty for reduced or terminated on-call on some measure of market; for example, the cost of on-call will equal a defined percentage of market median compensation (e.g., 50 percent) for the particular specialty. In cases where the physician is reducing or eliminating on-call obligation, the amount of compensation reduced or taken away from that physician is then reallocated among those physicians who continue to take on-call assignments.

In an indirect treatment of the financial impact of reduced on-call, some practices merely assume that the reduction in on-call obligations will, in fact, reduce the physician's production, and, in the context of a production-based compensation plan, the physician will naturally receive less compensation. Depending on the practice specialty and call schedule, however, this does not always work, because the physician who is able to cease on-call obligations will commonly have increased production levels because he or she is not as tired, does not have the same disruptions to regular schedule pre- and post-call days, and/or can perform more elective procedures. As a result, some practices will even consider reducing the physician's productivity credit by a defined level (e.g., a 25 percent reduction to the credit otherwise provided) or use a similar means to recognize this "opportunity gain" for the physician who has ceased participation in on-call activity.

Though infrequent, a second method of handling the financial impact of call reduction is to use positive incentives or rewards for call obligations, and thus naturally "withholding" these incentives for physicians who do not participate in the call schedule. Under such a scenario, the practice distributes a discrete portion of the compensation pool to physicians for their on-call obligations. It will typically also require physicians to continue on-call obligations for a defined time period.

On-call coverage requirements also will be typically addressed in specific arrangements that define the ground rules related to call reduction. These arrangements may allow for on-call obligations to be terminated or reduced at a specific age (e.g., 55, 60, or 65 years). The age requirement is commonly coupled with a defined number of years of service to the group. Most groups will also impose a cap or a limit on the total number of physicians who can be off-call at any one time. Also defined is the adverse financial impact to the physician (if any) for when on-call obligations are reduced, and the impact this has on partnership status and the "retirement time clock." Overall, although few physicians "love" doing on-call work, it is important to recognize that the practice's interests should predominate. For example, a practice could decide that reduction of on-call duty may be permitted as long as there are at least five full-time physicians to take on-call in the practice when covering two hospitals, or when the number off-call is below a defined percentage of the whole.

An example of a transition plan that outlines the treatment of reduced on-call obligations is provided in Exhibit 11.4. In this practice, the decision to reduce on-call obligations is viewed as an initial step in planning for retirement and/or practice termination, which raises a host of other issues that can be addressed by the practice in its transition plan. These other issues include physician status at the end of the off-call period (e.g., whether physicians can be rehired or not), fail-safe provisions (e.g., to ensure that there are sufficient numbers of physicians available for appropriate on-call schedules and to handle practice emergencies), practice noncompete (to address the terminating physician's ability to compete with the practice), and other similar issues. By addressing these issues via a transition plan, both the medical practice and the physician can better plan for the impacts of changes in practice patterns among the practice's physicians.

Compensation Implications

Physicians in transition must receive compensation for their services, but a delicate balance exists between crafting a transition arrangement that is too good or too bad for the physician in transition as opposed to the physicians who remain in full-time practice. If a transition arrangement is too "rich," then virtually every practice physician may want to move to a transition status. Thus, in crafting transition arrangements, attention to the overall interests of the group as a whole and protecting those who are working full-time and in a nontransitional manner should take priority. In practical terms, this means that the physician who is engaged in a transition arrangement will generally not receive compensation at the same level as those who are working full time.

The practice's compensation plan will dictate how that arrangement will actually impact the physician desiring transition. Exhibit 11.5 illustrates the basic relationship between different types of compensation plans by reference to the allocation of revenues and expenditures within the practice when the plan is put into play.

Regardless of the compensation methodology that is used, a physician in transition will (and generally should) receive lower compensation under the practice's compensa-

EXHIBIT 11.4   Transition Plan Example for Reduced On-Call Obligations

Transition Plan – Reduction in On-Call Activity

Physicians may elect to reduce on-call activity at some point in their career. This transition plan outlines the eligibility requirements and stipulations for such requests.

Physician Eligibility – Age and Tenure

Physicians with at least 15 years of service may cease weekend call at age 58; weeknight call at age 63. While physicians may elect to cease taking on-call, they are not required to do so. A physician who wishes to not have employment terminated before a particular age can elect to cease on-call at an age greater than the minimums outlined above.

Stipulations for On-Call Reduction

On-call reduction opportunities are contingent on the following:

Notification

Physicians must provide notice at least two years in advance of going off-call. If such notification is not received, the physician will be required to petition the executive committee/board, which will be under no obligation to grant such request.

Maximum Time Periods

The maximum period for time-off weekend call is four years.

The maximum period for time-off weekday call is two years.

Price for On-Call Reduction

The price for terminating on-call is $1,500 per day for primary on-call and $1,000 per day for secondary on-call. The price will have an automatic adjustment factor that is linked to the group's performance (e.g., changes in average compensation for shareholder physicians) to enable the price to increase over time. Funds deducted from physicians not taking on-call will be reallocated among shareholder physicians who take on-call.

Fail-Safe Provisions

There must be at least 10 physicians in the group who are available to take call (5 for primary on-call and 5 for secondary on-call). If there is an insufficient number of physicians in the group available to take call, the physician who recently has been granted on-call termination will be required to re-commence on-call activities, followed by the next most recent physician granted on-call termination, etc.

All physicians are also expected to take a reasonable amount of call in an emergency (e.g., if a physician must rotate out of the on-call schedule due to injury, disability, or death). For such purposes, a reasonable period of on-call will be requested of physicians who have terminated on-call activity (e.g., three months of full on-call responsibilities).

Physicians who are required to provide on-call services for more than three months during an off-call period can petition the executive committee/board to extend the period of time off on-call for the amount of time on-call in excess of three months.

Buy and Sell of On-Call Obligations

Buying and selling of on-call is not allowed. However, physicians can petition the executive committee/board for a limited exception to address personal needs/issues, and the executive committee can make short-term variations from basic on-call obligations.

Status at End of Period Off-Call

Employment as a shareholder/partner automatically terminates once a physician is off-call for a four-year period, at which time shareholder/partner status ceases and practice buy-out (including stock purchase and payment of deferred compensation) begins.

At the end of the four-year period, the physician and group can elect to enter into a year-to-year employment relationship, with physician compensation paid via a productivity or salary arrangement, although such an offer is not required or guaranteed. The group can decline to offer employment to the physician upon termination of a four-year period, or to not renew employment following termination of a contract term.

Health and Other Insurance

Each physician is generally responsible for managing his or her own ongoing access to health benefits following termination of employment. This can be accomplished by the physician's decision to manage the timing of termination from the practice and/or retirement, purchase of other insurance, etc.

The practice will, however, endeavor to provide access to insurance coverage for a limited time period following termination provided that: (1) the arrangement must have no direct cost to the group (meaning the physician will need to keep the group "whole" in terms of premium/stop-loss costs by not receiving full deferred compensation amount or otherwise); and (2) the continuation of coverage is for only a limited time period.

Practice Noncompete

A noncompete is viewed as essential to the practice's long-term viability. A noncompete will continue to be imposed via the employment agreement. The practice noncompete will *not* apply if:

- ▶ Physician terminates due to breach of agreement by employer; or
- ▶ Practice terminates physician's employment without cause.

---

tion plan. Yet, the mechanical means to achieve that practical objective – lower compensation – will vary depending upon the plan. And, as with all things, not all compensation plans will result in the same type of reduction. How the practice allocates revenues and expenditures – that is, the particular architecture it uses – will impact the level of compensation both before and after transition. As a result, a particular approach used to craft the transition arrangement will need to be considered.

By illustration, Exhibit 11.6 shows the level of compensation earned by a physician under a compensation system that uses a production-based allocation of revenues coupled with a modified cost accounting or combined equal share and utilization-based cost allocation (60 percent equal share; 40 percent based upon utilization) model (Revenue Element 4 with Expense Element 8). Under this example, production levels for all physicians in the practice, other than the physician in transition, remain con-

EXHIBIT 11.5 Compensation Plans and Transition Arrangements

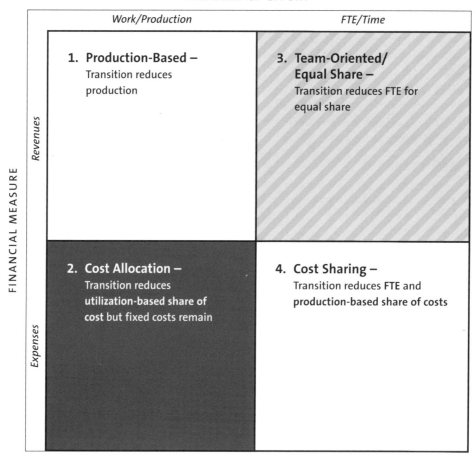

© 2006 Johnson & Walker Keegan

stant, but the transitioning physician's production decreases. Because the production decreases, the share of practice overhead that is allocated based on utilization also decreases (because the reduced production yields some reduced level of utilization). The result is a reduction of compensation of approximately $43,000. In this example, the transition arrangement is arguably "self-adjusting" in that the physician's reduced work results in some reduction in the physician's utilization of practice resources. However, because the physician continues to pay an equal share of the practice's fixed expenses (estimated at 60 percent of the total under the expense allocation system), despite the reduction in the utilization-based component of practice expenses, the compensation plan yields a reduced level of compensation.

EXHIBIT 11.6

Transition Mechanics:
Production-Based and Cost Allocation Compensation Plan*

	Before		Transition
Production	$550,000	**Production**	$475,000
% of Utilization	20%	% of Utilization	15%
FTE	1.00	FTE	0.75
Expenses		**Expenses**	
Utilization Share (40%)	$109,800	Utilization Share (40%)	$77,288
Fixed/Equal Share (60%)	$164,700	Fixed/Equal Share (60%)	$164,700
	$274,500		$241,988
Physician-Specific		Physician-Specific	
Direct Expenses	$50,400	Direct Expenses	$50,400
Compensation	$225,100	**Compensation**	$182,613

* Reduced production coupled with reduction of utilization-based component of expenses reduces compensation.

© 2006 Johnson & Walker Keegan

Conversely, Exhibit 11.7 uses the same data but a different compensation plan architecture in which the equal share component of practice operating expenses or overhead is, in fact, reduced based upon the physician's full-time equivalency (FTE) level. Moreover, in this example, 40 percent of the practice overhead costs are allocated based on production rather than utilization. Therefore, as the physician's production decreases, his or her share of overhead also decreases, but the reduction in expenses is more dramatic under this example than under the compensation plan used in Exhibit 11.6.

These two exhibits demonstrate the financial implications of different compensation plans under a transition arrangement. Under the model depicted in Exhibit 11.6, the practice's overhead allocation involves a pure equal share component (60 percent) without regard to individual physician FTE levels. It is also then combined with a utilization-based component for allocating practice expenditures (Expense Element 7). In contrast, Exhibit 11.7 reduces the equal share portion of the overhead allocation based on the physician's reduced FTE, and demonstrates a difference in compensation under this type of methodology for the physician in transition of approximately $23,000 in compensation as a result of the transition arrangement.

Exhibit 11.8 shows other variations of these same data using different approaches to revenue and expense allocation as part of the compensation plan for physicians in the transition arrangement. Exhibits 11.6, 11.7, and 11.8 highlight the importance of modeling transition arrangements as part of the existing and potential future compensation plans. They also illustrate the reality that different

EXHIBIT 11.7

Transition Mechanics: Production-Based and Cost Share Compensation Plan*

	Before			Transition
Revenues	$550,000	**Revenues**		$475,000
% of Production	18%	% of Production		16%
FTE	1.00	FTE		0.75
Revenues		**Revenues**		
Production Share (100%)	$550,000	Production Share (100%)		$77,288
Expenses		**Expenses**		
Production Share (40%)	$99,000	Production Share (40%)		$82,267
Fixed/Equal Share (60%)	$164,700	Fixed/Equal Share (60%)		$130,026
	$263,700			$212,293
Physician-Specific Direct Expenses	$50,400	Physician-Specific Direct Expenses		$50,400
Compensation	$235,900	**Compensation**		$212,307

* Reduced production coupled with reduced share of production-based and FTE share of fixed expenses reduces compensation.

© 2006 Johnson & Walker Keegan

compensation plans will result in different "bottom line" results regarding compensation for physicians in transition. Simply put, where a physician starts on the compensation plan matrix involving the combination of revenues and expenditures will influence the adjustment method that may be used as part of the transition arrangement, and the perceptions of the transition plan's fairness in "bottom line" terms, as depicted in Exhibit 11.8.

Central to all of the transition arrangements is the actual reality that the vast majority of practice operating costs are, in fact, fixed. And while the physician in transition may, in fact, receive or utilize a relatively smaller portion of certain practice expenditures or resources (e.g., time of certain support staff members or the use of medical and surgical supplies), the majority of all other practice operating costs (e.g., general administrative staff, business office, clinical support staff, medical records, building and occupancy, information technology, furniture and equipment, promotion, and others) will likely remain unchanged. Consequently, a reduction to a three-day workweek without a corresponding reduction in practice costs will negatively impact the practice and the physicians that are working a full-time schedule. Staffing expenditures continue to be incurred even though the physician is absent, because the telephones still need to be managed, prescriptions need to be refilled, patients will request their laboratory and test results, patients will call with medical questions, and other external patient flow processes will continue to occur. Additionally, when a physician is absent from the clinical setting, another physician in the practice must respond to clinical

EXHIBIT 11.8 Influence of Current State on Transition Mechanics

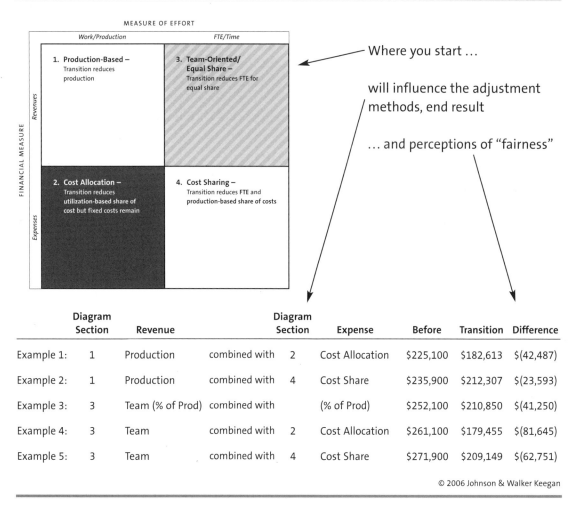

	Diagram Section	Revenue		Diagram Section	Expense	Before	Transition	Difference
Example 1:	1	Production	combined with	2	Cost Allocation	$225,100	$182,613	$(42,487)
Example 2:	1	Production	combined with	4	Cost Share	$235,900	$212,307	$(23,593)
Example 3:	3	Team (% of Prod)	combined with		(% of Prod)	$252,100	$210,850	$(41,250)
Example 4:	3	Team	combined with	2	Cost Allocation	$261,100	$179,455	$(81,645)
Example 5:	3	Team	combined with	4	Cost Share	$271,900	$209,149	$(62,751)

© 2006 Johnson & Walker Keegan

questions from patients, thus negatively impacting the productivity of full-time physicians who assume this coverage.

In some cases, a practice with a large number of part-time physicians will actually need more infrastructure than a practice that has full-time physicians. For example, staffing to support five full-time physicians will be different than staffing to support eight physicians who are essentially doing the work of five (e.g., 5.00 clinical FTEs). In this instance, eight schedules – not five – have to be managed; eight different practice styles – not five – must be supported. Likewise, the physicians on job-share arrangements will commonly have duplicate benefits and other costs, despite their reduced-time status.

When physicians are on productivity-based compensation plans, we will frequently see the physician who transitions to part-time status attempt to manage the same patient volume as his full-time colleagues. While some physicians can do this effortlessly – for instance, they may work at higher production levels than their colleagues – other physicians may incur overtime for staff or require more staff assigned to the physician in order to work at high volumes. In essence, a full-time practice is attempted in simply fewer clinic days or clinic sessions. It can also negatively impact patient perceptions of service delivery. This is why a number of medical practices have outlined patient volume expectations and compensation limits for part-time status – for example, the 50 percent physician is expected to see 50 percent of the patient volume and earn 50 percent of the level of his or her full-time colleagues.

The scenario analysis undertaken in connection with and examination of transition planning will typically involve modeling the transition arrangement under the practice's current or proposed compensation plan. Through that mechanism, consideration can be paid to whether the transition plan takes into account the appropriate level of "cost" that needs to be borne by the physician under the transition arrangement. Perhaps more important is the focus on the "cost" that may be borne by the physicians in the practice who remain. The actual result of the scenario analysis may involve the development of a new plan, or it may simply result in an understanding of the implications of transition arrangements on existing arrangements. In either case, the scenario analysis is essential to developing a true understanding of what the transition arrangement will mean both for the physician in transition and the rest of the practice.

Physician transition plans permit a practice to proactively plan for nonstandard physician work schedules, whether they are due to generational issues, illness, or simply a desire to alter a physician's work/life balance in a manner that is different from the norm established by the medical practice. They also permit physicians to plan for changes in their work life by articulating up front the impacts to a desire or need to go to part-time status, reduce on-call obligations, and the like. The key from our perspective is for a medical practice to develop a plan now – hopefully before it is needed – so that a precedent-setting decision based on any one individual physician's circumstances is not made that will be detrimental to the other physicians in the practice or to the future health of the medical practice itself.

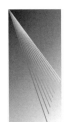

TWELVE

Industry Trends in Physician Compensation

eclining reimbursement and other pressures in the health care environment are leading to a number of key developments and trends in physician compensation systems today. This chapter reviews those broad trends, including the trends and directions of change in physician compensation systems, the factors influencing those changes, and the key issues being considered in connection with compensation plan development.

THE ISSUES AND CHALLENGES

Physician compensation plans are facing a number of challenges and issues on a variety of fronts. A review of market dynamics and pressures faced by physician compensation arrangements suggests that pressures are occurring on at least the following broad dimensions (see Exhibit 12.1):

1. **Individualistic vs. team-oriented models.** Many practices are facing the challenge of whether their compensation plan should promote the culture of

EXHIBIT 12.1 Industry Trends

► Individualistic vs. team orientation

► Cost sharing vs. cost accounting

► Ancillary services revenue generation and distribution

► Increased diversity of goals and preferences resulting in increased organizational complexity

► Performance variation resulting in greater potential for conflict

► Small, medium, and large practice distinctions – combined with the reality that many large groups are actually many small groups

► Private, hospital-affiliated, and academic similarities and differences

► Changing reimbursement mechanisms, including pay-for-performance

► Changing performance measures due to technology

► Legal and regulatory requirements and intervention

teamwork or individualism, or something in-between. In many settings, team-oriented models are under pressure by desires to move to more individualistic models.

2. **Cost sharing vs. cost accounting.** Consistent with the drive toward increased individualistic models, medical practices are examining the questions of practice expenses and to what degree physicians should share costs vs. increase direct individual responsibility for cost of practice through the use of cost accounting and similar methods.

3. **Ancillary services development, revenue generation, and distribution.** As reimbursement for professional services declines from both public and private payers, medical practices are increasingly looking at alternative revenue sources from ancillary services to pay practice overhead and stabilize, if not enhance, physician compensation levels. However, not every physician will have an equal opportunity, stake, or role in promoting and using ancillary services. In multispecialty practices in particular, different subsets of the practice may be the primary users and drivers of profitable (or not so profitable) ancillary services lines. The requirements of the Stark law and state self-referral laws notwithstanding, the fundamental questions of how to pay for and allocate the profits from ancillary services are increasingly a driving force for changes to medical practice compensation systems.

4. **Increased diversity and organizational complexity.** Medical practices today are no longer comprised solely of physicians with largely similar and homogeneous goals and desires. Practices today are more likely to be made up of a patchwork of physicians in different age brackets, different genders, different backgrounds, varying lifestyle goals, and widely varying perspectives regarding work, medical practice, and compensation. All of these changes and their corresponding diversity translate into increased organizational complexity and increased demands by physicians that the relationship between physicians and their work more clearly meet each individual's unique perspectives and goals.

5. **Performance variation resulting in greater potential for conflict.** A common outgrowth of the diversity among physicians is greater variation of work and production levels and, with that, significantly greater potential for conflict. Physicians have always worked at different levels. However, the naturally occurring variation in production and work levels, when combined with the cultural gulf between physicians with different lifestyle expectations, frequently will increase conflict between and among individual physicians and physician subspecialties.

6. **Distinctions based upon practice size.** The historic variations in compensation methodologies, ranging from largely team-oriented models with small group practices to more individualistic models as the practice grows in size,

and eventually returning to team-oriented models for extremely large mega-practices, continues to hold true in today's environment. Nonetheless, the diversity and increased desire to meet unique needs referenced above are translated into the methodologies used in medical practices of different sizes. As a result, even in medium to large medical practices, segmentation of the practice into smaller subpractices for compensation and sometimes other (e.g., governance) purposes is increasingly common. This is particularly the case as multispecialty practices strive to demonstrate that the benefits of remaining in a multispecialty setting are worth the perceived cost to physicians in certain highly sought-after medical and surgical subspecialties. These pressures are driving many multispecialty group practices to craft arrangements that attempt to balance the benefits of multispecialty practice with those of smaller, single specialty organizations.

7. **Blurring of private, hospital-affiliated, and academic compensation plans.** The compensation plan methodologies and models used in a variety of settings continue to blur, and the age-old positions about the "right way" to compensate physicians in a particular setting are quickly moving to the sidelines. As reimbursement declines and fiscal pressures continue in all sectors of health care, the key factors relating to physician compensation and practice success in the private practice setting – encouraging enhanced revenue generation and expense management – are increasingly serving as the guideposts for physician compensation plans in all settings.

8. **Changing reimbursement mechanisms.** The current emphasis for payer reimbursement is contingent payment based upon performance outcomes. The extent to which the pay-for-performance (P4P) and other similar methods of determining reimbursement levels from a health plan to a medical practice will be further translated into the practice's own compensation plan is not yet known. Also unknown is whether the measures used in these types of reimbursement strategies definitively measure "quality" per se.

From our perspective, the alignment of payer reimbursement strategies and medical practice compensation plans makes a great deal of sense, yet that would require practices to devote less attention to production, which has heretofore been one of the primary performance measures utilized in physician compensation plan design. As increasing levels of reimbursement are based on clinical and practice efficiency measures, the alignment of reimbursement methods (health plan to medical group) with distribution methods (medical group to physician) is a natural consequence.

9. **Changing performance measures due to technology.** Advances in both medical and information technology are leading to different forms of medical practice, including e-consults, telemedicine, and home-directed care (in the absence of the physician's physical presence), and other forms. It is likely that,

in the very near future, the actual measures of physician work and effort will need to expand to include these and other additional measures that recognize physician work beyond the traditional face-to-face physician-patient encounter.

10. **Legal and regulatory requirements and intervention.** The heightened scrutiny of physician compensation arrangements by legal and regulatory agencies regarding compensation will likely cause medical practices to continually evaluate their compensation plans in light of changing rules and requirements.

TRENDS IN PHYSICIAN COMPENSATION ARRANGEMENTS

The various factors referenced above are leading to a variety of broad trends in physician compensation arrangements. As with all things, the nature of changes to physician compensation plans frequently depends upon the nature of the plan as it stands today. Thus, the following general trends in physician compensation arrangements can be seen in today's evolving marketplace.

► TRENDS IN INDIVIDUALISTIC/PRODUCTION PLANS

Medical practices that use individualistic models focusing on a combination of physician production and revenue generation and physician-specific expense allocation are moving toward greater direct cost allocation as a means to increase individual physician responsibility and accountability. These practices are commonly moving from negotiated overhead arrangements or modified cost accounting to alternative cost allocation methodologies involving increasingly "strict" cost accounting methods.

Likewise, ancillary services revenues make up an increasingly large portion of medical practice revenue generation. Many practices that generate income from ancillary services are exploring how that income can be more directly allocated to the physicians responsible for its production. Now that the federal Stark law's requirements are relatively clear due to a final rule governing the law's application to physician compensation plans, medical practices and their advisors are exploring methodologies that will indirectly compensate physicians for a share of the practice revenues generated from ancillary services as required by the law, while attempting to create an appropriate reward and incentive structure that still provides some level of incentive for ancillary services production.

On the revenue front, medical practices relying on individualistic physician compensation plans continue to view cash as king and focus almost exclusively on net collections from professional and other services as the primary metric of production or work. In some cases, however, practices are recognizing the differences between payer mixes and are therefore adopting revenue allocation methods that combine net collections from professional services and work relative value units (WRVUs) as an appropriate and "fair" approach to rewarding physician work. Some practices – single specialty practices in particular – are using homegrown methods such as time value units that approximate relative value units (RVUs) but that are tailored to the unique culture and perceived needs of the particular practice and specialty.

► TRENDS IN TEAM-ORIENTED PLANS

Many medical practices continue to have team-oriented plans, with the team orientation expressed through a substantial equal share component, either in the allocation of revenues, expenses, or both. Many of those practices, however, are revisiting the percentage of compensation that is based on the equal share component to determine if an appropriate alignment of incentives is warranted.

On the revenue side in particular, the virtues of teamwork promoted through a substantially equal share component are increasingly coming under pressure due to the variations in production and diversity of physician preferences related to work and lifestyle. As a result, equal share portions of revenue allocation are being modified to increase individual responsibility and accountability for physicians' personal work levels. Equal share arrangements are also being modified to accommodate special circumstances, such as physician preferences related to on-call obligations, physician part-time work, and transition or retirement arrangements, including extended periods of sabbatical or similar leave.

For example, some medical practices that historically had a 100 percent equal share team-oriented compensation system are shifting to blended team-oriented plans that combine an equal share component (to promote teamwork) with individual production components that focus on physician-specific net collections from professional services, as well as on WRVUs. Thus, a 40/40/20 plan, defined as 40 percent equal share, 40 percent production measured by net collections, and 20 percent production measured by WRVUs, might be considered a means to more appropriately balance team orientation (e.g., equal share), revenue generation (e.g., net collections), and work levels that mitigate the effects of payer mix (e.g., WRVUs).

These practices are also coupling the new plan methodology with more explicit performance expectations that outline requirements related to weeks worked, minimum levels of production, on-call obligations, and related performance requirements. These performance expectations may simply make explicit the expectations and requirements that were previously implicit – but that may have been forgotten (or, in some cases, abused) by one or more physicians. By making the performance expectations explicit, the practice now has a benchmark against which to evaluate individual physician performance and, implicitly, the power (if not the responsibility) to make adjustments if individual physicians fail to meet the agreed upon standards.

► TRENDS IN MULTISPECIALTY PRACTICES

The above-referenced trends and factors affecting physician compensation occur in all practice types, yet multispecialty practices face their own unique set of challenges. For the most part, changes in physician compensation plans in multispecialty practices are generally designed to: (1) promote increased responsibility, accountability, and choice by individual physicians; and (2) approximate the culture and preferences found in single specialty practices.

As a result of these goals, multispecialty practices are increasingly focused on the allocation of costs to individual specialty-based departments and divisions. Likewise, as increased accountability and responsibility prevail, specialist physicians' willingness to overtly provide financial support to primary care is coming under stress. Methodologies that previously involved sharing of income or increased expense sharing are being challenged on the grounds that they are not truly reflective of medical practice economics today.

In multispecialty practices, with the virtual elimination of the gatekeeper model in most markets and where there is typically a preponderance of primary care leadership of the medical practice delivery system, specialist physician dissatisfaction is of concern. The satisfaction of specialist physicians is increasingly important to multispecialty practice survival and success. Most multispecialty practices have developed significant levels of ancillary services – only some of which can actually be used by primary care physicians in support of patient care. Given the debt service on facilities and equipment, and the costs of personnel in multispecialty practices, the continued involvement and support of specialist physicians are required to support practice overhead levels and generate ancillary services income. Multispecialty practices are working to change revenue-expenditure allocation methods to meet the difficult task of balancing the needs of specialist physicians with practice financial goals.

The trend toward increased cost allocation and cost accounting also translates into cost allocation to ancillary services departments. Closer review of the true profitability of particular service lines – laboratory, diagnostic imaging, and others – is occurring with increased frequency. As a result, practices are allocating a portion of general administrative overhead to ancillary services departments as a means to ensure that the departments themselves bear their own fair share of practice overhead.

With the growth of ancillaries, the importance of the Stark law's "rule of five" that affects the level upon which ancillary services revenues or profits may be distributed within the practice is also growing in importance. Multispecialty practices are increasingly confronted with challenges related to the allocation of ancillary services revenues and profits. Many are finding themselves having to address the specialists' assertion that "I'd make more money if I was out on my own."

As a result of these factors, multispecialty practices that use true team-oriented methodologies in which the practice's net profits are allocated through the physician compensation plan (without the use of any form of explicit cost allocation methodology) are becoming increasingly rare. Instead, more individualistic models, either at the individual physician or subpractice level, are being utilized. These models involve increased levels of cost allocation and cost accounting. And while most practice operating costs continue to be fixed, significant battles are occurring over the costs that have some variability based upon production or utilization. Thus, medical practices are considering, for example:

- ► Allocating business office costs (e.g., professional fee billing) based upon claims volume of the physician or specialty/department.

- ► Moving rent costs from equal share allocation methods to square footage or combined equal share and number of exam room–based methodologies.

- ► Allocating direct operating expenses that benefit individual physicians (e.g., non-physician providers, professional liability insurance premiums, health insurance costs, continuing medical education [CME], and similar expenses) directly to individual physicians.

- ► Allocating ancillary services revenues and profits to separate service lines (e.g., laboratory and diagnostic imaging subject to the Stark law, diagnostic imaging not subject to the Stark law, physical therapy, complimentary and alternative services, etc.). Each service line is then subject to its own allocation methodology with only the profits (if any) allocated among the physicians who actually utilize the services and are responsible for profit generation, to the extent possible and as allowed by the Stark law's "rule of five."

Despite the level of increased granularity in ancillary services allocation, outright utilization of ancillary services (and, therefore, individual physician contribution to ancillary services profitability) will often vary widely even within a single medical practice. By illustration, Exhibit 12.2 reflects the ratio of ancillary services production to professional services production within a particular medical practice. Certain physicians have relatively high levels of ancillary services utilization in relation to the levels of professional service work performed. Others have dramatically lower levels – in some instances, almost one-half the level of ancillary services usage for each dollar of professional service net collections.

In such circumstances, historic methodologies allocating ancillary services on an equal share or similar basis will frequently be viewed as unfair. This is because the physician who has relatively low levels of ancillary services usage (perhaps due to a significantly healthier and younger patient base) will be perceived as benefiting disproportionately from the methodology. Conversely, physicians with relatively high levels of ancillary services ordering due to their patient base or approach to practice will benefit less – even though they still have certain physician responsibilities with respect to such services. Of course, the physicians with higher levels of ancillary services utilization could be overutilizing these services (e.g., churning), while physicians with lower utilization could be practicing high quality care at low cost. This distinction is admittedly difficult to determine, contributing to problematic perceptions of the "fairness" with which ancillary revenue is distributed.

The Stark II final rule's clarification that medical practices may use "pods" comprised of five or more physicians to determine and pay ancillary services income and profits is providing greater flexibility to multispecialty practices. The practices must still

EXHIBIT 12.2   The Ancillary Revenue Challenge

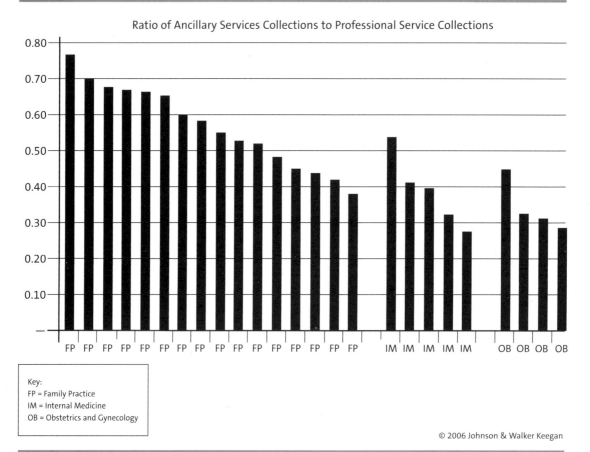

Ratio of Ancillary Services Collections to Professional Service Collections

Key:
FP = Family Practice
IM = Internal Medicine
OB = Obstetrics and Gynecology

© 2006 Johnson & Walker Keegan

ensure that ancillary services income is only allocated indirectly based upon physician referral patterns, but the "rule of five" allows for significantly greater flexibility. Practices can create subpractices or pods of five or more physicians for the distribution of ancillary profits using any number of factors, including, for example, a ratio of professional services production to ancillary services usage. They also can fund different pods and allocate profits to different pods using wholly acceptable criteria. In this process, they can award those that clearly have a higher utilization rate while not providing the same level of financial reward to those at the lowest end of the spectrum.

► TRENDS IN HOSPITAL-AFFILIATED PRACTICES

Hospital-affiliated practices tend to involve either direct employment or captive group practice models. The methodologies referenced above that are used in single specialty and multispecialty settings can also be used in captive practice models, where the group practice is owned and operated (either directly or indirectly) by a hospital or health system, but the practice bills for services in its own right.

In hospital-employment models, however, physicians are direct W-2 employees of the hospital. Therefore, the compensation methodologies used in more typical group practice settings cannot be used, because a group practice does not exist in a legal sense, even if the physicians and hospital attempt to create one for operational, cultural, and other purposes. Nonetheless, in the employment setting, the majority of hospitals are still attempting to mimic the economics and realities of private practice to the extent possible. They use a combination of base plus incentive, set dollar amounts per WRVU or graduated dollar amounts per WRVU, to approximate private practice realities. However, as noted in Chapter 9, these organizations are precluded from distributing designated health services (DHS) revenue to their physicians and are held to a different standard regarding issues of reasonableness of compensation levels paid to physicians.

A common ultimate goal of the hospital-affiliated compensation system is to mimic the private practice setting, while also affording greater protection and benefits by being in a hospital-affiliated practice. Moreover, in many practices, an increased emphasis has been placed on managing costs to the extent feasible. The challenge being faced by hospital-affiliated systems is to recognize and appreciate the contribution of individual physicians to the success of the overall system.

For example, many hospitals have used WRVUs and have paid a set dollar amount per WRVU based upon physician production. Such methods have been viewed as simple, easy to understand, and useful in that they do not discriminate based upon payer mix. Yet, even these models are increasingly being questioned for a variety of reasons, including the fact that the models do not consider practice operating costs. Furthermore, they pay the same level of compensation for both the first and last unit of work, therefore presenting an artificial economic environment that is inconsistent with the financial realities of medical practices.

As a result, an alternative model being explored by many health systems is one that uses graduated dollar value – whether measured based on WRVUs, percentage of professional services gross charges, or some other factor – to pay for work and performance. This methodology is demonstrated in some of the compensation plan examples in Chapter 14 (see Hospital Examples 5 and 6). It recognizes that the level of true profit from the first unit of production is less than the profit from the last unit of production due to the need to pay fixed operating costs. That is, physicians performing at a low level of production will not receive the same level of compensation per unit of production as their colleagues who produce at higher levels. In some cases, graduated compensation methods not only tailor the payment per unit of work based upon physician specialty and work levels, but also based on full- and part-time physician status.

► TRENDS IN ACADEMIC PRACTICE PLANS

The approaches described above in private practices and hospital-affiliated practices are also increasingly being used in academic settings. With the increased pressures on reimbursement in academic medicine, academic practices are drawing from single specialty and multispecialty practice models as a means to increase productivity and decrease clinical practice operating costs.

In an academic environment, however, the emphasis is on school-wide physician compensation plans coupled with department physician compensation plans, and individual physician income levels consistent with these plans. This environment also emphasizes the institution's funds flow and tax system. Thus, the dean's office, the faculty practice plan, and department financial support generated by faculty member clinical productivity are increasingly focused upon in the context of faculty compensation and related funds flow models.

Specialist physicians in academic settings are increasingly using individualistic or XYZ compensation models (discussed in Chapter 15). Such models are common, given the relatively higher level of production and revenue-generating potential for specialists. For many subspecialty practices (e.g., orthopedics, cardiology, oncology), the individualistic models involving significant cost allocation also tend to mirror trends in private practice settings.

Primary care physicians in academic settings are, however, increasingly facing fiscal challenges. Pressures are rising related to primary care revenue generation and operating expenses, and therefore to compensation levels and to the need for financial support from other components of the academic enterprise. The result is a shift from outright subsidies for primary care to systems that pay primary care physicians for defined work efforts and products while also focusing attention on "controllable" costs.

► REEMERGENCE OF GAINSHARING

Much of this book has focused on compensation arrangements in which physicians situated in a group practice, hospital, or another organization are paid for their professional services. Yet, "gainshare" programs involving physicians and hospitals represent a potential emerging "state-of-the-art" compensation arrangement.

"Gainsharing" generally describes a contractual arrangement involving a hospital and a group of physicians directed at the promotion of hospital cost savings. Gainsharing arrangements are not new, but they were effectively prohibited until recently due to a July 1999, Office of the Inspector General (OIG) "Special Advisory Bulletin" that effectively prohibited all gainsharing arrangements based on the application of the Medicare Civil Monetary Penalties statute, which prohibits hospitals from paying physicians to reduce or limit services to Medicare and Medicaid beneficiaries under the physician's care.

In February 2005, the OIG issued six new advisory opinions detailing gainsharing arrangements. In the opinions, the six arrangements were found to be acceptable because they were structured in a way that would minimize the risk of violating federal fraud and abuse laws.

The gainshare arrangements that were reviewed and approved involved cardiologists and cardiac surgeons, but other surgical and medical specialties could potentially participate in carefully structured arrangements. Nonetheless, they highlight the features that the OIG is likely to view to be important for a legally acceptable gainsharing arrangement. Those features include:

► Limiting the duration of the gainshare program (e.g., one year) and the amount of compensation that can be paid under the arrangement (e.g., defining a compensation cap);

► Distributing payments from successful cost-savings programs to physician participants on a per capita (per physician) basis, rather than on a utilization basis or some other methodology;

► Ensuring that the cost-saving actions that are the focus of the gainsharing program can be separately identified and closely tracked in order to promote transparency and accountability;

► Making sure that the program is based on valid clinical/medical support and expertise that conclude that the program is unlikely to have an adverse impact on quality or patient care;

► Applying the program to all payers and all procedures, rather than limiting the program's application to a distinct subset of the patient population, such as patients enrolled in Medicare or other programs;

► Creating floors as part of the program related to the use of certain items and services, with the determination of such floors based upon assessments of good clinical practice and historic usage patterns;

► Ensuring that participating physicians continue to have access to the same devices and supplies that were available before the program was created; and

► Providing full disclosure of the gainshare arrangement to patients in connection with surgeries and procedures that are the focus and subject of the program.

These program features are likely to be essential to a legally appropriate gainsharing program.

Gainshare programs are likely to grow with increased frequency in light of the recent OIG advisory opinions, and due to the fact that the Internal Revenue Service (IRS) had previously approved similar programs – thus eliminating uncertainty related to laws regarding tax-exempt organizations. However, the OIG did not specifically consider whether the gainshare arrangements would meet the Stark law's requirements; therefore, the lack of an affirmative approval of a gainshare arrangement in light of the Stark law's requirements may serve as a speed bump to any rapid development and expansion of such programs. Barring congressional action to clarify the regulatory environment and provide positive encouragement of gainsharing arrangements, such arrangements will likely be developed and implemented on largely an incremental basis – and will likely also be subject to heightened scrutiny.

The key industry trends discussed in this chapter are apparent in physician compensation plans and are a direct result of the significant challenges and changes facing medical practices today. Due to changes in the reimbursement environment, medical practices are increasingly focused on actual revenues (e.g., net collections from professional services) and cost management and cost allocation strategies to align compensation with the financial realities of the medical practice. Battles over technical components and ancillary services revenues are increasingly fought, as these represent expanded revenue streams to compensate for the declines in reimbursement for professional services production. Performance measures used in compensation plans are expanding beyond clinical production to ensure alignment with contingent reimbursement strategies, such as pay-for-performance, and/or to encourage physicians to adopt and integrate new technologies. There are movements to revisit the benefits of integrated systems and a general "push back" related to providing ongoing revenue sharing and support to primary care by medical and surgical specialists. All of this is occurring in a complex health care environment subject to increasing challenges from legal mandates and the need to recruit and retain physicians in scarce specialties and underprovided markets.

The industry trends add to the complexity of compensation planning in the medical practice and often lead to increasingly sophisticated compensation plan methodologies adopted by today's medical practices.

Compensation Plan Examples

"And no two compensation plans are exactly alike. The challenges facing medical practices and their compensation plans are as varied and complex as the practices themselves."

JOHNSON & KEEGAN, 2006

INTRODUCTION – COMPENSATION PLAN EXAMPLES

Part III of this book presents case examples of compensation plans. It deals with the practical question of *how* an organization determines and pays for the services of individual physicians – the compensation plan's methodology and technical dimensions. The following chapters describe compensation plans that may be used by group practices, hospital-affiliated and hospital-employed practices, academic practices, and other organizations to pay physicians or groups of physicians for their services.

► THE COMPENSATION PLAN MATRIX AND PLAN ARCHITECTURES

Of course, there are literally hundreds of different compensation plans that are used throughout the country, and no two plans are exactly the same. However, the range of different compensation plan architectures can be described through the use of the compensation plan matrix and arrayed on a continuum ranging from team-oriented to individualistic plans. The compensation plan matrix and the array of plan architectures using elements of the matrix were discussed in detail in Chapters 5 and 6, but a brief refresher will be useful.

The compensation plan matrix is again provided in Exhibit III.1. This matrix builds on the cultural and financial dimensions of compensation plans. The matrix contains nine distinct elements that refer to the treatment of revenues and expenses in a compensation plan and to the general impact the plans have on practice culture.

The nine elements in the compensation plan matrix can, in turn, be used individually or in combination to describe 18 basic compensation plan architectures or frameworks that represent the basic compensation plan methodological options. These architectures can, in turn, be arrayed on a continuum of plan architectures that range from those that are the most team-oriented to those that are the most individualistic. The array of plan architectures is again presented in Exhibit III.2.

As a general matter, the most *team-oriented* plans tend to pay practice expenses "off the top" and use the compensation plan to distribute a pool of funds, but they *do not* assign or allocate shares of overhead to individual physicians. Conversely, the most *individualistic* plans tend to treat physicians as largely separate profit-and-loss centers; therefore, they tend to involve both a pure production-based allocation of practice revenues, coupled with an explicit allocation of practice operating costs to individual physicians.

Plans that are in the *"middle ground"* lie between these two extremes in that they blend aspects of team-oriented and individualistic approaches through any number of methodologies, commonly including a sharing of revenues combined with various approaches to expense allocation. In reality, most compensation plans actually tend to involve a middle ground approach.

EXHIBIT III.1 The Compensation Plan Matrix

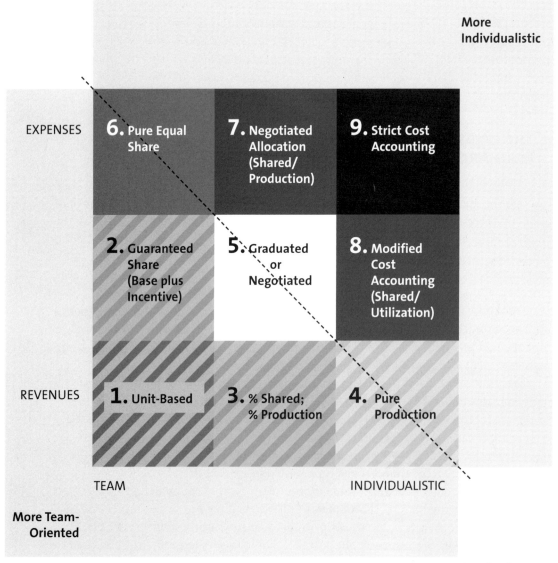

The matrix and array contain the full range of common approaches to physician compensation, including:

► Equal share plans;

► Base plus incentive plans;

EXHIBIT III.2 Array of Compensation Plan Architectures

Architecture	A	B	C	D	E	F	G	H	I	J	K	L	M	N	O	P	Q	R
Revenue Element	1	2	3	4	5	2	3	2	3	2	3	2	3	4	4	4	4	4
Expense Element						6	6	7	7	8	8	9	9	5	6	7	8	9
			TEAM					MIDDLE GROUND							INDIVIDUALISTIC			

© 2006 Johnson & Walker Keegan

► Straight salary plans; and

► Productivity-based plans.

However, the use of the matrix, coupled with the array of plan architectures, allows for a more detailed understanding of the variations between and among these common approaches by addressing the financial and cultural dimensions of compensation in greater detail.

The following chapters provide detailed compensation plan examples that build on the compensation plan matrix in Exhibit III.1 and that are classified by reference to the array in Exhibit III.2. The plan architectures are further presented by reference to the type of organization that will typically consider and use such a methodology. They specifically distinguish between plans used in: (1) bona fide "Group Practices" vs. (2) other settings, such as hospitals, and in other types of relationships.

This distinction is important, because the legal requirements of the Stark law provide that certain approaches to compensation may *only* be used in bona fide Group Practices. *Specifically*, although physicians in all settings may be compensated for the designated health services (DHS)[1] that they personally perform, only physicians in bona fide Group Practices that comply with the Stark law's exception for in-office ancillary services may indirectly benefit from the DHS referrals they make to their medical practices. As a result, these organizations generally have a wider range of compensation plan options than those available for use in other entities. Conversely, physicians in settings outside of Group Practices may not be compensated, directly or indirectly, for their DHS referrals.[2]

The different treatment provided to Group Practices by the Stark law means that physician compensation plans may generally be divided into two distinct camps:

► Those that may be used with physicians working in and for bona fide Group Practices; and

► Those that can be used to pay physicians providing services to other organizations.

Because of this, it is important to recognize that the compensation plans described in the following chapters for use in non-Group Practice settings (e.g., hospital employment and academic practice models) *can* also generally be used in a Group Practice setting, but not the reverse. That is, many of the compensation plans outlined for use in a Group Practice setting may generally *not* be available *in their pure form* for use in a non-Group Practice setting (e.g., hospital, academic institution) because under the Stark law, Group Practices enjoy considerably greater flexibility in their compensation methods and practices. Many of these Group Practice plans may be adapted for use in these other settings, but many will not be appropriate in a hospital or academic setting without some additional adjustment and refinement.

The next three chapters are organized along this Stark law treatment distinction. Chapter 13 presents case examples of compensation plans in bona fide Group Practices. In Chapter 14, we provide examples of compensation plans for physicians who are situated in hospital-affiliated and hospital-employed practices (those that are not considered bona fide Group Practices pursuant to the Stark law). The compensation plan examples in both of these chapters can be candidates for the clinical portion of compensation for faculty in academic institutions, although this will commonly require some variation and adjustment. However, in addition to these examples, in Chapter 15 we also share specific faculty practice plan examples to recognize the complexity of funds flow strategies and issues of alignment inherent in academic medicine.

Because of space constraints and model complexity, the individual plan examples that are included in this text illustrate the basic architectures using hypothetical data as applied to a relatively small number of physicians. Keep in mind that the purpose of the examples is to illustrate the mathematical calculations and models. The same basic methods can be adapted for use in larger organizations, for individual subsets of larger organizations, and on a specialty, departmental, or location-specific basis (subject to legal constraints). Moreover, methodological features used in one model example can frequently be incorporated into others. For this reason, each of the plan architectures and the various details illustrated in each can be viewed as building blocks designed to illustrate concepts. Those building blocks can be mixed and combined to create any number of alternative compensation plans and models.

Notes

1. DHS are generally defined as items and services within the following broad categories that may be paid for under the Medicare program: clinical laboratory services; physical therapy, occupational therapy, and speech-language pathology services; radiology and certain other imaging services; radiation therapy services and supplies; durable medical equipment and supplies; parenteral and enteral nutrients, equipment, and supplies; prosthetics, orthotics, and prosthetic devices and supplies; home health services; and inpatient and outpatient hospital services. Although other provisions of federal law apply the law's self-referral prohibition to Medicaid, no formal guidance has yet been published related to such services. With respect to certain categories of DHS, CMS provides a definitive listing of services that are defined as DHS (and, for example, those diagnostic services that are not included in the list will not be defined

as DHS). No such exclusive listing is provided for the other DHS categories. Identification of the particular DHS being ordered or referred by individual physicians is an essential part of developing a legally compliant compensation plan.

2. Moreover, even where a physician is part of a bona fide Group Practice, under certain circumstances other laws and rules may impose additional restrictions on the compensation that may be paid to physicians, and how that compensation may be determined. For example, a bona fide Group Practice might be owned by a hospital, an academic institution, or another entity that is either a provider of services and/or a tax-exempt enterprise. In such circumstances, the Stark law and other laws (i.e., laws governing exempt organizations, the anti-kickback law, and others) would also apply. See Chapter 9, "The Legal Element," for a detailed review of these complex issues.

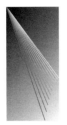

THIRTEEN

Compensation Plans in Bona Fide Group Practices

Compensation plans in bona fide Group Practices, including those that are physician-owned, as well as Group Practices that are owned and operated by third parties (e.g., hospitals and in some faculty practice plans), vary from one another based on multiple factors, including plan goals, design principles, group culture, and other group-specific factors.

In this chapter, we share case study examples of compensation plans that have generally been adopted and used by private practice medical Group Practices that rely upon and comply with the Stark law's exception for "in-office ancillary services." This exception allows physicians to make referrals for designated health services (DHS) within their medical group and enables physicians in the Group Practice to indirectly receive income or profits from DHS furnished through the practice. It is this ability to benefit from DHS referrals that primarily distinguishes these "Group Practice" compensation plans from those that can be used in other settings and relationships.

These same methods may also be used in other settings (e.g., with hospital-affiliated Group Practices or academic Group Practices) – provided that, in each instance, the practice entity constitutes a bona fide Group Practice as that term is defined in the Stark law (previously defined in Chapter 9, "The Legal Element"). Variations of these plans may also potentially be used in other settings, such as hospital employment arrangements; however, care must be taken to ensure that the plans are structured appropriately. Physicians who are employed by a hospital are subject to different compensation standards as they relate to DHS referrals, as discussed in Chapter 9.

The following plan architectures describe compensation plans that may be used in bona fide Group Practices. These plans are arrayed on a continuum that combines the elements referenced in the compensation plan matrix from team-oriented to individualistic models. In this chapter, we present five architectures that are team-oriented, five that are individualistic, and additional "middle ground" architectures. These architectures are situated on our array of plan architectures that were described in Chapters 5 and 6. We again present the compensation plan matrix and the array of plan architectures in Exhibits 13.1 and 13.2. The basic descriptions of these architectures follow.

EXHIBIT 13.1 The Compensation Plan Matrix

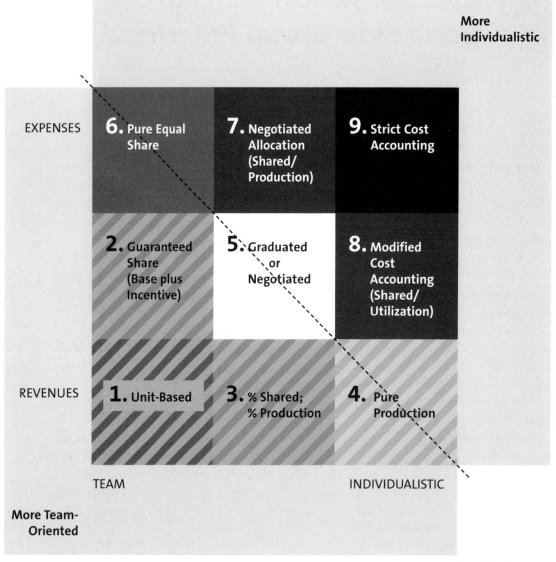

© 2006 Johnson & Walker Keegan

Team-Oriented Architectures

- ► Group Practice Architecture A – Unit-Based Plans;
- ► Group Practice Architecture B – Guaranteed Share (Base Plus Incentive) Plans;
- ► Group Practice Architecture C – Combined Equal Share and Production-Based Income Allocation Plans;
- ► Group Practice Architecture D – Pure Production Plans; and

EXHIBIT 13.2 Array of Compensation Plan Architectures

Architecture	A	B	C	D	E	F	G	H	I	J	K	L	M	N	O	P	Q	R
Revenue Element	1	2	3	4	5	2	3	2	3	2	3	2	3	4	4	4	4	4
Expense Element						6	6	7	7	8	8	9	9	5	6	7	8	9
	TEAM					MIDDLE GROUND								INDIVIDUALISTIC				

© 2006 Johnson & Walker Keegan

▶ Group Practice Architecture E – Graduated or Negotiated Revenue (or Income) Allocation Plans.

Individualistic Architectures

▶ Group Practice Architecture N – Pure Production with Negotiated or Graduated Expense Allocation Plans;

▶ Group Practice Architecture O – Pure Production with Equal Share Expense Allocation Plans;

▶ Group Practice Architecture P – Pure Production with Negotiated Expense Allocation Plans (Production-Based Expense Allocation);

▶ Group Practice Architecture Q – Pure Production with "Modified" Cost Accounting Plans; and

▶ Group Practice Architecture R – Pure Production with "Strict" Cost Accounting Plans.

With respect to each plan, we outline the basic nature of the plan, describe the type of practices and physician specialties that are known to use the plan type, describe the methodological steps associated with the plan's calculation, and provide observations on potential plan strengths and weaknesses along six dimensions, recognizing that there is no "perfect" plan. The six dimensions evaluated for each plan are those that are generally present in better-performing compensation plans. They include:

Measure: Selection of a measure(s) that is clear and understandable;

Productivity focus: Strength of the plan's focus on clinical productivity;

Financial: Fiscal viability of the plan;

Simplicity: Level of simplicity represented by the plan;

Alignment: Alignment of the plan with the medical practice's goals; and

Fairness: Issues of equity that may be of concern to physicians.

As noted above, because of space constraints and plan complexity, individual plan examples generally illustrate the basic architecture being described using hypothetical data involving a relatively small number of physicians. Keep in mind that the purpose of the examples is to illustrate the mathematical calculations and models; the same basic methods can be adapted for use in large organizations, for individual subsets of large organizations, and on a specialty, departmental, or location-specific basis. In addition, while the case examples are presented to illustrate how an architecture works overall, the methodological features and technical dimensions illustrated in one plan example can frequently be incorporated into other plans and models, serving as building blocks that can be mixed and matched to create any number of alternative compensation plans.

TEAM-ORIENTED ARCHITECTURES AND EXAMPLES

We begin our review of the models with the most basic architectures at the "team-oriented" end of the array of plan architectures listed in Exhibit 13.2 – Architectures A through E. These basic architectures illustrate plans that do not expressly consider practice expenses in a mathematical sense, but that instead pay practice operating costs "off the top" and allocate what remains (practice net income) on an agreed upon manner through the compensation plan.

Our compensation plan examples begin at the far left side of the array with the most team-oriented architecture (Architecture A), which uses a pure unit-based approach to revenue or income distribution (Revenue Element 1), with no express expense treatment. We follow this by moving inward on the continuum to review the following architecture examples:

- ▶ Architecture B – team-oriented plans using a guaranteed share of practice revenues or income (Revenue Element 2), with no express expense treatment;

- ▶ Architecture C – plans using a combined equal share and production-based approach to revenue or income distribution (Revenue Element 3), with no express expense treatment;

- ▶ Architecture D – plans that use pure production in the allocation of practice revenues or income (Revenue Element 4), with no express expense treatment; and

- ▶ Architecture E – plans involving a mixed system that uses a graduated or negotiated approach to revenue or income allocation (Revenue Element 5), with expenses considered indirectly.

▶ GROUP PRACTICE ARCHITECTURE A – UNIT-BASED PLANS
Revenue Element 1

Overview

This plan architecture uses the most "team-oriented" approach to physician compensation (Revenue Element 1 in Exhibit 13.1) by paying each physician a compensation level that is determined on a "per unit" basis. The most common examples of unit-based plan types involve pure equal share models and straight salary plans. Other variations include those that pay on an hourly, per shift or per diem (per day) basis, or even those that pay compensation as a defined percentage of work unit (e.g., percentage of net collections from professional services, percentage of gross professional services charges).

Central to each of these team-oriented plans in a Group Practice setting is the fact that there is no express consideration of practice expenses as part of the individual physician compensation methodology. Instead, the plan divides up the pool of funds available for compensation on some agreed upon "per unit" basis (e.g., each physician receives an equal share of practice income after payment of expenses).

Application

Single specialty medical practices often find unit-based plans to be useful in promoting a team or "group practice" orientation. This plan architecture can also be adopted for use in departments or divisions of multispecialty groups. Unit-based plans commonly work best in medical groups or in subdivisions of medical groups in which the physicians: (1) have similar work levels; (2) tend to perform many of the same types of services and procedures (without actual or de facto subspecialization); or (3) are heavily dependent upon external referrals for practice volume.

Thus, such plans are commonly used in single specialty general internal medicine groups, medical subspecialty practices and departments within multispecialty groups (e.g., hematology, oncology, gastroenterology, pulmonary medicine, rheumatology), surgical practices (e.g., general orthopedic surgery, cardiovascular surgery, vascular surgery, general surgery, urology), and in hospital-based departments (e.g., emergency medicine, pathology, and radiology). Unit-based plans are also used in hospital-affiliated arrangements, as discussed in Chapter 14 and as illustrated by plan Examples 1 through 3 in that chapter.

Methodology – Unit-Based Plans

The basic steps in a unit-based plan using a pure equal share plan are described in Example A-1 at the end of this section. Following this example, four variations of the basic architecture involving unit-based plans are then presented (Examples A-2 through A-5). Examples A-1 through A-5 are also illustrated in Exhibits 13.3 through 13.7.

Example A-1 – Basic Example of Architecture A:
Pure Equal Share Variation

Step 1. Determine the Practice's "Net Income" (Revenues Net of Expenses)
Pool practice revenues and deduct practice expenses, excluding physician-specific direct expenses.

Step 2. Allocate Net Income on an Equal Share Basis

The formula used to allocate net income in this example is a pure equal share allocation formula. Net revenue from the Group Practice as a whole is allocated to each physician based on a pure equal share basis. Thus, if the practice has 12 physicians, each physician receives 1/12 (or 8.33 percent) of the total practice income.

Step 3. Determine Physician-Specific Compensation

In this example, each physician's equal share of practice income is reduced by the actual cost of physician-specific direct expenses (e.g., health insurance costs, life insurance, etc.), although many practices include these physician-specific direct expenses as part of the practice's overall operating costs (rather than directly allocating them to individual physicians). The primary value with directly tracking and allocating direct expenses to the physician who benefits from them is to help ensure that the physician truly understands how much contribution he or she is making to the practice and, correspondingly, the benefit (cash compensation plus fringe benefits) he or she is receiving from the practice.

The basic mathematical formula to determine each physician's cash compensation is as follows:

> Practice-Specific Equal Share (Available for Compensation and Direct Benefits)
> − Physician-Specific Direct Expenses
> ─────────────────────────────────
> Physician Cash (Take Home) Compensation

Step 4. Adjust Compensation Based on Previous "Draws" and Pay Bonus

Although this plan architecture uses a pure equal share methodology, practice physicians are commonly paid a periodic advance or "draw" on the total compensation based on the amount they are expected to receive. The amount paid as a draw is then reconciled with the amount earned through the pure equal share component on a quarterly, annual, or other periodic basis. The difference is then paid to the physician in the form of a bonus.

Potential variations of Architecture A are shown in Examples A-2 through A-5 (illustrated in Exhibits 13.4 through 13.7). These variations involve the general approaches that follow.

Example A-2

This example adjusts the equal share component based on full-time equivalency (FTE) level, such that physician A (in this example, a part-time physician with a .75 FTE) receives a reduced equal share of practice income.

Example A-3

This variation of the basic equal share plan pays a portion of practice net income based on the number of days worked in the practice. Under this plan option, practice net income is divided by the total number of days worked in the practice by all practice physicians to determine an amount of net income per day of service (Step 2). This per diem income amount is multiplied by the number of days of service to determine each physician's share of practice income from which each physician's direct expenses are subtracted in the same manner as illustrated in Examples A-1 and A-2 (Step 3). This plan illustrates a salary advance or draw that is also based on a predefined amount per day (Step 4), along with a reconciliation of the amount earned to the amount paid through the draw to determine an end-of-year bonus amount. Such per diem arrangements will commonly be use in emergency medicine, urgent care, hospitalist, and similar groups.

Example A-4

This fourth example builds on plans that are commonly used in hospital employment arrangements but applies such models in a Group Practice context. This plan awards practice income net of expenses based on a defined dollar amount per work relative value unit (WRVU) of clinical service. Thus, it determines practice net income (Step 1) but allocates that income among practice physicians on a per WRVU basis such that each physician receives the same amount of compensation per unit of work (measured by WRVUs) (Steps 2 and 3). From this amount is deducted the physician's direct benefit costs and other expenses as in the other examples to determine the total W-2 compensation earned during the year (Step 3). The amounts previously advanced on a per WRVU basis (based on estimates and budgets in the practice) are then compared to the amount earned to determine the physician's bonus (shown here on an end-of-year basis) (Step 4).

Example A-5

This fifth example is a straight salary plan that links salary levels to production during a previous time period. In Example A-5 (Exhibit 13.7), a physician's production during one fiscal year determines the salary that will be paid during the following fiscal year. The salary constitutes the "per unit" payment for the physician's service. These plans obviously consider production and work levels, but without the direct and immediate feedback mechanism that more clearly links current-period compensation to current-period production.

Each of these plans can also be coupled with any number of additional variations, including requirements linked to minimum performance expectations (e.g., a predefined number of days or weeks worked per year, a minimum number of patient visits or WRVUs generated, or otherwise). See Chapters 10 and 14 for a discussion of performance expectations, and plan examples reported in Chapter 14, for illustrations of how performance expectations can be incorporated into physician compensation plans.

Exhibit 13.8 provides an assessment of Group Practice Architecture A.

EXHIBIT 13.3

Example A-1 – Group Practice Architecture A –
Unit-Based Plan (Pure Equal Share)*
Revenue Element 1

Step 1	Determine practice net income.	Total					
	Net Collections from Professional Services	$2,975,000					
	Total Operating Expenses	$(1,338,750)					
		$1,636,250					

Step 2	Allocate net income on equal share basis.		Dr. A	Dr. B	Dr. C	Dr. D	Dr. E
	FTE	5.00	1.00	1.00	1.00	1.00	1.00
	Share per FTE	$327,250					
	Equal Share (before physician-specific direct expenses)		$327,250	$327,250	$327,250	$327,250	$327,250

Step 3	Determine physician-specific compensation.		Dr. A	Dr. B	Dr. C	Dr. D	Dr. E
	Direct Expenses		$(50,400)	$(52,390)	$(48,983)	$(54,000)	$(59,400)
	W-2 Compensation Earned		$276,850	$274,860	$278,267	$273,250	$267,850

Step 4	Adjust based on previous draws and pay bonus.		Dr. A	Dr. B	Dr. C	Dr. D	Dr. E
	Advance/Draw Paid		$(170,000)	$(170,000)	$(170,000)	$(170,000)	$(170,000)
	Bonus (end of year)		$106,850	$104,860	$108,267	$103,250	$97,850

* Hypothetical numbers presented for illustrative purposes only. Numbers may not total in all cases due to rounding.

© 2006 Johnson & Walker Keegan

EXHIBIT 13.4

Example A-2 – Group Practice Architecture A –
Unit-Based Plan (Pure Equal Share, Adjusted for Part-Time FTE)*
Revenue Element 1

	Total	Dr. A	Dr. B	Dr. C	Dr. D	Dr. E
Step 1	**Determine practice net income.**					
Net Collections from Professional Services	$2,975,000					
Total Operating Expenses	$(1,338,750)					
	$1,636,250					
Step 2	**Allocate net income on equal share per FTE basis.**					
FTE	4.75	0.75	1.00	1.00	1.00	1.00
Share per FTE	$344,474					
Equal Share (before physician-specific direct expenses)		$258,355	$344,474	$344,474	$344,474	$344,474
Step 3	**Determine physician-specific compensation.**					
Direct Expenses		$(50,400)	$(52,390)	$(48,983)	$(54,000)	$(59,400)
W-2 Compensation Earned		$207,955	$292,084	$295,491	$290,474	$285,074
Step 4	**Adjust based on previous draws and pay bonus.**					
Advance/Draw Paid		$(170,000)	$(170,000)	$(170,000)	$(170,000)	$(170,000)
Bonus (end of year)		$37,955	$122,084	$125,491	$120,474	$115,074

* Hypothetical numbers presented for illustrative purposes only. Numbers may not total in all cases due to rounding.

EXHIBIT 13.5

Example A-3 – Group Practice Architecture A –
Unit-Based Plan (Per Diem [per Day] Compensation)*
Revenue Element 1

	Total	Dr. A	Dr. B	Dr. C	Dr. D	Dr. E
Step 1 **Determine practice net income.**						
Net Collections from Professional Services	$2,975,000					
Total Operating Expenses	$(1,338,750)					
	$1,636,250					
Step 2 **Allocate net income on equal share (per diem) basis.**						
Days Worked (per year)	1,046	209	185	230	200	222
Per Diem Amount	$1,564					
Equal Amount Per Diem (before physician-specific direct expenses)		$326,937	$289,394	$359,787	$312,859	$347,273
Step 3 **Determine physician-specific compensation.**						
Direct Expenses		$(50,400)	$(52,390)	$(48,983)	$(54,000)	$(59,400)
W-2 Compensation Earned		$276,537	$237,004	$310,804	$258,859	$287,873
Step 4 **Adjust based on previous draws and pay bonus.**						
Advance/Draw per Day	$1,000	$(209,000)	$(185,000)	$(230,000)	$(200,000)	$(222,000)
Bonus (end of year)		$67,537	$52,004	$80,804	$58,859	$65,873

* Hypothetical numbers presented for illustrative purposes only. Numbers may not total in all cases due to rounding.

EXHIBIT 13.6

Example A-4 – Group Practice Architecture A – Unit-Based Plan (Dollars per WRVU)*
Revenue Element 1

Step 1	**Determine practice net income.**					
		Total				
	Net Collections from Professional Services	$2,975,000				
	Total Operating Expenses	$(1,338,750)				
		$1,636,250				

			Dr. A	**Dr. B**	**Dr. C**	**Dr. D**	**Dr. E**
Step 2	**Allocate net income on equal share (per WRVU) basis.**						
	Total WRVU	41,534	8,503	6,309	8,892	9,738	8,092
	Dollars per WRVU	$39.40					
	Equal Amount per WRVU (before physician-specific direct expenses)		$334,979	$248,546	$350,304	$383,633	$318,788
Step 3	**Determine physician-specific compensation.**						
	Direct Expenses		$(50,400)	$(52,390)	$(48,983)	$(54,000)	$(59,400)
	W-2 Compensation Earned		$284,579	$196,156	$301,321	$329,633	$259,388
Step 4	**Adjust based on previous draws and pay bonus.**						
	Advance/Draw per WRVU	$25.00	$(212,575)	$(157,725)	$(222,300)	$(243,450)	$(202,300)
	Bonus (end of year)		$72,004	$38,431	$79,021	$86,183	$57,088

* Hypothetical numbers presented for illustrative purposes only. Numbers may not total in all cases due to rounding.

EXHIBIT 13.7

Example A-5 –
Group Practice Architecture A – Unit-Based Plan (Straight Salary)*
Revenue Element 1

Step 1 Determine practice specialty for salary purposes.
Practice Specialty: General Internal Medicine†

Step 2 Establish salary levels by range of production (measured by WRVU).

Low WRVU	High WRVU	Salary for Range
Under 2,800		$99,600
2,800	3,199	$116,200
3,200	3,599	$132,800
3,600	3,999	$149,400
4,000	4,799	$166,000
4,800	5,199	$182,600
5,200	5,599	$199,200
5,600	5,999	$215,800
6,000	Over 6,000	$232,400

Step 3 Assess physician production level (WRVU) for prior 12 month period.

	WRVU
Dr. A	3,678
Dr. B	4,893
Dr. C	4,102
Dr. D	4,409
Dr. E	2,909
Dr. F	3,789

Step 4 Assign physician salary based on production.

	Salary
Dr. A	$149,400
Dr. B	$182,600
Dr. C	$166,000
Dr. D	$166,000
Dr. E	$116,200
Dr. F	$149,400

* Hypothetical numbers presented for illustrative purposes only. Numbers may not total in all cases due to rounding.
† Different production and salary arrangements developed for each practice specialty.

EXHIBIT 13.8   Assessment of Group Practice Architecture A – Unit-Based Plans

Dimension	Strengths	Weaknesses
Measure	Promotes team and group practice orientation. Encourages "one-for-all-and-all-for-one" orientation. Nonlinkage to ancillary services revenue generation promotes Stark law compliance. Helps prevent cherry-picking and similar behaviors commonly seen in production-oriented plans. Neutralizes impact of payer mix.	May allow for "free rider" physicians with differing production or work levels.
Productivity	Strong production orientation can still be promoted through group practice culture of productivity (as opposed to directly through compensation plan model).	Does not measure or reward differences in individual production. Tends to work best in practices with largely homogeneous production levels and work styles. Productivity culture may be difficult to maintain when there are wide variations in physician work/life expectations due to age, gender, existing financial resources, and values.
Financial		Does not directly promote individual physician attention to cost of practice issues. Requires sound financial management at the group level.
Simplicity	Ease of administration.	
Alignment	Encourages group practice orientation. Teamwork through equal shares or similar per unit compensation method.	May not promote attention to individual physician performance. Generally requires linkage with performance expectations.
"Fairness"	Works well in homogeneous practices where physicians have similar work levels and services and/or are dependent upon external referrals.	Physicians may perceive plan as inequitable given differences in work levels, payer mix, or otherwise.

© 2006 Johnson & Walker Keegan

► GROUP PRACTICE ARCHITECTURE B – GUARANTEED SHARE OF REVENUES OR INCOME (BASE SALARY) PLUS INCENTIVE PLANS
Revenue Element 2

Overview

Group Practice Architecture B uses the second most team-oriented approach to physician compensation (Revenue Element 2 of Exhibit 13.1) by paying each physician a share of practice revenue or income that is entirely or largely guaranteed in the form of a base salary coupled with an incentive component or payment.

Base salary or guaranteed payments under this plan type can be determined based on any number of grounds, such as physician discipline or specialty, seniority or years in the practice, clinical FTE, or a combination of these and other factors that are consistently applied. The base salary is paid and effectively guaranteed. See Chapter 14, plan Examples 4 and 7, for other ways to use Architecture B that involve a guaranteed salary arrangement used in a hospital or academic medical center context. As with all pure team-oriented models, there is no express consideration of practice expenses as part of the physician-specific compensation methodology.

The incentive component of this Architecture B can be linked to any number of incentive measures, including clinical production (e.g., as measured by net collections, WRVUs, or other measures), quality, cost of service, patient satisfaction, and others. In a Group Practice context, incentive measures that focus on quality, satisfaction, and other measures are commonly funded in advance, or are "pre-funded," through the allocation of a defined level of practice income, and are then awarded to individual physicians based on performance measures.

Incentive measures may also be more "additive" in nature, as would be expected with "pay-for-performance" (P4P) reimbursement systems. Under these systems, the overall reimbursement received by a physician and/or medical practice may be contingent upon performance in relation to quality, safety, practice efficiency, information technology utilization, or other measures that are determined and defined by external parties (e.g., third-party payers) rather than by the Group Practice itself. In cases where the incentive is provided on an additive basis, then the practice must still allocate that additional reimbursement (net of practice expenses) on an agreed upon basis. See Chapter 8 for a discussion of P4P and incentive-based reimbursement. The use of nonclinical production measures for physician compensation is discussed in Chapter 10, and examples of plan architectures using qualitative and other nonclinical production-based incentive measures can be found in Chapter 14.

Application

Base plus incentive and similar compensation plans using Architecture B are commonly found in multispecialty practices, hospital-based employment models, and academic practices. They are also used in some single specialty, physician-owned Group Practices. Such plans are commonly used in both small (e.g., fewer than 10 physicians) and large (e.g., more than 100 physicians) multispecialty groups and some faculty practice plans. The incentive component of plans using this Architecture B can also be adapted and applied to any of the other architectures by prefunding the incentive component and awarding incentives on quality, satisfaction, or other grounds, or by allocating additional third-party reimbursement (including that received via P4P, managed care, or other reimbursement systems) based on such measures.

Methodology – Plans with Guaranteed Share of Revenues or Income (Base Salary) Plus Incentives

A basic example of a base salary plus production incentive plan is provided in Example B-1 below, followed by three variations of this basic model (Examples B-2, B-3, and B-4). Examples B-1, B-2, B-3, and B-4 are also illustrated in Exhibits 13.9, 13.10, 13.11, and 13.12, respectively, shown at the end of this section.

Example B-1 – Basic Example of Architecture B: Base Salary Plus Production Incentive

Step 1. Determine Physician Base Salary Levels

Establish base salary levels that will constitute a portion of the physician's compensation that is entirely or largely guaranteed. Base salary levels may be determined through any number of means, including practice specialty or discipline, a combination of specialty and FTE level, or other methods. The base salary is typically set at no more than 60 to 80 percent of the total anticipated compensation. This guaranteed base salary then effectively becomes a portion of the Group Practice's total expenses that must be considered in conjunction with the determination of amounts available for incentive compensation. Example B-1 shows base salaries linked to market levels of compensation (using Medical Group Management Association [MGMA] median or other data as the measure of "market"). Example B-1 also reflects production for individual physicians measured by net collections from professional services, although other measures of production can also be employed.

Step 2. "Prefund" Nonclinical Production Portion of the Incentive Pool

In a physician-owned Group Practice setting, all or a large portion of the total incentive compensation is commonly paid to physicians based on a production basis (e.g., individual production as a percentage of total production). When a portion of incentive is allocated based on performance in relation to quality, patient satisfaction, cost control, or other goals, that portion is commonly prefunded by setting aside a portion of practice net income to be distributed through such incentive measures. Step 2 in Example B-1 shows the establishment of a nonclinical production-based incentive pool linked to quality that is predefined and funded on a flat dollar per physician basis (in this example, $10,000 per each physician); however, other methods can also be used, including a set percentage of base salary, fluctuating pools based on P4P reimbursement mechanisms, and others.

Step 3. Determine the Practice's Net Income Before Determining the Production-Based Incentive

The base salary payments and amounts set aside for payment of nonclinical production-based incentive compensation can be viewed as part of the practice's expense structure that must be deducted before awarding of production-based incentive compensation. Accordingly, the plan methodology must deduct such "expense" amounts from practice revenues in Step 3 to determine the amount available that can be awarded via the production incentive payments.

Step 4. Determine Physician-Specific Compensation

In this example, each individual physician's compensation equals the sum of the physician's base salary, plus the physician's share of the nonclinical production-based incentive compensation (e.g., based on quality, patient satisfaction, and/or other criteria), plus the physician's share of the production-based incentive. In this example, the production-based incentive is awarded on a straight percentage of production basis (with production measured by net collections from professional services).

Examples of methods to award such nonclinical production incentive measures are discussed in Chapter 10, "Special Issues in Physician Compensation." Example B-1 shows that the amount available for physician compensation is reduced by the actual cost of physician-specific direct expenses (e.g., health insurance costs, life insurance, etc.). However, many base plus incentive models include such direct expenses in practice overhead such that the combination of base plus incentive payments equals total compensation.

Step 5. Reconcile to the Base Salary Previously Paid, and Pay the Bonus

The base salary portion of compensation is commonly paid in accordance with a practice's regular pay schedule (e.g., every two weeks or monthly) as a means to provide a stable level of compensation to practice physicians. The amount actually paid through the base salary is then reconciled with the amount earned through the formula (base salary plus incentive payments) on a quarterly, annual, or other periodic basis. The difference is then paid to the physician in the form of a bonus.

Given that the base salary is typically viewed as largely a guaranteed payment, it is possible for a physician to receive a base salary only and no incentive compensation. Practices that adopt compensation systems that involve guaranteed payments will also commonly define other requirements to address performance outliers and, in some cases, reduction of future guaranteed payments based upon practice deficiencies and deficits.

Potential variations of Architecture B are shown in examples B-2 through B-4. These variations involve the following general approaches:

Example B-2

In this example (see Exhibit 13.10), the base salary levels are adjusted by specialty based on FTE level, such that physicians C and E (in this example, part-time physicians with a .80 FTE and .75 FTE, respectively) receive reduced base salaries due to their reduced time commitment. This example also demonstrates prefunding of the quality incentive portion based on a predefined dollar amount per physician FTE (rather than per physician).

Example B-3

Unlike Examples B-1 and B-2, this example uses a practice-defined base salary by physician specialty, rather than linking the base salary to a percentage of market data (Step 1). This example also allocates the production-based incentive portion based on each physician's percentage of WRVUs to total practice WRVUs.

Example B-3 (see Exhibit 13.11) also illustrates a P4P incentive that is awarded by third-party payers based on clinical indicators and practice efficiency. The funds are shown in Step 2, with the award actually being made in Step 4. The method used to award the P4P or quality reward would be an additional step and would potentially use methods such as those described in Chapter 8. This example also shows a reconciliation of the amount earned to the amount paid through the base salary to determine an end-of-year or other bonus amount, but it includes the physician-specific direct expenses of each physician (e.g., health insurance and other costs) as part of practice overhead, rather than directly assigning these costs to each physician.

Example B-4

Example B-4 (see Exhibit 13.12) uses the same allocation method as Example B-2 but adds to this an ancillary services overall profits pool. The profits pool is distributed among the Group Practice's physicians on an equal share per FTE basis, but not every physician in the practice participates in the pool. Specifically, because in this example the practice includes a general surgeon (with typically low levels of ancillary services utilization), the revenues and expenses from ancillary services (e.g., laboratory, dexascans, etc.) are tracked to a separate ancillary services profit-and-loss center and are allocated among some, but not all, of the practice's physicians.

This example illustrates a Stark law compliant compensation method using an overall profit shares methodology, an equal share allocation method (adjusted for FTE level), and the allocation of profits among any subset of the Group Practice comprised of five or more physicians (in this example, eight of nine physicians). Under this methodology, the physicians in the Group Practice share in ancillary services income but on a basis that is only indirectly related to the volume or value of their referrals. Example B-4 also treats all ancillary services the same – regardless of the payer – and, in doing so, adopts a conservative approach to compliance with the Stark law.

As with other team-oriented models, each of these options can also be coupled with any number of additional variations, including requirements linked to minimum performance expectations (e.g., a predefined number of days or weeks worked per year, or a minimum number of patient visits or WRVUs generated). See Chapters 10 and 14 for a discussion of performance expectations. Plan examples are given in Chapter 14 to illustrate how performance expectations can be incorporated into compensation plans. The measures of professional services production for purposes of the incentive component can also vary (e.g., using gross charges, net collections, WRVUs, or other measures).

In multispecialty groups, the concept of primary care support and revenue sharing can also be implemented in such models. To illustrate this concept, a multispecialty group might assess a "tax" against specialty physician revenues and pay proceeds from that tax to primary care (or other) physicians who achieve specific performance expectations or requirements. For example, physicians who achieve median or higher production targets might receive all or part of the incentive payment. Such a system could include a guaranteed base, plus an incentive component linked to individual physician production.

Exhibit 13.13 provides an assessment of Group Practice Architecture B.

EXHIBIT 13.9

Example B-1 –
Group Practice Architecture B – Guaranteed Share (Base Salary) Plus Incentive Plan*
Revenue Element 2

	Total	Dr. A Gen IM	Dr. B Gen IM	Dr. C Gen IM	Dr. D Gen IM	Dr. E FP w/OB	Dr. F FP w/OB	Dr. G Pulm	Dr. H Rheum	Dr. I Gen Surg
Step 1 Assemble production information.										
Median (MGMA) by Specialty		$160,000	$160,000	$160,000	$160,000	$155,000	$155,000	$225,000	$190,000	$280,000
% of Market for Base	70%									
Base Salary (% of market)	$1,151,500	$112,000	$112,000	$112,000	$112,000	$108,500	$108,500	$157,500	$133,000	$196,000
Net Collections from Professional Services	$3,975,000	$480,000	$425,000	$376,000	$400,000	$346,000	$410,200	$458,900	$438,000	$640,900
Physician % to Total Net Collections		12.08%	10.69%	9.46%	10.06%	8.70%	10.32%	11.54%	11.02%	16.12%

Step 2 Determine quality incentive pool per physician.	
incentive pool per physician	$10,000
Number of Physicians	9
Total Quality Incentive Pool	$90,000

Step 3 Determine income for production incentive.	
Revenues	$3,975,000
Expenses	
Nonphysician Overhead	$(2,186,250)
Base Salaries (from above)	$(1,151,500)
Quality Incentive Pool (from above)	$(90,000)
Production-Based Incentive	$547,250

Step 4 — Determine physician-specific compensation.

	Total									
Base Salary	$1,151,500	$112,000	$112,000	$112,000	$112,000	$108,500	$108,500	$157,500	$133,000	$196,000
Quality Incentive Pool Award†	$90,000	$9,000	$10,800	$5,400	$16,200	$900	$7,200	$9,000	$27,000	$4,500
Physician % to Total Net Collections (from above)		12.08%	10.69%	9.46%	10.06%	8.70%	10.32%	11.54%	11.02%	16.12%
Production Incentive Award	$547,250	$66,083	$58,511	$51,765	$55,069	$47,635	$56,473	$63,178	$60,301	$88,235
Total Compensation (before physician-specific direct expenses)		$187,083	$181,311	$169,165	$183,269	$157,035	$172,173	$229,678	$220,301	$288,735
Direct Expenses		$(50,400)	$(52,390)	$(48,983)	$(54,000)	$(40,000)	$(43,000)	$(48,981)	$(50,940)	$(50,009)
W-2 Compensation Earned		$136,683	$128,921	$120,182	$129,269	$117,035	$129,173	$180,697	$169,361	$238,726

Step 5 — Determine end-of-year bonus.

Base Salary Paid		$112,000	$112,000	$112,000	$112,000	$108,500	$108,500	$157,500	$133,000	$196,000
Bonus (end of year)		$24,683	$16,921	$8,182	$17,269	$8,535	$20,673	$23,197	$36,361	$42,726

* Hypothetical numbers presented for illustrative purposes only. Numbers may not total in all cases due to rounding.
† The specific criteria used to reward the quality incentive are not specified in this example; see Chapter 8, "Pay-for-Performance (P4P) and Physician Compensation" and Chapter 10, "Special Issues in Physician Compensation."

Key:
FP w/OB = Family Practice with Obstetrics
FP w/o OB = Family Practice without Obstetrics
Gen IM = General Internal Medicine
Gen Surg = General Surgery
Pulm = Pulmonary Medicine
Rheum = Rheumatology

© 2006 Johnson & Walker Keegan

EXHIBIT 13.10 — Example B-2 – Group Practice Architecture B – Guaranteed Share (Base Salary) Plus Incentive Plan, Adjusted for FTE*
Revenue Element 2

		Total	Dr. A Gen IM	Dr. B Gen IM	Dr. C Gen IM	Dr. D Gen IM	Dr. E FP w/OB	Dr. F FP w/OB	Dr. G Pulm	Dr. H Rheum	Dr. I Gen Surg
Step 1	**Assemble production information.**										
	Median (MGMA) by Specialty		$160,000	$160,000	$160,000	$160,000	$155,000	$155,000	$225,000	$190,000	$280,000
	FTE Level	8.55	1.00	1.00	0.80	1.00	0.75	1.00	1.00	1.00	1.00
	% of Market for Base	70%									
	Base Salary (% of market) x FTE	$1,101,975	$112,000	$112,000	$89,600	$112,000	$81,375	$108,500	$157,500	$133,000	$196,000
	Net Collections from Professional Services	$3,975,000	$480,000	$425,000	$376,000	$400,000	$346,000	$410,200	$458,900	$438,000	$640,900
	Physician % to Total Net Collections		12.08%	10.69%	9.46%	10.06%	8.70%	10.32%	11.54%	11.02%	16.12%
Step 2	**Determine quality incentive pool per FTE.**	$10,000									
	Number of FTE	8.55									
	Total Quality Incentive Pool	$85,500									
Step 3	**Determine income for production incentive.**										
	Revenues	$3,975,000									
	Expenses										
	Nonphysician Overhead	$(2,186,250)									
	Base Salaries (from above)	$(1,101,975)									
	Quality Incentive Pool (from above)	$(85,500)									
	Production-Based Incentive	$601,275									

Step 4 — Determine physician-specific compensation.

	Total									
Base Salary	$1,101,975	$112,000	$112,000	$89,600	$112,000	$81,375	$108,500	$157,500	$133,000	$196,000
Quality Incentive Pool Award†	$85,500	$8,550	$10,260	$5,130	$15,390	$855	$6,840	$8,550	$25,650	$4,275
Physician % to Total Net Collections (from above)		12.08%	10.69%	9.46%	10.06%	8.70%	10.32%	11.54%	11.02%	16.12%
Production Incentive Award	$601,275	$72,607	$64,287	$56,875	$60,506	$52,337	$62,049	$69,415	$66,254	$96,945
Total Compensation (before physician-specific direct expenses)		$193,157	$186,547	$151,605	$187,896	$134,567	$177,389	$235,465	$224,904	$297,220
Direct Expenses		$(50,400)	$(52,390)	$(48,983)	$(54,000)	$(40,000)	$(43,000)	$(48,981)	$(50,940)	$(50,009)
W-2 Compensation Earned		$142,757	$134,157	$102,622	$133,896	$94,567	$134,389	$186,484	$173,964	$247,211

Step 5 — Determine end-of-year bonus.

Base Salary Paid		$112,000	$112,000	$89,600	$112,000	$81,375	$108,500	$157,500	$133,000	$196,000
Bonus (end of year)		$30,757	$22,157	$13,022	$21,896	$13,192	$25,889	$28,984	$40,964	$51,211

* Hypothetical numbers presented for illustrative purposes only. Numbers may not total in all cases due to rounding.

† The specific criteria used to reward the quality incentive are not specified in this example; see Chapter 8, "Pay-for-Performance (P4P) and Physician Compensation" and Chapter 10, "Special Issues in Physician Compensation."

Key:
FP w/OB = Family Practice with Obstetrics
FP w/o OB = Family Practice without Obstetrics
Gen IM = General Internal Medicine
Gen Surg = General Surgery
Pulm = Pulmonary Medicine
Rheum = Rheumatology

EXHIBIT 13.11

Example B-3 – Group Practice Architecture B – Guaranteed Share (Base Salary) Plus Incentive Plan, Additive P4P Quality Bonus Pool*
Revenue Element 2

	Total	Dr. A Gen IM	Dr. B Gen IM	Dr. C Gen IM	Dr. D Gen IM	Dr. E FP w/OB	Dr. F FP w/OB	Dr. G Pulm	Dr. H Rheum	Dr. I Gen Surg
Step 1 **Assemble production information.**										
Base Salary	$1,160,000	$115,000	$115,000	$115,000	$115,000	$115,000	$115,000	$140,000	$130,000	$200,000
WRVU by Physician	44,629	5,614	4,907	4,002	4,156	3,987	4,204	5,872	4,325	7,562
Physician % of WRVU		13%	11%	9%	9%	9%	9%	13%	10%	17%
Step 2 **Total the external P4P award.†**	$173,271									
Step 3 **Determine income for production incentive.**										
Revenues (excluding P4P payment)†	$4,675,000									
Expenses										
Nonphysician Overhead	$(2,571,250)									
Base Salaries (from above)	$(1,160,000)									
Physician Direct Expenses	$(438,703)									
Production-Based Incentive	$505,047									
Step 4 **Determine physician-specific compensation.**										
Base Salary	$1,160,000	$115,000	$115,000	$115,000	$115,000	$115,000	$115,000	$140,000	$130,000	$200,000
P4P Payment‡	$173,271	$1,733	$24,258	$13,862	$32,921	$5,198	$17,327	$25,991	$34,654	$17,327
Physician % of WRVU (from above)		13%	11%	9%	9%	9%	9%	13%	10%	17%
Production Incentive Award	$505,047	$63,531	$55,530	$45,289	$47,032	$45,119	$47,575	$66,451	$48,944	$85,576
W-2 Compensation Earned		$180,264	$194,788	$174,151	$194,953	$165,317	$179,902	$232,442	$213,598	$302,903

Step 5 Determine end-of-year bonus.

Base Salary Paid	$115,000	$115,000	$115,000	$115,000	$115,000	$140,000	$130,000	$200,000
Bonus (end of year)	$65,264	$79,788	$59,151	$79,953	$50,317	$64,902	$92,442	$83,598	$102,903

* Hypothetical numbers presented for illustrative purposes only. Numbers may not total in all cases due to rounding.

† Assumes additional P4P award received from third-party payers.

‡ The specific criteria used to reward the P4P award are not specified in this example; see Chapter 8, "Pay-for-Performance (P4P) and Physician Compensation," for examples.

Key:
FP w/OB = Family Practice with Obstetrics
FP w/o OB = Family Practice without Obstetrics
Gen IM = General Internal Medicine
Gen Surg = General Surgery
Pulm = Pulmonary Medicine
Rheum = Rheumatology

EXHIBIT 13.12

Example B-4 – Group Practice Architecture B – Guaranteed Share (Base Salary) Plus Incentive Plan, Adjusted for FTE with Ancillary Profits Pool*
Revenue Element 2

		Total	Dr. A Gen IM	Dr. B Gen IM	Dr. C Gen IM	Dr. D Gen IM	Dr. E FP w/OB	Dr. F FP w/OB	Dr. G Pulm	Dr. H Rheum	Dr. I Gen Surg
Step 1	**Assemble production information.**										
	Median (MGMA) by Specialty		$160,000	$160,000	$160,000	$160,000	$155,000	$155,000	$225,000	$190,000	$280,000
	FTE Level	8.55	1.00	1.00	0.80	1.00	0.75	1.00	1.00	1.00	1.00
	% of Market for Base	70%									
	Base Salary (% of market) x FTE	$1,101,975	$112,000	$112,000	$89,600	$112,000	$81,375	$108,500	$157,500	$133,000	$196,000
	Net Collections from Professional Services	$3,975,000	$480,000	$425,000	$376,000	$400,000	$346,000	$410,200	$458,900	$438,000	$640,900
	Physician % to Total Net Collections		12%	11%	9%	10%	9%	10%	12%	11%	16%
Step 2	**Determine ancillary profits pool.**										
	Ancillary Services Revenues	$450,870									
	Ancillary Services Expenses	$(345,000)									
	Total Ancillary Services Profits	$105,870									
Step 3	**Determine income for production incentive.**										
	Revenues (excluding ancillary)	$3,975,000									
	Expenses (excluding ancillary)										
	Nonphysician Overhead	$(2,186,250)									
	Base Salaries (from above)	$(1,101,975)									
	Production-Based Incentive	$686,775									

Step 4 — Determine physician-specific compensation.

	Total									
Base Salary	$1,101,975	$112,000	$112,000	$89,600	$112,000	$108,500	$81,375	$157,500	$133,000	$196,000
Physician % to Total Net Collections (from above)		12%	11%	9%	10%	10%	9%	12%	11%	16%
Production Incentive Award	$686,775	$82,931	$73,429	$64,963	$69,109	$70,872	$59,780	$79,286	$75,675	$110,731
Ancillary Participation by Specialty & FTE†	7.55	1.00	1.00	0.80	1.00	1.00	0.75	1.00	1.00	0.00
Ancillary Services Profits Share†	$105,870	$14,023	$14,023	$11,218	$14,023	$14,023	$10,517	$14,023	$14,023	$—
Total Compensation (before physician-specific direct expenses)		$208,954	$199,451	$165,781	$195,132	$193,394	$151,672	$250,808	$222,697	$306,731
Direct Expenses		$(50,400)	$(52,390)	$(48,983)	$(54,000)	$(43,000)	$(40,000)	$(48,981)	$(50,940)	$(50,009)
W-2 Compensation Earned		$158,554	$147,061	$116,798	$141,132	$150,394	$111,672	$201,827	$171,757	$256,722

Step 5 — Determine end-of-year bonus.

Base Salary Paid	$112,000	$112,000	$89,600	$112,000	$108,500	$81,375	$157,500	$133,000	$196,000
Bonus (end of year)	$46,554	$35,061	$27,198	$29,132	$41,894	$30,297	$44,327	$38,757	$60,722

* Hypothetical numbers presented for illustrative purposes only. Numbers may not total in all cases due to rounding.
† Ancillary services profits allocated on equal share, adjusted by FTE among all physicians other than general surgery.

Key:
FP w/OB = Family Practice with Obstetrics
FP w/o OB = Family Practice without Obstetrics
Gen IM = General Internal Medicine
Gen Surg = General Surgery
Pulm = Pulmonary Medicine
Rheum = Rheumatology

© 2006 Johnson & Walker Keegan

EXHIBIT 13.13 Assessment of Group Practice Architecture B –
Guaranteed Share of Revenues or Income (Base Salary) Plus Incentive

Dimension	Strengths	Weaknesses
Measure	Promotes team and group practice orientation through base salary component. Nonlinkage to ancillary services revenue generation promotes Stark law compliance. Provides guaranteed payments that can be linked to practice discipline. Allows for combined measurement of production and other incentive measures, such as quality, patient satisfaction, and others.	May allow for "free rider" physicians with differing production or work levels. Inherent challenges in measuring quality, satisfaction, and other "subjective" issues through incentive measure.
Productivity	Strong production orientation can still be promoted through incentive measures.	Production portion of compensation may be insufficient to truly motivate performance.
Financial	Portion of income is stable, portion is production-oriented.	Does not promote individual physician attention to cost of practice issues. Requires sound financial management at the group level.
Simplicity	Ease of administration. Relatively straightforward and understandable.	Base or "guaranteed" payments must be established via some means, resulting in potential questions regarding the perceived "fairness" of plan. Incentive measure may add significant complexity.
Alignment	Encourages group practice orientation. Teamwork promoted through base salary or other "guaranteed" payments.	May not promote sufficient attention to individual physician performance. Linkage with performance expectations is generally required.
"Fairness"	Works well in practices where physicians are generally working at similar levels, when compared to peers in the same practice specialty (e.g., at or above median for specialty).	Physicians may perceive plan as inequitable given differences in work levels, payer mix, or otherwise.

© 2006 Johnson & Walker Keegan

► GROUP PRACTICE ARCHITECTURE C – COMBINED EQUAL SHARE AND PRODUCTION ALLOCATION OF REVENUES OR INCOME PLANS
Revenue Element 3

Overview

This plan type uses the third most team-oriented approach to physician compensation (Revenue Element 3 only, in Exhibit 13.1). It allocates practice net income on a combined equal share and production basis. In a Group Practice setting, this plan can help promote teamwork and group practice perspective via the equal share component, while also allowing for a consideration of differences in production levels due to work variation, payer mix, practice subspecialty or the like. Thus, this model combines both a team and production orientation, but it does so without any express consideration of practice operating expenses (other than physician-specific direct expense costs).

Architecture C (as well as other architectures) can also include additional incentive measures, including those relating to quality, cost of service, patient satisfaction, and other measures. See Chapters 8 and 10, and the discussion regarding Architecture B related to the funding and awarding of these types of quality and other measures in the compensation architecture, including how such measures can be developed and used in conjunction with emerging "P4P" reimbursement systems.

Application

Combined equal share and production-based models are commonly found in single specialty practices or in divisions of multispecialty Group Practices. They are commonly used within a single specialty to address the increasing subspecialization and the need to differentiate compensation levels based on subspecialty activity. Common physician specialties in which such plans are used include primary care; medical subspecialties such as cardiology, pulmonary medicine, and medical oncology; and surgical specialties such as orthopedics, general surgery, cardiovascular surgery, vascular surgery, urology, and others. These plans are also used in hospital-based specialties, including emergency medicine, radiology, pathology, and hospitalist groups.

A common issue to be addressed in these Group Practices relates to the level of compensation that should be considered "equal share" vs. the amount that should vary based on individual physician performance. The portion of revenue or income that is divided on an equal share basis generally ranges from a high of 75 percent to a low of 25 percent. Factors that impact the level of revenues or income that is identified for equal share treatment commonly include:

► The degree of variation between physician production levels;

► Differences in payer mix;

► The current level of revenue or income sharing in the practice at the time the new compensation plan is being developed; and/or

► Outreach and "home-base" practice environments (e.g., in cardiology practices in which interventional physicians are located at the hospital, and noninvasive cardiologists are in outreach locations).

When an equal share portion of revenues or income is applied to all physicians in a multispecialty group practice, the level of sharing on an equal share basis is generally relatively slight (e.g., less than 10 percent).

Methodology – Combined Equal Share and Production Plans

A basic plan example for Architecture C is presented below for an orthopedic surgery practice (Example C-1), followed by three variations on the basic approach (Examples C-2 through C-4). Note that this architecture can apply to single specialty groups, to a specific specialty within a multispecialty group, or to a multispecialty group more generally. Examples C-1 through C-4 are illustrated in Exhibits 13.14 through 13.17, respectively, shown at the end of this section.

Example C-1 – Basic Example of Architecture C: Equal Share and Production-Based Plan Variation

Step 1. Determine Physician Production, FTE, and Other Levels
Assess and determine physician production using a standard method (e.g., net collections or gross charges from professional services, WRVUs, or other measures). Example C-1 includes physician FTE levels such that the equal share portion of the plan is adjusted by the physician FTE level. In Example C-1, production levels for individual physicians are measured and reported as net collections from professional services, although other production measures (e.g., WRVUs) may also be used.

Step 2. Determine Net Practice Income
In a physician-owned Group Practice, determine the total amount of income available for payment of physician compensation and benefits. This is a simple calculation involving the subtraction of practice overhead expenses (excluding physician salaries and physician-specific direct expenses) from total practice revenues to yield a net income number that is also referred to in Example C-1 as the "compensation pool."

Step 3. Allocate Net Income Based on Equal Share and Production
The total practice net income is allocated such that a predefined portion is assigned on an equal share per physician basis, and the remaining is assigned based on a percentage of production. Example C-1 (see Exhibit 13.14) uses a 25 percent equal share/75 percent production allocation method. Other common variations involve 50 percent equal share/50 percent production allocation or 75 percent equal share/25 percent production allocation methods. The precise allocation percentage varies depending on a number of factors (as discussed above). Example C-1 also adjusts the equal share portion based on each physician's FTE level (e.g., a .80 FTE physician receives 80 percent of an equal share allocation).

Step 4. Determine Physician-Specific Compensation

In this basic example, each individual physician's compensation equals the sum of the physician's equal share portion of practice net income, plus the physician's production-based share of practice net income. As in other examples, Example C-1 illustrates the direct allocation of employee benefits and similar expenses to each individual physician.

The basic mathematical formula used in this architecture is as follows:

Practice Revenues
− Practice Overhead Expenses
———————————————
Compensation Pool

Physician-Specific Compensation Equals:

Equal Share Portion (Adjusted by FTE)
+ Production-Based Portion
− Physician-Specific Direct Expenses
———————————————
Physician Cash (Take Home) Compensation

Step 5. Reconcile to the Advance Previously Paid, and Pay the Bonus

In this example, an advance or draw on total compensation is commonly paid in accordance with a practice's regular pay schedule (e.g., every two weeks or monthly) as a means to provide a stable level of compensation to practice physicians. The amount actually paid through the advance or draw is then reconciled with the amount earned through the formula on a quarterly, annual, or other periodic basis. The difference is then paid to the physician in the form of a bonus. The advance or draw in this case is, in practical terms, "at risk" in that it is not a guaranteed payment as in those examples using Architecture B (discussed previously). Accordingly, in plans such as this, which use an advance or draw on total anticipated compensation, the compensation plan must generally also consider practice "deficits" or "overpayments" when the actual amount earned under the plan is *less* than the amount advanced via the draw mechanism. In such circumstances, subsequent advances or draw amounts are typically reduced to repay the deficit, and the draw amount may also be reduced to help prevent subsequent deficits.

Potential variations of Architecture C are shown in Examples C-2 through C-4 and are described below.

Example C-2

Example C-2 (illustrated in Exhibit 13.15) adjusts the equal share and production portions to a 50 percent/50 percent treatment. It also uses an ancillary services profits pool that is allocated on a largely equal share basis among practice physicians, with the exception of Drs. C and H. This example shows that Dr. H (a spine surgeon at 1.0 FTE) and Dr. C (a general orthopedic surgeon at .8 FTE) participate in the ancillary services profits at lower levels given their practice specialties and time commitments to the practice. The distribution of net profits from ancillary services is based on two methods: (1) 25 percent based on professional service production (individual physician production as a percentage of total production); and (2) 75 percent based on a pro rata share. The spine surgeon and the part-time physician each receive lower levels of pro rata participation in the ancillary services profits.

The awarding of different levels of ancillary profits is acceptable under the Stark law, because compensation is still not directly related to referrals. Likewise, the productivity portion of the ancillary services distribution is based on the physicians' personally performed services and on services "incident to" such services – in this case, as measured by net collections from professional services. It is not related to the volume of ancillary services production and therefore is not directly related to ancillary referrals.

Example C-3

This variation of the basic plan measures production through a combination of net collections from professional services and WRVUs in an effort to take payer mix into consideration. This example includes a P4P award bonus that is aligned with reimbursement by third-party payers. The P4P award is illustrated in Step 3, with the award actually being distributed to practice physicians in Step 4C. The method used to award the P4P dollars is an additional step and can potentially use other methods such as those described in Chapter 8.

In example C-3 (see Exhibit 13.16), the compensation pool is allocated based on a 60 percent equal share basis, with 40 percent allocated based on production. The 40 percent production portion is allocated in Step 4B based on two methods. In this example, one-half of the production portion (20 percent of the total compensation pool) is allocated based on the individual physician's net collections from professional services as a percentage to total net collections from professional services. The remaining half of the production portion (20 percent of the total compensation pool) is allocated based on the individual physician's WRVUs as a percentage of total WRVUs. This dual treatment of production is used as a means to balance payer mix fluctuations among the physicians. Step 4C in this example reflects the treatment of a P4P pool allocated in two ways. Fifty percent of the pool is allocated on an equal share basis, adjusted for physician FTE level. The remaining 50 percent is allocated for production based on individual physician net collections as a percentage to total net collections.

Consistent with other plan examples, a reconciliation of the amount earned to the amount paid is conducted to determine a bonus amount that is paid to the physician at the end of year or on another agreed upon time frame.

Example C-4

In Example C-4 (see Exhibit 13.17), production is measured through the use of net collections from professional services, but the plan also includes an "equal share" portion in the allocation of net collections. The equal share portion is designed as a means to reasonably shift some level of "support" from specialists to primary care physicians in the Group Practice, to recognize the "multiplier" effect of primary care referrals to specialties, and/or to ensure competitive levels of primary care compensation to aid recruitment and retention. This is accomplished by the "sharing" of revenues before allocation of income as a means of shifting the level of production credited to each physician. This model example uses a small (5 percent) of equal share reallocation of net collections, with adjustments for FTE levels. This plan example should not be interpreted to mean that this "revenue-sharing" approach is required in each multispecialty practice. It should be noted that, in many practices, primary care physicians are expected to function as their own financially viable cost center. Here, too, the particular practice culture will impact the compensation plan that is likely to be viewed as acceptable for a particular practice.

As with other team-oriented plans, each of these options can also be coupled with any number of additional variations, including requirements linked to minimum performance expectations, different measures of production, different combinations of equal share and production (e.g., 10 percent equal share/90 percent production, 20 percent equal share/80 percent production, 60 percent equal share/40 percent production, etc.), and multiple measures based upon practice goals and incentive objectives. See Chapters 10 and 14 for a discussion of performance expectations, and plan examples in Chapter 14 for illustrations of how performance expectations can be incorporated into compensation plans.

Exhibit 13.18 provides an assessment of Group Practice Architecture C.

EXHIBIT 13.14

Example C-1 – Group Practice Architecture C – Combined Equal Share (25%) and Production (75%) Income Allocation Plan*
Revenue Element 3

		Total	Dr. A Gen Ortho	Dr. B Gen Ortho	Dr. C Gen Ortho	Dr. D Foot/Ankle	Dr. E Hand	Dr. F Sports	Dr. G Sports	Dr. H Spine
Step 1	**Assemble production information.**									
	FTE Level	7.80	1.00	1.00	0.80	1.00	1.00	1.00	1.00	1.00
	Net Collections from Professional Services	$6,907,387	$750,000	$825,000	$700,350	$815,000	$856,004	$958,000	$1,025,012	$978,021
	Physician % to Total Net Collections		11%	12%	10%	12%	12%	14%	15%	14%
Step 2	**Determine practice net income.**									
	Revenues	$6,907,387								
	Expenses									
	Nonphysician Overhead	$(3,108,324)								
	Compensation Pool	$3,799,063								
Step 3	**Determine physician-specific compensation.**									
	Equal Share Component (25%)	$949,766								
	Equal Share (adjusted by FTE)		$121,765	$121,765	$97,412	$121,765	$121,765	$121,765	$121,765	$121,765
	Production Share Component (75%)									
	Physician % to Total Net Collections (from above)		11%	12%	10%	12%	12%	14%	15%	14%
	Production Share	$2,849,297	$309,375	$340,313	$288,894	$336,188	$353,102	$395,175	$422,817	$403,434

Step 4	**Determine total compensation (before physician-specific direct expenses).**	$431,140	$462,077	$386,306	$457,952	$474,866	$516,940	$544,582	$525,198
	Direct Expenses	$(50,400)	$(52,390)	$(48,983)	$(54,000)	$(40,000)	$(43,000)	$(48,981)	$(50,940)
	W-2 Compensation Earned	$380,740	$409,687	$337,323	$403,952	$434,866	$473,940	$495,601	$474,258
Step 5	**Determine end-of-year bonus.**								
	Advance/Draw Paid	$300,000	$300,000	$300,000	$300,000	$300,000	$300,000	$300,000	$300,000
	Bonus (end of year)	$80,740	$109,687	$37,323	$103,952	$134,866	$173,940	$195,601	$174,258

* Hypothetical numbers presented for illustrative purposes only. Numbers may not total in all cases due to rounding.

Key:
Gen Ortho = General Orthopedic Surgery

© 2006 Johnson & Walker Keegan

EXHIBIT 13.15

Example C-2 – Group Practice Architecture C –
Combined Equal Share (50%) and Production (50%) Income Allocation, with Ancillary Services Profits Pool Plan*
Revenue Element 3

		Total	Dr. A Gen Ortho	Dr. B Gen Ortho	Dr. C Gen Ortho	Dr. D Foot/Ankle	Dr. E Hand	Dr. F Sports	Dr. G Sports	Dr. H Spine
Step 1	**Assemble production information.**									
	FTE Level	7.80	1.00	1.00	0.80	1.00	1.00	1.00	1.00	1.00
	Net Collections from Professional Services	$6,907,387	$750,000	$825,000	$700,350	$815,000	$856,004	$958,000	$1,025,012	$978,021
	Physician % to Total Net Collections		11%	12%	10%	12%	12%	14%	15%	14%
	Participation in Ancillary Profits	7.05	1.00	1.00	0.80	1.00	1.00	1.00	1.00	0.25
Step 2	**Determine practice net income (excluding ancillary).**									
	Revenues (excluding ancillary)	$6,907,387								
	Expenses (excluding ancillary) Nonphysician Overhead	$(3,108,324)								
	Compensation Pool	$3,799,063								
Step 3	**Determine ancillary services profits pool (e.g., MRI and X-ray).**									
	Ancillary Services Revenues	$1,890,290								
	Ancillary Services Expenses	$(1,209,936)								
		$680,354								
Step 4	**Determine physician-specific compensation.**									
	Ancillary Services Profits Pool	$510,266								

	Total								
Equal Share (with adjustments) (75%)†	7.05	1.00	1.00	0.80	1.00	1.00	1.00	1.00	0.25
		$72,378	$72,378	$57,902	$72,378	$72,378	$72,378	$72,378	$18,095
Production Share (25%)	$170,089	$18,468	$20,315	$17,246	$20,069	$21,078	$23,590	$25,240	$24,083
Compensation Pool									
Equal Share Component (50%)	$1,899,531	$243,530	$243,530	$194,824	$243,530	$243,530	$243,530	$243,530	$243,530
Production Share Component (50%)									
Physician % to Total Net Collections (from above)		11%	12%	10%	12%	12%	14%	15%	14%
Production Share	$1,899,531	$206,250	$226,875	$192,596	$224,125	$235,401	$263,450	$281,878	$268,956
Step 5 **Determine total compensation (ancillary share + equal share + production share).**									
Total Compensation (before physician-specific direct expenses)		$540,626	$563,098	$462,568	$560,101	$572,387	$602,948	$623,026	$554,663
Direct Expenses		$(50,400)	$(52,390)	$(48,983)	$(54,000)	$(40,000)	$(43,000)	$(48,981)	$(50,940)
W-2 Compensation Earned		$490,226	$510,708	$413,585	$506,101	$532,387	$559,948	$574,045	$503,723
Step 6 **Determine end-of-year bonus.**									
Advance/Draw Paid		$300,000	$300,000	$300,000	$300,000	$300,000	$300,000	$300,000	$300,000
Bonus (end of year)		$190,226	$210,708	$113,585	$206,101	$232,387	$259,948	$274,045	$203,723

* Hypothetical numbers presented for illustrative purposes only. Numbers may not total in all cases due to rounding.

† Pro rata shares adjusted for Drs. C and H. See narrative description for additional information.

Key:
Gen Ortho = General Orthopedic Surgery

EXHIBIT 13.16

Example C-3 – Group Practice Architecture C – Combined Equal Share (60%) and Production (40%) Income Allocation, with P4P Incentive Pool Plan*

Revenue Element 3

		Total	Dr. A Gen Ortho	Dr. B Gen Ortho	Dr. C Gen Ortho	Dr. D Foot/Ankle	Dr. E Hand	Dr. F Sports	Dr. G Sports	Dr. H Spine
Step 1	Assemble production information.									
	FTE Level	7.80	1.00	1.00	0.80	1.00	1.00	1.00	1.00	1.00
	Net Collections from Professional Services	$6,907,387	$750,000	$825,000	$700,350	$815,000	$856,004	$958,000	$1,025,012	$978,021
	Physician % to Total Net Collections		11%	12%	10%	12%	12%	14%	15%	14%
	Professional Services Production (WRVUs)	65,078	7,284	7,952	6,700	8,011	8,450	8,741	9,531	8,409
	Physician % to Total WRVUs		11%	12%	10%	12%	13%	13%	15%	13%
Step 2	Determine practice net income (excluding ancillary).									
	Revenues (excluding ancillary)	$6,907,387								
	Expenses (excluding ancillary) Nonphysician Overhead	$(3,108,324)								
	Compensation Pool	$3,799,063								
Step 3	Determine pay-for-performance award (awarded by third-party payers).	$324,500								
Step 4	Determine physician-specific compensation.									
Step 4A	Equal Share per FTE (60%)	$2,279,438	$292,236	$292,236	$233,788	$292,236	$292,236	$292,236	$292,236	$292,236

Step 4B	**Production Share (40% total)**									
Physician % to Total Net Collections (from above)			11%	12%	10%	12%	12%	14%	15%	14%
Collections Share (20% of total)	$759,813		$82,500	$90,750	$77,039	$89,650	$94,160	$105,380	$112,751	$107,582
Physician % to WRVU Share (from above)			11%	12%	10%	12%	13%	13%	15%	13%
WRVU Share (20% of total)	$759,813		$85,044	$92,843	$78,225	$93,532	$98,657	$102,055	$111,278	$98,179
			$459,779	$475,828	$389,052	$475,417	$485,053	$499,670	$516,265	$497,996
Step 4C	**P4P Pool**									
Equal Share per FTE (50% of P4P pool)	$162,250	7.80	1.00	1.00	0.80	1.00	1.00	1.00	1.00	1.00
			$20,801	$20,801	$16,641	$20,801	$20,801	$20,801	$20,801	$20,801
Production Share (50% of P4P pool)	$162,250									
Physician % to Total Net Collections (from above)			11%	12%	10%	12%	12%	14%	15%	14%
			$17,617	$19,379	$16,451	$19,144	$20,107	$22,503	$24,077	$22,973
			$38,418	$40,180	$33,092	$39,945	$40,908	$43,304	$44,878	$43,774
Step 5	**Determine total compensation (equal share + production share + P4P share).**									
Total Compensation (before physician-specific direct expenses)			$413,154	$423,166	$343,919	$421,831	$427,304	$440,920	$449,865	$443,592
Direct Expenses			$(50,400)	$(52,390)	$(48,983)	$(54,000)	$(40,000)	$(43,000)	$(48,981)	$(50,940)
W-2 Compensation Earned			$362,754	$370,776	$294,936	$367,831	$387,304	$397,920	$400,884	$392,652
Step 6	**Determine end-of-year bonus.**									
Advance/Draw Paid			$300,000	$300,000	$300,000	$300,000	$300,000	$300,000	$300,000	$300,000
Bonus (end of year)†			$62,754	$70,776	$(5,064)	$67,831	$87,304	$97,920	$100,884	$92,652

* Hypothetical numbers presented for illustrative purposes only. Numbers may not total in all cases due to rounding.
† Deficit in case of Dr. C would be addressed by reduction in compensation paid during future periods, reduction in future advances, or both.

Key:
Gen Ortho = General Orthopedic Surgery

© 2006 Johnson & Walker Keegan

EXHIBIT 13.17

Example C-4 – Group Practice Architecture C –
Combined Equal Share and Production
(Net Collections as Production Measure) Plan*
Revenue Element 3

Step 1 Assemble practice net income (including ancillary).

Total Net Collections	$14,389,420
Expenses	
Nonphysician Overhead	$(8,345,864)
Compensation Pool	$6,043,556

Step 2 Determine physician production percentage.

Physician	Specialty	FTE	Professional Services Net Collections	5% Equal Share FTE	Adjusted Collections	Physician % to Total Adjusted Collections
Dr. A	Family Practice	1	$365,502	$26,054	$391,556	3.77%
Dr. B	Family Practice	1	$315,387	$26,054	$341,440	3.28%
Dr. C	Family Practice	1	$411,133	$26,054	$437,187	4.21%
Dr. D	Internal Medicine	0.8	$370,260	$20,843	$391,103	3.76%
Dr. E	Internal Medicine	0.75	$318,255	$19,540	$337,795	3.25%
Dr. F	Internal Medicine	1	$365,378	$26,054	$391,432	3.77%
Dr. G	Internal Medicine	1	$346,002	$26,054	$372,055	3.58%
Dr. H	Internal Medicine	0.9	$324,904	$23,448	$348,352	3.35%
Dr. I	Internal Medicine	0.75	$301,120	$19,540	$320,661	3.08%
Dr. J	Internal Medicine	0.8	$317,171	$20,843	$338,014	3.25%
Dr. K	Rheumatology	1	$354,851	$26,054	$380,905	3.66%
Dr. L	Cardiology	1	$548,233	$26,054	$574,287	5.52%
Dr. M	Cardiology	1	$864,741	$26,054	$890,795	8.57%
Dr. N	Pulmonary Medicine	1	$437,646	$26,054	$463,700	4.46%
Dr. O	Gastroenterology	1	$745,059	$26,054	$771,113	7.42%
Dr. P	Gastroenterology	1	$870,637	$26,054	$896,691	8.63%
Dr. Q	General Surgery	1	$474,023	$26,054	$500,076	4.81%
Dr. R	General Surgery	1	$643,668	$26,054	$669,722	6.44%
Dr. S	General Orthopedic Surgery	1	$734,352	$26,054	$760,406	7.31%
Dr. T	General Orthopedic Surgery	1	$792,103	$26,054	$818,157	7.87%
Total		19	$9,900,426	$495,021	$10,395,447	100.00%

Step 3   **Allocate compensation pool on % to total basis.**   ($6,043,556 Total)

Physician	Compensation Pool	Direct Benefit Cost	W-2 Compensation
Dr. A	$227,637	$(36,822)	$190,815
Dr. B	$198,502	$(37,872)	$160,630
Dr. C	$254,165	$(43,292)	$210,873
Dr. D	$227,374	$(38,984)	$188,390
Dr. E	$196,383	$(41,292)	$155,091
Dr. F	$227,565	$(40,292)	$187,273
Dr. G	$216,300	$(40,312)	$175,988
Dr. H	$202,520	$(23,623)	$178,897
Dr. I	$186,421	$(30,121)	$156,300
Dr. J	$196,510	$(35,632)	$160,878
Dr. K	$221,445	$(41,002)	$180,443
Dr. L	$333,871	$(46,523)	$287,348
Dr. M	$517,878	$(49,523)	$468,355
Dr. N	$269,579	$(42,512)	$227,067
Dr. O	$448,298	$(48,563)	$399,735
Dr. P	$521,305	$(49,652)	$471,653
Dr. Q	$290,727	$(50,121)	$240,606
Dr. R	$389,353	$(48,212)	$341,141
Dr. S	$442,074	$(49,325)	$392,749
Dr. T	$475,648	$(47,563)	$428,085
Total	$6,043,556	$(841,238)	$5,202,318

* Hypothetical numbers presented for illustrative purposes only. Numbers may not total in all cases due to rounding.

EXHIBIT 13.18 Assessment of Group Practice Architecture C – Combined Equal Share and Production Plans

Dimension	Strengths	Weaknesses
Measure	Promotes team and group practice orientation through equal share component. Allows for combined measurement of production and other incentive measures, such as quality, patient satisfaction, and others. Can use any number of measures to balance work and payer mix (e.g., WRVUs, net collections, gross charges, etc.).	Determinations required regarding equal share portion. Equal share portion selected may continually be questioned or renegotiated.
Productivity	Strong production orientation can be promoted by direct production measure. Combination of equal share and production can be used to address physician transition or part-time issues and other variations in physician work/life expectations due to age, existing financial resources, and values.	Inherent conflict is likely between physicians who prefer larger (or smaller) production portions of compensation.
Financial	Portion of income is stable, portion is production-oriented.	Physicians are likely to have varying perceptions of the "overhead" each is "paying" (in the form of income forgone). Does not promote direct individual physician attention to cost of practice issues. Requires sound financial management at the group level.
Simplicity	Ease of administration. Relatively simple and easy to understand.	Equal share portion of income must be established via some means, and perceived "fairness" may be questioned.

Dimension	Strengths	Weaknesses
Alignment	Encourages group practice orientation. Teamwork is promoted through the equal share portion. Individual physician production is promoted through production portion.	Depending upon the equal share portion, may not promote attention to individual physician performance. Linkage with performance expectations generally helpful, though not required (e.g., to allow for reduction of equal share when less than 1.0 FTE).
"Fairness"	Works well in single specialty practices where physicians have some degree of overlap, but where work levels may also diverge. Some level of equal share is relatively common in multispecialty practices in order to promote internal referrals.	Physicians may perceive plan as inequitable given differences in work levels, payer mix, or otherwise.

© 2006 Johnson & Walker Keegan

▶ GROUP PRACTICE ARCHITECTURE D – PURE PRODUCTION-BASED PLANS
Revenue Element 4

Overview

In Group Practice Architecture D, net income of the Group Practice is allocated on a pure production basis. This architecture is team-oriented in that it does not expressly assign practice operating expenses as part of the compensation equation, but instead uses Revenue Element 4 to reward compensation based on a pure production basis. This method rewards production at the individual level but also promotes teamwork by paying practice expenses at the aggregate level and not assigning such expenses to any individual physician. Thus, while this architecture does promote teamwork, it is more individualistic in nature than Architectures A, B, or C.

Application

Single specialty medical practices may see this plan as a good blend of group and individual focus, while rewarding and encouraging production. The plan is also used in some small- to medium-size multispecialty groups, although the use of such models in a pure form is increasingly difficult due to differing levels of production and ancillary services usage by different practice specialties. With appropriate modifications, plans of this nature are also commonly used in individual departments and divisions of multispecialty groups and in faculty practice plans.

Methodology – Pure Production-Based Plans

The basic plan methodology for a multispecialty practice is depicted below in Example D-1 (illustrated in Exhibit 13.19). In this example, the Group Practice consists of primary care, medical specialties, and surgical specialties. Two additional plan variations are presented in order of increasing complexity to demonstrate compensation plans employing this architecture (Examples D-2 and D-3 are illustrated in Exhibits 13.20 and 13.21), shown at the end of this section.

Example D-1 – Basic Example of Architecture D: Pure Production Plan Using Net Income

Step 1. Determine Practice "Net Income" (Revenues Net of Expenses)
In this example, all revenue – including "incident to" and ancillary services revenue – is pooled, and all practice expenses, excluding physician-specific direct expenses, are deducted to create a "compensation pool" that is then allocated among physicians in the Group Practice.

Step 2. Allocate Net Income

Net income of the practice is allocated on a straight individual physician production basis as a percentage of total production. Production can be measured through a single measure (as in this example) through gross charges from professional services (excluding ancillary services), or through a mixed allocation method, such as a portion based on each individual physician's WRVUs as a percentage of total WRVUs, combined with a portion based on individual net collections from professional services as a percentage of total net collections (e.g., 40 percent/60 percent split). Variations of the basic approach to this architecture are provided in Examples D-2 and D-3, as well as variations that take into account differing approaches to support primary care physicians within a multispecialty Group Practice.

Although Example D-1 does not furnish production credit for "incident to" services, such services can, in fact, be included in determining each physician's production for purposes of productivity bonuses under the Stark law's in-office ancillary services exception. See Chapter 9 for a more complete review of these concepts.

Step 3. Determine Physician-Specific Compensation

Practice-Specific Amount Available for Compensation and Physician Direct Expenses
− Physician-Specific Direct Expenses
───────────────────────────────────────
Physician Cash (Take Home) Compensation

Variations of Architecture D are shown in Examples D-2 and D-3.

Example D-2

This plan variation (illustrated in Exhibit 13.20) uses adjusted gross charges as the basis for measuring production. For such purposes, adjusted gross charges are measured by applying the specialty-specific gross collection rate as a means to adjust to the specialty-specific payer mix, rather than applying the group-wide collection percentage.

Example D-3

Under this plan (illustrated in Exhibit 13.21), net income from the practice is allocated on a combined percentage of WRVUs and percentage of net collections from professional services basis. Thus, physician production is measured through two different metrics. For purposes of the Stark law, this plan uses a "productivity bonus" methodology so that each physician's "production" for bonus purposes can be determined based on the WRVUs or net collections generated through the physician's personally performed services, as well as on services that are "incident to" the physician's personally performed services. Accordingly, this measure of production can include WRVUs and net collection production "credit" for services that are incident to services of the physician (i.e., services of nurses working under physician supervision, or physical therapy services furnished and billed on an "incident to" basis).

These and other models can, through a combination of measures (e.g., net collections from professional services and WRVUs), neutralize or minimize payer mix discrepancies among physicians. The plans used in Architecture D (as well as other architectures) can also include bonus pools that are awarded by third-party payers based on clinical indicators or quality, administrative efficiency, and other measures, as might be seen in a P4P reimbursement environment. Such bonus pools can also be created, however, within a Group Practice by withholding a portion of net collections to "fund" a bonus pool that rewards physicians based on quality, patient satisfaction, or other measures.

As with other team-oriented models, each of these options in Architecture D can also be coupled with any number of additional variations, including requirements linked to minimum performance expectations, different measures of production, and multiple measures based upon practice goals and incentive objectives. See Chapters 10 and 14 for a discussion of performance expectations, and plan examples in Chapter 14 for illustrations of how performance expectations can be incorporated into compensation plans.

Exhibit 13.22 presents the strengths and weaknesses of Architecture D.

EXHIBIT 13.19

Example D-1 – Group Practice Architecture D –
Pure Production (Professional Services Gross Charges) Plan*
Revenue Element 4

Step 1 Assemble practice net income (including ancillary).

Total Net Collections	$14,389,420
Expenses	
Nonphysician Overhead	$(8,345,864)
Compensation Pool	$6,043,556

Step 2 Determine physician production percentage.

Physician	Specialty	Professional Services Gross Charges	Physician % to Total Gross Charges
Dr. A	Family Practice	$562,311	2.93%
Dr. B	Family Practice	$485,210	2.53%
Dr. C	Family Practice	$632,512	3.30%
Dr. D	Internal Medicine	$569,631	2.97%
Dr. E	Internal Medicine	$489,623	2.56%
Dr. F	Internal Medicine	$562,120	2.93%
Dr. G	Internal Medicine	$532,310	2.78%
Dr. H	Internal Medicine	$499,852	2.61%
Dr. I	Internal Medicine	$463,262	2.42%
Dr. J	Internal Medicine	$487,956	2.55%
Dr. K	Rheumatology	$563,256	2.94%
Dr. L	Cardiology	$1,245,985	6.50%
Dr. M	Cardiology	$1,965,321	10.26%
Dr. N	Pulmonary Medicine	$754,562	3.94%
Dr. O	Gastroenterology	$1,585,232	8.27%
Dr. P	Gastroenterology	$1,852,420	9.67%
Dr. Q	General Surgery	$1,128,625	5.89%
Dr. R	General Surgery	$1,532,543	8.00%
Dr. S	General Orthopedic Surgery	$1,562,452	8.15%
Dr. T	General Orthopedic Surgery	$1,685,326	8.80%
Total		$19,160,509	100.00%

Step 3 **Allocate compensation pool on % to total basis.** ($6,043,556 Total)

Physician	Physician Allocation of Gross Charges	Direct Benefit Cost	W-2 Compensation
Dr. A	$177,363	$(36,822)	$140,541
Dr. B	$153,044	$(37,872)	$115,172
Dr. C	$199,505	$(43,292)	$156,213
Dr. D	$179,671	$(38,984)	$140,687
Dr. E	$154,436	$(41,292)	$113,144
Dr. F	$177,302	$(40,292)	$137,010
Dr. G	$167,900	$(40,312)	$127,588
Dr. H	$157,662	$(23,623)	$134,039
Dr. I	$146,121	$(30,121)	$116,000
Dr. J	$153,910	$(35,632)	$118,278
Dr. K	$177,661	$(41,002)	$136,659
Dr. L	$393,005	$(46,523)	$346,482
Dr. M	$619,896	$(49,523)	$570,373
Dr. N	$238,002	$(42,512)	$195,490
Dr. O	$500,010	$(48,563)	$451,447
Dr. P	$584,285	$(49,652)	$534,633
Dr. Q	$355,988	$(50,121)	$305,867
Dr. R	$483,391	$(48,212)	$435,179
Dr. S	$492,824	$(49,325)	$443,499
Dr. T	$531,581	$(47,563)	$484,018
Total	$6,043,556	$(841,238)	$5,202,318

* Hypothetical numbers presented for illustrative purposes only. Numbers may not total in all cases due to rounding.

© 2006 Johnson & Walker Keegan

EXHIBIT 13.20

Example D-2 – Group Practice Architecture D –
Pure Production (Adjusted Charges) Plan *
Revenue Element 4

Step 1 **Assemble practice net income (including ancillary).**

Total Net Collections	$14,389,420
Expenses	
Nonphysician Overhead	$(8,345,864)
Compensation Pool	$6,043,556

Step 2 **Determine physician production percentage.**

Physician	Specialty	Professional Services Gross Charges	Specialty Collection %	Adjusted Gross Charges	Physician % to Total Adjusted Gross Charges
Dr. A	Family Practice	$562,311	65%	$365,502	3.69%
Dr. B	Family Practice	$485,210	65%	$315,387	3.19%
Dr. C	Family Practice	$632,512	65%	$411,133	4.15%
Dr. D	Internal Medicine	$569,631	65%	$370,260	3.74%
Dr. E	Internal Medicine	$489,623	65%	$318,255	3.21%
Dr. F	Internal Medicine	$562,120	65%	$365,378	3.69%
Dr. G	Internal Medicine	$532,310	65%	$346,002	3.49%
Dr. H	Internal Medicine	$499,852	65%	$324,904	3.28%
Dr. I	Internal Medicine	$463,262	65%	$301,120	3.04%
Dr. J	Internal Medicine	$487,956	65%	$317,171	3.20%
Dr. K	Rheumatology	$563,256	63%	$354,851	3.58%
Dr. L	Cardiology	$1,245,985	44%	$548,233	5.54%
Dr. M	Cardiology	$1,965,321	44%	$864,741	8.73%
Dr. N	Pulmonary Medicine	$754,562	58%	$437,646	4.42%
Dr. O	Gastroenterology	$1,585,232	47%	$745,059	7.53%
Dr. P	Gastroenterology	$1,852,420	47%	$870,637	8.79%
Dr. Q	General Surgery	$1,128,625	42%	$474,023	4.79%
Dr. R	General Surgery	$1,532,543	42%	$643,668	6.50%
Dr. S	General Orthopedic Surgery	$1,562,452	47%	$734,352	7.42%
Dr. T	General Orthopedic Surgery	$1,685,326	47%	$792,103	8.00%
Total		$19,160,509		$9,900,426	100.00%

Step 3   **Allocate compensation pool on % to total basis.**   ($6,043,556 Total)

Physician	Compensation Pool	Direct Benefit Cost	W-2 Compensation
Dr. A	$223,115	$(36,822)	$186,293
Dr. B	$192,523	$(37,872)	$154,651
Dr. C	$250,969	$(43,292)	$207,677
Dr. D	$226,019	$(38,984)	$187,035
Dr. E	$194,274	$(41,292)	$152,982
Dr. F	$223,039	$(40,292)	$182,747
Dr. G	$211,211	$(40,312)	$170,899
Dr. H	$198,332	$(23,623)	$174,709
Dr. I	$183,814	$(30,121)	$153,693
Dr. J	$193,612	$(35,632)	$157,980
Dr. K	$216,613	$(41,002)	$175,611
Dr. L	$334,660	$(46,523)	$288,137
Dr. M	$527,867	$(49,523)	$478,344
Dr. N	$267,154	$(42,512)	$224,642
Dr. O	$454,809	$(48,563)	$406,246
Dr. P	$531,467	$(49,652)	$481,815
Dr. Q	$289,359	$(50,121)	$239,238
Dr. R	$392,917	$(48,212)	$344,705
Dr. S	$448,274	$(49,325)	$398,949
Dr. T	$483,527	$(47,563)	$435,964
Total	$6,043,556	$(841,238)	$5,202,318

* Hypothetical numbers presented for illustrative purposes only. Numbers may not total in all cases due to rounding.

© 2006 Johnson & Walker Keegan

EXHIBIT 13.21

Example D-3 – Group Practice Architecture D –
Pure Production (Measured by WRVUs and Net Collections) Plan*
Revenue Element 4

Step 1   Assemble practice net income (including ancillary).

Total Net Collections	$14,389,420
Expenses	
Nonphysician Overhead	$(8,345,864)
Compensation Pool	$6,043,556

Step 2   Determine physician production percentage.

Physician	Specialty	Professional Services Net Collections	Physician % to Total Collections	WRVU from Professional Services	Physician % to Total WRVU
Dr. A	Family Practice	$365,502	3.69%	4,623	3.64%
Dr. B	Family Practice	$315,387	3.19%	3,856	3.03%
Dr. C	Family Practice	$411,133	4.15%	4,865	3.83%
Dr. D	Internal Medicine	$370,260	3.74%	4,520	3.56%
Dr. E	Internal Medicine	$318,255	3.21%	4,123	3.24%
Dr. F	Internal Medicine	$365,378	3.69%	4,852	3.82%
Dr. G	Internal Medicine	$346,002	3.49%	4,756	3.74%
Dr. H	Internal Medicine	$324,904	3.28%	4,129	3.25%
Dr. I	Internal Medicine	$301,120	3.04%	3,852	3.03%
Dr. J	Internal Medicine	$317,171	3.20%	3,256	2.56%
Dr. K	Rheumatology	$354,851	3.58%	4,796	3.77%
Dr. L	Cardiology	$548,233	5.54%	8,956	7.05%
Dr. M	Cardiology	$864,741	8.73%	10,425	8.20%
Dr. N	Pulmonary	$437,646	4.42%	7,958	6.26%
Dr. O	Gastroenterology	$745,059	7.53%	9,136	7.19%
Dr. P	Gastroenterology	$870,637	8.79%	10,658	8.39%
Dr. Q	General Surgery	$474,023	4.79%	5,968	4.70%
Dr. R	General Surgery	$643,668	6.50%	6,325	4.98%
Dr. S	General Orthopedic Surgery	$734,352	7.42%	9,789	7.70%
Dr. T	General Orthopedic Surgery	$792,103	8.00%	10,236	8.05%
Total		$9,900,426	100.00%	127,079	100.00%

Step 3   Allocate compensation pool on physician % to total basis;
50% measured by net collections; 50% by WRVUs.   ($6,043,556 Total)

Physician	Collection Pool	WRVU Pool	Compensation Before Benefits	Direct Benefit Cost	W-2 Compensation
Dr. A	$111,557	$109,929	$221,487	$(36,822)	$184,665
Dr. B	$96,261	$91,691	$187,952	$(37,872)	$150,080
Dr. C	$125,485	$115,684	$241,168	$(43,292)	$197,876
Dr. D	$113,010	$107,480	$220,490	$(38,984)	$181,506
Dr. E	$97,137	$98,040	$195,177	$(41,292)	$153,885
Dr. F	$111,520	$115,374	$226,894	$(40,292)	$186,602
Dr. G	$105,606	$113,092	$218,697	$(40,312)	$178,385
Dr. H	$99,166	$98,182	$197,349	$(23,623)	$173,726
Dr. I	$91,907	$91,596	$183,503	$(30,121)	$153,382
Dr. J	$96,806	$77,424	$174,230	$(35,632)	$138,598
Dr. K	$108,307	$114,043	$222,349	$(41,002)	$181,347
Dr. L	$167,330	$212,962	$380,292	$(46,523)	$333,769
Dr. M	$263,934	$247,893	$511,827	$(49,523)	$462,304
Dr. N	$133,577	$189,231	$322,808	$(42,512)	$280,296
Dr. O	$227,405	$217,243	$444,647	$(48,563)	$396,084
Dr. P	$265,733	$253,434	$519,167	$(49,652)	$469,515
Dr. Q	$144,680	$141,911	$286,591	$(50,121)	$236,470
Dr. R	$196,458	$150,401	$346,859	$(48,212)	$298,647
Dr. S	$224,137	$232,770	$456,907	$(49,325)	$407,582
Dr. T	$241,763	$243,399	$485,162	$(47,563)	$437,599
Total	$3,021,778	$3,021,778	$6,043,556	$(841,238)	$5,202,318

* Hypothetical numbers presented for illustrative purposes only. Numbers may not total in all cases due to rounding.

EXHIBIT
13.22

Assessment of Practice Architecture D – Pure Production-Based Plans

Dimension	Strengths	Weaknesses
Measure	Rewards physician production and work based on physician personal production measures. Allows for use of production from professional services (and "incident to" services) using Stark law compliant productivity bonus methodology.	Potential conflict regarding "overhead" contribution by different specialties.
Productivity	Encourages and directly rewards individual production.	May lead to competition for patients or other inappropriate behavior.
Financial	Rewards individuals for additional work levels. Can use multiple measures to address payer mix considerations.	May not promote appropriate attention to cost of practice issues. Depending on the measure selected, may lead to issues related to revenue cycle performance.
Simplicity	Ease of administration. Understandable system.	May lead to confusion regarding "overhead paid" by individual physicians.
Alignment	Encourages both individual and group practice orientation.	Works best where there are similar levels of production and limited (or largely uniform) levels of ancillary services usage. May be difficult to implement and/or maintain in multispecialty practices with inconsistent ancillary services generation between or among practice specialties.
"Fairness"	Can be perceived as fair where production levels are relatively consistent, or where mutual interdependence and referral relationships are recognized and acknowledged in a multispecialty setting.	Physicians may perceive plan as inequitable given differences in payer mix and ancillary services utilization.

▶ GROUP PRACTICE ARCHITECTURE E – GRADUATED OR NEGOTIATED REVENUE (OR INCOME) ALLOCATION PLANS
Revenue Element 5

Overview

This team-oriented plan uses Element 5 of Exhibit 13.1 involving a graduated or negotiated approach to practice revenue or income allocations, but without regard to a direct method of allocating practice expenses (as in individualistic plans). Thus, plans using this basic Architecture E are team-oriented, because they still do not use an express allocation of practice costs. However, they are also near the "middle ground" of plan types, because they effectively apply some form of "tax" or other approach that effectively (albeit indirectly) approximates overhead in some manner. A similar middle ground approach is also described in Architecture N.

Application

This plan type can be used by single specialty or multispecialty practices. Similar plans are also used in hospital employment and similar structural models.

Methodology – Plan with Graduated or Negotiated Revenue (or Income) Allocation

The basic plan methodology for Architecture E is first presented (Example E-1), followed by a variation of this plan with enhanced complexity and sophistication (Example E-2).

Example E-1 – Basic Architecture E: Graduated Revenue Allocation Plan

Example E-1 (illustrated in Exhibit 13.23) is a plan that provides direct production credit to individual physicians for the professional services net revenues they generate. Example E-1 also allocates ancillary services income, net of expenses, through an overall profits pool, using each physician's WRVUs on a percentage to total basis to allocate net ancillary services profits as allowed by the Stark law. The sum of these two amounts (personal production net collections, plus a percentage of ancillary services profits) is then applied to a "tiered" percentage that serves as a surrogate for practice operating expenses.

Step 1. Allocate Professional Services Net Collections

In this example, professional services production is measured by net collections, with each physician allocated his or her professional services net collections amount.

Step 2. Determine Ancillary Services Profits Pool, and Allocate Income

Ancillary services are treated as a separate profit (or loss) center, and net income from ancillary services (ancillary services revenues minus ancillary services allocated expenses) is tracked to a single cost center. The net income or profits from ancillary services are then allocated among group physicians based on each physician's respective percentage share of WRVUs. Note that other measures of production, such as gross charges or net collections from professional services could also be used. Under the Stark law, physicians in Group Practices may be paid a productivity bonus, with physician production measured by including each physician's personally performed services *plus* services that are properly billed "incident to" the physician's personally performed services.

Step 3. Determine the Physician's Allocated Revenues

Add the amounts calculated based on Steps 1 and 2 to derive the physician's allocated revenues. The mathematical formula is as follows:

Physician's Professional Services Net Revenues
+ Physician's Share of Ancillary Profits
_____
Allocated Revenues for Each Physician

Step 4. Apply Allocated Revenues to Practice "Tier" Methodology to Determine Physician-Specific Compensation

The total allocated revenues are effectively "taxed" or assessed at different levels to pay practice overhead costs (excluding physician compensation and direct benefits). The assessment levels generally vary and are "tiered" as a means to generate sufficient funds to pay practice costs. In this example, the following thresholds are applied to allocated revenue:

Allocated Revenue	Assessment
Up to $250,000	60 percent
$250,001 to $400,000	55 percent
$400,001 to $600,000	50 percent
$600,001 and above	45 percent

The exact assessment levels, thresholds, and tiers will be determined based on a practice's financial conditions and budget; therefore, the numbers, thresholds, and percentages used in this example should be considered an illustration of this architecture only, with exact dollars, thresholds, and percentages based on financial modeling specific to each medical group. Adequate funds are required to pay practice operating costs, and the tier methodology could potentially result in the retention of too little or an excessive amount of funds to pay such costs. Where the tier tax results in an insufficient amount to pay practice overhead, the actual funds available to pay physician compensation and direct expenses will be reallocated on a percent to total basis using each physician's total allocated amount available for compensation for the basis for such an allocation. Likewise, where the tier retains excessive amounts of funds to pay overhead costs, the excess (less amounts retained for reserves or other purposes) will be reallocated on a similar basis. Example N-1 (Exhibit 13.43) illustrates a similar approach.

Step 5. Subtract Physician-Specific Direct Benefits from the Allocated Revenue to Determine Individual Physician Compensation Levels

A variation of Architecture E is shown in Example E-2. Other variations of this basic model are also illustrated in Chapter 14 dealing with hospital-based plans.

Example E-2

Example E-2 (illustrated in Exhibit 13.24) builds on concepts similar to those of E-1, except that it pays different amounts based on different ranges of WRVU production in comparison to market, with the WRVU conversion factors also based on market rates of compensation per WRVU by practice specialty. Thus, Example E-2 pays or "credits" a defined dollar amount per WRVU up to a defined level (e.g., up to 80 percent of the market median), a higher amount per WRVU up to another tier, defined as 80 percent of median to median, and still higher amounts for WRVU production in excess of the median (e.g., above the median to 120 percent of the median, and above 120 percent of median production).

The compensation per WRVU levels are set for each specialty based on market data, using market median data as the reference points. In this model, the practice is effectively encouraging all physicians to perform at no less than median levels of WRVU production by specialty; hence the use of a fewer dollars per WRVU conversion factor for production below the median. It also awards production in excess of the median.

The specific steps involved in Example E-2 are outlined below.

Step 1. Determine WRVU Thresholds by Specialty

In this example, the thresholds are 80 percent of the median, median, and 120 percent of the median. These levels generally approximate the 25th percentile, the 50th percentile, and the 75th percentile of benchmarks for many specialties.

Step 2. Assign Dollars per WRVU by Production and by Specialty

In this step, the market median compensation per WRVU for each specialty is first determined (Step 2A). Then a tiered approach is used to index from this market median based on WRVU production levels (Step 2B).

Step 3. Determine Compensation Credit Based on Individual Physician Production

The threshold dollars per WRVU are applied to each physician's actual WRVUs to determine "compensation credit" based on their individual production levels. For example, the first 3,389 WRVUs for Dr. A in the example are credited with $28.91 per WRVU, the next 847 (3,390–4,236) with $33.04 per WRVU, etc.

Step 4. Compute the Percentage to Total of "Compensation Credit" for Each Physician

In Step 4, the allocated compensation per WRVU identified in Step 3 is totaled for each physician, then the physician's "compensation credit" as a percentage to total "compensation credits" is computed. This percentage represents each physician's share of the compensation pool or net practice income based on this plan.

Step 5. Determine Practice Net Income (all sources)

Step 6. Compute Each Physician's Share of Practice Net Income
In Step 6, the percentages identified in Step 4 are applied to practice net income (professional services revenue less practice operating expenses) to derive each physician's share of practice net income, which in this case is paid as W-2 compensation.

In a Group Practice, such a compensation plan requires special adjustment in light of the fact that practice overhead costs are not directly considered in providing compensation credit to individual physicians using the graduated dollars per WRVU approach. Thus, if a Group Practice has excessive operating costs, the actual compensation available for physician compensation may be less than that shown in each physician's allocated compensation per WRVU (Step 3).

Alternatively, as in this example, if the practice is highly successful, then the funds available for compensation defined as practice net income will be greater than those calculated as "compensation credit" to the physician – meaning that practice physicians may actually earn more than their "compensation credit."

As with other plan architectures, Architecture E involving graduated systems can also include bonus pools or awards that are paid by third parties based on clinical, quality, practice efficiency, and other measures as might be seen in a P4P reimbursement environment. Bonus pools and incentives linked to quality and other measures can also be created through practice income by withholding a portion of the practice net income in order to "fund" an incentive pool that rewards physicians based on these or similar measures.

These examples can also be coupled with any number of additional variations, including requirements linked to minimum performance expectations, different measures of production, and other measures based upon practice goals and incentive objectives. See Chapters 10 and 14 for a discussion of performance expectations, and plan examples in Chapter 14 for illustrations of how performance expectations can be incorporated into compensation plans.

Exhibit 13.25 presents the strengths and weaknesses of Architecture E.

EXHIBIT 13.23

Example E-1 – Group Practice Architecture E –
Graduated Revenue Allocation Plan*
Revenue Element 5

		Total	Dr. A FP w/o OB	Dr. B FP w/o OB	Dr. C FP	Dr. D IM
Step 1	Allocate physician professional services net revenues.					
	Net Collections from Professional Services	$5,227,559	$385,502	$365,387	$411,133	$395,260
Step 2	Determine ancillary services profits pool (e.g., MRI and X-ray).					
	Ancillary Services Revenues	$1,890,290				
	Ancillary Services Expenses	$(1,209,936)				
		$680,354				
	Actual WRVU Production	60,090	4,147	3,459	4,364	4,055
	Physician % to Total WRVU		6.90%	5.76%	7.26%	6.75%
	Share of Ancillary Services Profits	$680,354	$46,954	$39,164	$49,412	$45,908
Step 3	Determine total allocated revenues.	$5,907,913	$432,456	$404,551	$460,545	$441,168
Step 4	Apply percentages to allocated revenues (surrogate for overhead).					
	Up to and including $250,000	60%	$(150,000)	$(150,000)	$(150,000)	$(150,000)
	$250,001–$400,000	55%	$(82,500)	$(85,003)	$(82,500)	$(82,500)
	$400,001–$600,000	50%	$(16,228)		$(30,272)	$(20,584)
	Over $600,000	45%				
	Total		$(248,728)	$(235,003)	$(262,772)	$(253,084)
	Total Amount Available for Compensation	$2,584,686	$183,728	$169,548	$197,772	$188,084
Step 5	Determine physician-specific direct expenses.		$(36,822)	$(37,872)	$(43,292)	$(38,984)
Step 6	Determine total W-2 compensation (net of benefits).		$146,906	$131,676	$154,480	$149,100

* Hypothetical numbers presented for illustrative purposes only. Numbers may not total in all cases due to rounding.

Key:
Card Inv = Cardiology: Invasive
Card Non-Inv = Cardiology: Noninvasive
FP = Family Practice
FP w/o OB = Family Practice without Obstetrics
IM = Internal Medicine
Pulm = Pulmonary Medicine
Rheum = Rheumatology

© 2006 Johnson & Walker Keegan

	Dr. E IM	Dr. F IM	Dr. G IM	Dr. H IM	Dr. I Rheum	Dr. J Card Non-Inv	Dr. K Card Inv	Dr. L Pulm
	$325,255	$397,378	$375,002	$367,171	$354,851	$548,233	$864,741	$437,646
	3,699	4,353	4,266	2,921	4,302	8,034	9,352	7,139
	6.16%	7.24%	7.10%	4.86%	7.16%	13.37%	15.56%	11.88%
	$41,876	$49,280	$48,305	$33,070	$48,711	$90,963	$105,883	$80,827
	$367,131	$446,658	$423,307	$400,241	$403,563	$639,196	$970,624	$518,473
	$(150,000)	$(150,000)	$(150,000)	$(150,000)	$(150,000)	$(150,000)	$(150,000)	$(150,000)
	$(64,422)	$(82,500)	$(95,319)	$(82,633)	$(82,500)	$(82,500)	$(82,500)	$(82,500)
		$(23,329)			$(1,781)	$(100,000)	$(100,000)	$(59,236)
						$(17,638)	$(166,781)	
	$(214,422)	$(255,829)	$(245,319)	$(232,633)	$(234,281)	$(350,138)	$(499,281)	$(291,736)
	$152,709	$190,829	$177,988	$167,609	$169,281	$289,058	$471,343	$226,736
	$(41,292)	$(40,292)	$(40,312)	$(35,632)	$(41,002)	$(46,523)	$(49,523)	$(42,512)
	$111,417	$150,537	$137,676	$131,977	$128,279	$242,535	$421,820	$184,224

EXHIBIT 13.24

Example E-2 – Group Practice Architecture D – Graduated Dollars per WRVU Plan*
Revenue Element 5

		Total	Dr. A FP w/OB	Dr. B FP w/OB	Dr. C FP	Dr. D IM
Step 1	**Assign WRVU thresholds by specialty.†**					
	80% of Median‡		3,389	3,389	3,154	3,264
	Median†		4,236	4,236	3,943	4,080
	120% of Median‡		5,083	5,083	4,732	4,896
Step 2	**Assign compensation per WRVU by production target.****					
Step 2A	Market Median $ per WRVU by Specialty		$41.30	$41.30	$39.13	$42.12
Step 2B	Apply Percentage to Median $ per WRVU					
	Under 80% of Median	70%	$28.91	$28.91	$27.39	$29.48
	80% of Median to Median	80%	$33.04	$33.04	$31.30	$33.70
	Above Median to 120% of Median	100%	$41.30	$41.30	$39.13	$42.12
	Over 120% of Median	120%	$49.56	$49.56	$46.96	$50.54
Step 3	**Determine "compensation credit" based on production.**					
Step 3A	Actual WRVUs during Compensation Period		4,126	4,526	4,325	2,751
Step 3B	Assign Dollars Based on Graduated Levels					
	Up to 80% of Median		$97,970	$97,970	$86,402	$81,110
	80% of Median to Median		$24,357	$27,991	$24,686	
	Above Median to 120% of Median			$11,977	$14,948	
	Over 120% of Median					
	Total Allocated Compensation/WRVU	$2,036,874	$122,327	$137,939	$126,036	$81,110
Step 4	**Determine percentage of allocated compensation/WRVU.**	100.00%	6.01%	6.77%	6.19%	3.98%
Step 5	**Determine practice net income (all sources).**					
	Net Collections	$5,014,559				
	Total Operating Expenses	$(2,484,986)				
	Practice Net Income (comp. pool)	$2,529,573				

Dr. E IM	Dr. F IM	Dr. G IM	Dr. H IM	Dr. I Rheum	Dr. J Card Inv	Dr. K Card Non-Inv	Dr. L Pulm
3,264	3,264	3,264	3,264	3,207	6,648	5,251	4,471
4,080	4,080	4,080	4,080	4,009	8,310	6,564	5,589
4,896	4,896	4,896	4,896	4,811	9,972	7,877	6,707
$42.12	$42.12	$42.12	$42.12	$49.64	$51.86	$49.80	$43.38
$29.48	$29.48	$29.48	$29.48	$34.75	$36.30	$34.86	$30.37
$33.70	$33.70	$33.70	$33.70	$39.71	$41.49	$39.84	$34.70
$42.12	$42.12	$42.12	$42.12	$49.64	$51.86	$49.80	$43.38
$50.54	$50.54	$50.54	$50.54	$59.57	$62.23	$59.76	$52.06
3,564	3,865	4,962	2,985	4,085	10,546	8,124	6,231
$96,236	$96,236	$96,236	$88,010	$111,444	$241,336	$183,057	$135,772
$10,109	$20,251	$27,496		$31,841	$68,953	$52,302	$38,792
		$34,370		$3,773	$86,191	$65,377	$27,850
		$3,336			$35,721	$14,773	
$106,345	$116,487	$161,438	$88,010	$147,058	$432,201	$315,509	$202,415
5.22%	5.72%	7.93%	4.32%	7.22%	21.22%	15.49%	9.94%

continued on next page

Exhibit 13.24 – Example E-2 continued

		Total	Dr. A FP w/OB	Dr. B FP w/OB	Dr. C FP	Dr. D IM
Step 6	**Determine share of compensation pool based on percentage of allocated comp/WRVU (from above).**	$2,529,573	$151,917	$171,305	$156,523	$100,730
	Total W-2 Compensation (physician-specific direct expenses paid by practice)††		$151,917	$171,305	$156,523	$100,730

* Hypothetical numbers presented for illustrative purposes only. Numbers may not total in all cases due to rounding.

† Uses market benchmarks for illustrative purposes. Group-specific, combined group, and market-based or other measures can be used.

‡ 80% and 120% of median approximate to 25th and 75th percentiles in many medical practice specialties based on MGMA compensation data. Exact percentages of median for thresholds would be determined.

** Uses market benchmarks to assign dollars per WRVU. Model designed to encourage minimum production at no less than median levels; hence reduced dollars for production below median.

†† Illustration assumes that practice pays physician-specific direct expense costs (e.g., health insurance, etc.) and that costs are already included in practice operating expe

```
Key:
Card Inv = Cardiology: Invasive
Card Non-Inv = Cardiology: Noninvasive
FP = Family Practice
FP w/OB = Family Practice with Obstetrics
FP w/o OB = Family Practice without Obstetrics
IM = Internal Medicine
Pulm = Pulmonary Medicine
Rheum = Rheumatology
```

Dr. E IM	Dr. F IM	Dr. G IM	Dr. H IM	Dr. I Rheum	Dr. J Card Inv	Dr. K Card Non-Inv	Dr. L Pulm
$132,068	$144,664	$200,488	$109,298	$182,629	$536,746	$391,827	$251,377
$132,068	$144,664	$200,488	$109,298	$182,629	$536,746	$391,827	$251,377

EXHIBIT 13.25 Assessment of Group Practice Architecture E – Plan with Graduated or Negotiated Revenue (or Income) Allocation

Dimension	Strengths	Weaknesses
Measure	Promotes team and group practice orientation by encouraging overall production. Can use any number of measures of production to balance work and payer mix (e.g., WRVUs, or professional services net collections or gross charges, etc.).	Award based upon work may have little to no direct relationship to actual financial performance.
Productivity	Encourages production beyond a base, target, or "floor" level due to the graduated tiers of dollars per WRVU, varying "tax" levels on net collections, or similar means.	May lead to competition for patients.
Financial	Tiers or "tax" levels encourage physician productivity, with tax levels lower as production increases. Allocation of ancillary revenue and expense to form profit-and-loss pool can be used to reflect financial realities of ancillary activity.	Tiers or "tax" levels as applied to allocated revenues or other measures may not provide sufficient funds to pay overhead costs. Close monitoring and management are required to ensure that practice expenditures do not exceed practice revenues and that physician compensation levels are competitive. Approach to overhead may not provide appropriate attention to cost of practice issues. WRVU method of determining production credit is payer-neutral, which may not permit adequate attention to payer mix or reimbursement required to fund the compensation pool.
Simplicity	Relatively easy to administer once tiers are determined.	Tiers or other "tax" levels that are applied to revenues must be determined, requiring financial modeling, negotiation, and agreement.

Dimension	Strengths	Weaknesses
Alignment	Encourages individual and group practice orientation. Tiers or similar "tax" mechanisms can be viewed to approximate (although imperfectly) practice operating expenses associated with different production levels.	Minimum production and work levels may not be met absent formal performance expectations.
"Fairness"	"Tax" levels and tiers can be tailored to reflect financial realities of different practice specialties. See Architecture N for a similar approach to cost of practice issues.	Can be perceived as unfair by physicians with lower levels of production by specialty, since taxation is graduated downward.

INDIVIDUALISTIC ARCHITECTURES AND EXAMPLES

Having reviewed the basic "team-oriented" compensation plan architectures by reviewing Architectures A through E above, we will now turn to the opposite end of the array to review the basic "individualistic" architectures. This discussion will begin with the far right end of the array of architectures with the most individualistic architecture (**Architecture R**), which uses both a pure production approach to revenue allocation (Revenue Element 4, as depicted in Exhibit 13.1), and a pure or "strict" approach to overhead expense allocation based on utilization (Expense Element 9, as depicted in Exhibit 13.1).

We will follow this example by moving inward on the array to review the following architecture examples:

- ► **Architecture Q** – combining pure production revenue allocation (Revenue Element 4) with modified cost accounting expense allocation systems (Expense Element 8);

- ► **Architecture P** – using pure production (Revenue Element 4) with negotiated expense allocation based on production (Expense Element 7);

- ► **Architecture O** – combining pure production (Revenue Element 4) with a pure "equal share" expense allocation system (Expense Element 6); and

- ► **Architecture N** – involving a mixed system that combines pure production (Revenue Element 4) on the revenue side of the equation with a negotiated or graduated expense allocation system (e.g., market norms or otherwise) (Expense Element 5).

► GROUP PRACTICE ARCHITECTURE R – "STRICT" COST ACCOUNTING PLANS
Revenue Element 4 and Expense Element 9

Overview

This plan uses agreed upon methods to allocate revenues and expenses across physicians in a single medical practice. The Group Practice in Example R-1 uses a "strict" cost accounting methodology to allocate practice income and expenses and to determine physician compensation.

Application

This plan type is commonly used by a variety of practices, including primary care, medicine subspecialty groups such as oncology and gastroenterology, surgical groups such as orthopedic surgery, and multispecialty groups.

Methodology

In strict cost accounting compensation plans, agreed upon cost allocation methods are used to allocate each individual component of practice expense, with the basic objective being to allocate each element as directly as possible based upon actual or estimated resource utilization. For this reason, unlike the "modified" cost accounting plans discussed in Group Practice Example Q below, which typically distribute practice overhead through three or four categories and methods, strict cost accounting might use any number of methodologies to allocate practice expenses at the individual physician level.

The basic mathematical plan in a strict cost accounting plan involves the following steps:

Step 1. Allocate revenues on a pure production basis;

Step 2. Allocate expenditures using a strict cost accounting approach;

Step 3. Allocate ancillary services income or profits; and

Step 4. Determine physician-specific compensation.

Although this provides a rough outline of the basic steps, when it comes to strict cost accounting, "the devil is in the details." And so, these steps are reviewed in greater detail below.

Example R-1 – Detail of an Individualistic, Strict Cost Accounting Plan

Step 1. Determine Production Levels of Physicians and Divisions

In this step, production and other measures relating to individual physicians and the Group Practice as a whole are determined. These measures are used in subsequent steps as part of the revenue and/or cost allocation process. In Example R-1 (illustrated in Exhibit 13.26 at the end of this section), revenue production is measured by professional services net collections at the individual physician level. However, production as measured by patient encounters is used as a surrogate for utilization in the expense allocation, with a recognition of the differences in encounters between two divisions in the Group Practice (in this example, the South Division and the East Division) as discussed in Step 3 below. See Chapter 7, "Measuring Physician Work and Effort," for more information on the types of production and other measures, including the strengths and weaknesses of each.

Step 2. Allocate Revenues on a Pure Production Basis

In a strict cost accounting plan, revenues (e.g., net collections from professional services) are generally allocated directly to the physician responsible for revenue production to the extent possible. This includes professional services and the professional component of ancillary services that are personally performed by the physician. This allocation is on an individual physician basis and/or on a practice location or departments basis.

Ancillary services are treated as separate profit-and-loss centers for purposes of allocating net income using a Stark law compliant method (discussed in Step 4 below). An example of common types of revenue or net collections allocation methods is provided in Exhibit 13.27.

Step 3. Allocate Expenditures

In a strict cost accounting plan, practice operating expenses are allocated among individual physicians (or potentially to practice locations, departments, divisions, and/or specialties) based on resource utilization to the extent possible. Expenses that cannot be traced to a particular location, specialty, and/or physician (e.g., general and administrative expenses) are allocated using various methods. The method available involves a series of alternatives, such as:

- ► Equal per capita or per physician (without regard to differences in FTE levels);

- ► Equal based on physician FTE level;

- ► Percentage of utilization (with utilization measured by encounters [e.g., defined as ambulatory encounters only, or the sum of ambulatory plus hospital and/or surgical encounters], net collections or another surrogate measure); and

- ► Combination of equal share (based on an estimated 50 percent of the total "fixed" costs), and the remaining portion based on percentage of utilization.

An example of the types of expense allocation methods that might be used for individual expense items is presented in Exhibit 13.28. Note that alternative methods can be, and commonly are, used in connection with strict cost accounting plans. Exhibit 13.29 presents expense allocations regarding personnel and other general expenses.

Step 4. Allocate Ancillary Services Income or Profits

Revenue or profits from ancillary services, including DHS subject to the Stark law, must be allocated in a legally compliant manner. In this example, ancillary services are treated as a separate profit-and-loss center to which Group Practice overhead expenses (referenced above) are also allocated on a direct or other agreed upon basis. For such purposes, practice overhead that is assigned to the ancillary services line may be limited (e.g., equipment and direct personnel costs only), or treated more expansively (e.g., to include an allocation of general overhead costs, etc).

After the allocation of ancillary services revenues and share of expenses, the profit from the ancillary services line may only be allocated among physicians in a bona fide Group Practice through a manner that is *indirectly* related to the physicians' referrals for such services. In this example, such profits are allocated on a percent of total encounters basis, although other methods are also available, as discussed in Chapter 9, "The Legal Element." The result is an amount available for physician-specific compensation and physician-specific direct expenses.

Step 5. Determine Funds Available for Physician Compensation and Physician-Specific Direct Expenses

The calculations referenced above will yield a net income amount for each physician, essentially calculated as revenue attributed to the physician, less operating expenses plus ancillary profits.

Step 6. Calculate Physician-Specific Direct Expenses

As with the other more general overhead expense items, expenses that are allocated on a "direct" or physician-specific basis can be tracked to the individual physician. These will commonly include the types of expenses depicted in Exhibit 13.30.

Step 7. Calculate Physician Income after Direct Expenses

The mathematical formula used to calculate physician take-home compensation is as follows:

Physician-Specific Amount Available for Compensation and Direct Expenses
− Physician-Specific Direct Expenses
_____
Physician Cash (Take Home) Compensation

For a summary of the strengths and weaknesses of Architecture R, refer to Exhibit 13.31.

EXHIBIT 13.26

Example R-1 – Group Practice Architecture R – Pure Production and Strict Cost Accounting Plan*
Revenue Element 4 and Expense Element 9

Step 1	Assemble production information.	Total			Smith	Johnson
	Physician	9.00			1.00	1.00
	Physician FTE	8.75			1.00	1.00
	Ambulatory Encounters	5,158			206	504
	Physician % to Total Ambulatory Encounters				4%	10%
	Surgeries	2,172			188	266
	Total Ambulatory and Surgical Encounters	7,331			394	770
	Physician % to Total Encounters – All Divisions	100%			5%	11%
	Physician % to Total Encounters – South Division	100%			11%	21%
	Physician % to Total Encounters – East Division	100%				
	Net Collections from Professional Services	$4,127,816			$378,545	$524,376
	Physician % to Total Net Collections	100%			9%	13%

Step 2	Determine revenue.	Total	Allocation	Smith	Johnson
	Net Collections from Professional Services	$4,127,816	Direct	$378,545	$524,376
	Nonphysician Provider Net Collections	$173,002	Physician Use	$—	$32,203
	Ancillary Net Collections – Professional Component	$155,864	Direct to Performing Physician	$13,342	$62,145
	Interest Income	$46,897	Equal per FTE	$5,360	$5,360
	Other Income	$34,059	Direct	$10,221	$4,512
	Total Revenue	$4,537,638		$407,468	$628,595

Step 3	Determine operating expenses.				
	GENERAL OPERATING EXPENSES				
	Accounting	$(18,636)	Equal per Physician	$(2,071)	$(2,071)
	Advertising	$(4,525)	Equal per Physician	$(503)	$(503)
	Bank Charges	$(6,325)	Equal per Physician	$(703)	$(703)
	Biomedical Waste	$(2,763)	% Ambulatory Encounters	$(110)	$(270)
	Business Promotion	$(2,618)	Equal per Physician	$(291)	$(291)
	Cell Phones (admin)	$(2,400)	Equal per Physician	$(267)	$(267)
	Computer (admin)	$(87,036)	Equal per Physician	$(9,671)	$(9,671)
	Contract Services	$(2,618)	Equal per Physician	$(291)	$(291)
	Drugs and Medical Supplies	$(6,150)	% Ambulatory Encounters	$(246)	$(601)
	Dues and Licenses	$(10,794)	Equal per Physician	$(1,199)	$(1,199)
	Food/Entertainment	$(596)	Equal per Physician	$(66)	$(66)
	Insurance – General Liability	$(1,837)	Equal per Physician	$(204)	$(204)

Wilson	Einstein	Bornsten	Porter	Mathews	Patel	Kant
1.00	1.00	1.00	1.00	1.00	1.00	1.00
1.00	1.00	1.00	1.00	0.75	1.00	1.00
1,149	813	1,032	509	300	490	155
22%	16%	20%	10%	6%	9%	3%
228	293	309	273	168	271	176
1,377	1,106	1,341	782	468	761	331
19%	15%	18%	11%	6%	10%	5%
	31%	37%				
37%			21%	13%	20%	9%
$376,499	$356,821	$413,753	$637,903	$434,281	$532,153	$473,486
9%	9%	10%	15%	11%	13%	11%

Wilson	Einstein	Bornsten	Porter	Mathews	Patel	Kant
$376,499	$356,821	$413,753	$637,903	$434,281	$532,153	$473,486
$7,019	$—	$—	$24,991	$40,893	$32,442	$35,455
$13,645	$32,121	$24,512	$1,024	$3,212	$4,512	$1,351
$5,360	$5,360	$5,360	$5,360	$4,020	$5,360	$5,360
$230	$500	$9,852	$164	$2,580	$5,000	$1,000
$402,752	$394,802	$453,476	$669,441	$484,986	$579,467	$516,652
$(2,071)	$(2,071)	$(2,071)	$(2,071)	$(2,071)	$(2,071)	$(2,071)
$(503)	$(503)	$(503)	$(503)	$(503)	$(503)	$(503)
$(703)	$(703)	$(703)	$(703)	$(703)	$(703)	$(703)
$(616)	$(436)	$(553)	$(273)	$(161)	$(263)	$(83)
$(291)	$(291)	$(291)	$(291)	$(291)	$(291)	$(291)
$(267)	$(267)	$(267)	$(267)	$(267)	$(267)	$(267)
$(9,671)	$(9,671)	$(9,671)	$(9,671)	$(9,671)	$(9,671)	$(9,671)
$(291)	$(291)	$(291)	$(291)	$(291)	$(291)	$(291)
$(1,370)	$(969)	$(1,231)	$(607)	$(358)	$(584)	$(185)
$(1,199)	$(1,199)	$(1,199)	$(1,199)	$(1,199)	$(1,199)	$(1,199)
$(66)	$(66)	$(66)	$(66)	$(66)	$(66)	$(66)
$(204)	$(204)	$(204)	$(204)	$(204)	$(204)	$(204)

continued on next page

Exhibit 13.26 – Example R-1 continued

	Total	Allocation	Smith	Johnson
Insurance – Malpractice (corp)	$(11,299)	Equal per Physician	$(1,255)	$(1,255)
Interest/Penalties/Fees	$(742)	Equal per Physician	$(82)	$(82)
Laundry and Uniforms	$(450)	Equal per Physician	$(50)	$(50)
Lease Equipment	$(1,996)	Equal per Physician	$(222)	$(222)
Legal Expense	$(8,750)	Equal per Physician	$(972)	$(972)
Medical Expense Benefits – Flex	$(1,430)	Equal per Physician	$(159)	$(159)
Mileage Reimbursement (admin)	$(985)	Equal per Physician	$(109)	$(109)
Miscellaneous Expense	$(685)	Equal per Physician	$(76)	$(76)
Office Supplies	$(16,070)	Equal per Physician	$(1,786)	$(1,786)
Pagers and Answering Service	$(16,520)	Equal per Physician	$(1,836)	$(1,836)
Postage	$(8,467)	Equal per Physician	$(941)	$(941)
Rent – Common	$(12,692)	Equal per Physician	$(1,410)	$(1,410)
Rent – Division Specific	$(100,488)	Direct to Division	$(14,451)	$(14,451)
Repairs and Maintenance	$(35,782)	Equal per Physician	$(3,976)	$(3,976)
Subscriptions and Books	$(1,232)	Equal per Physician	$(137)	$(137)
Taxes	$(3,519)	Equal per Physician	$(391)	$(391)
Telephone	$(17,520)	Equal per Physician	$(1,947)	$(1,947)
Subtotal – General Operating Expenses	$(384,927)		$(45,421)	$(45,936)
SUPPORT STAFF EXPENSES				
Salaries				
Administrative Staff	$(99,272)	Equal per Physician	$(11,345)	$(11,345)
Billing Staff	$(139,349)	50% Equal FTE/50% Claims Volume†		
50% of Total (from above)	$(69,675)	Equal per FTE	$(7,963)	$(7,963)
50% of Total (from above)	$(69,675)	% of Claims Volume	$(3,745)	$(7,319)
Clinical Staff	$(25,471)	% of Total Encounters	$(1,369)	$(2,676)
Nonclinical Staff – South	$(11,818)	Direct Division/ % of Total Encounters	$(1,289)	$(2,520)
Nonclinical Staff – East	$(15,021)	Direct Division/ % of Total Encounters	$—	$—
Scheduling Staff – South	$(56,380)	Direct Division/ % of Total Encounters	$(6,152)	$(12,022)
Scheduling Staff – East	$(126,142)	Direct Division/ % of Total Encounters	$—	$—
Subtotal – Nonphysician Employee Allocated Salary	$(473,454)		$(31,863)	$(43,845)
BENEFITS AND OTHER EXPENSES				
Education – Employees	$(15,234)	% of Allocated Salary	$(1,025)	$(1,411)
Insurance Disability – Employees	$(23,542)	% of Allocated Salary	$(1,584)	$(2,180)
Insurance Health – Employees	$(57,600)	% of Allocated Salary	$(3,876)	$(5,334)
Payroll Taxes – Employees	$(59,182)	% of Allocated Salary	$(3,983)	$(5,481)
Profit-Sharing Contribution – Employees	$(102,450)	% of Allocated Salary	$(6,895)	$(9,488)
Workers Compensation – Employees	$(14,204)	% of Allocated Salary	$(956)	$(1,315)
Subtotal – Employee Benefits	$(272,211)		$(18,320)	$(25,209)
Total Operating Expenses	$(1,130,592)		$(95,604)	$(114,990)

Wilson	Einstein	Bornsten	Porter	Mathews	Patel	Kant
$(1,255)	$(1,255)	$(1,255)	$(1,255)	$(1,255)	$(1,255)	$(1,255)
$(82)	$(82)	$(82)	$(82)	$(82)	$(82)	$(82)
$(50)	$(50)	$(50)	$(50)	$(50)	$(50)	$(50)
$(222)	$(222)	$(222)	$(222)	$(222)	$(222)	$(222)
$(972)	$(972)	$(972)	$(972)	$(972)	$(972)	$(972)
$(159)	$(159)	$(159)	$(159)	$(159)	$(159)	$(159)
$(109)	$(109)	$(109)	$(109)	$(109)	$(109)	$(109)
$(76)	$(76)	$(76)	$(76)	$(76)	$(76)	$(76)
$(1,786)	$(1,786)	$(1,786)	$(1,786)	$(1,786)	$(1,786)	$(1,786)
$(1,836)	$(1,836)	$(1,836)	$(1,836)	$(1,836)	$(1,836)	$(1,836)
$(941)	$(941)	$(941)	$(941)	$(941)	$(941)	$(941)
$(1,410)	$(1,410)	$(1,410)	$(1,410)	$(1,410)	$(1,410)	$(1,410)
$(8,537)	$(14,451)	$(14,451)	$(8,537)	$(8,537)	$(8,537)	$(8,537)
$(3,976)	$(3,976)	$(3,976)	$(3,976)	$(3,976)	$(3,976)	$(3,976)
$(137)	$(137)	$(137)	$(137)	$(137)	$(137)	$(137)
$(391)	$(391)	$(391)	$(391)	$(391)	$(391)	$(391)
$(1,947)	$(1,947)	$(1,947)	$(1,947)	$(1,947)	$(1,947)	$(1,947)
$(41,136)	$(46,470)	$(46,848)	$(40,030)	$(39,669)	$(39,997)	$(39,418)
$(11,345)	$(11,345)	$(11,345)	$(11,345)	$(8,509)	$(11,345)	$(11,345)
$(7,963)	$(7,963)	$(7,963)	$(7,963)	$(5,972)	$(7,963)	$(7,963)
$(13,089)	$(10,513)	$(12,747)	$(7,433)	$(4,448)	$(7,234)	$(3,146)
$(4,785)	$(3,843)	$(4,660)	$(2,717)	$(1,626)	$(2,644)	$(1,150)
$—	$(3,620)	$(4,389)	$—	$—	$—	$—
$(5,562)	$—	$—	$(3,159)	$(1,890)	$(3,074)	$(1,337)
$—	$(17,269)	$(20,938)	$—	$—	$—	$—
$(46,707)	$—	$—	$(26,524)	$(15,874)	$(25,812)	$(11,226)
$(89,451)	$(54,553)	$(62,042)	$(59,141)	$(38,320)	$(58,071)	$(36,168)
$(2,878)	$(1,755)	$(1,996)	$(1,903)	$(1,233)	$(1,869)	$(1,164)
$(4,448)	$(2,713)	$(3,085)	$(2,941)	$(1,905)	$(2,888)	$(1,798)
$(10,883)	$(6,637)	$(7,548)	$(7,195)	$(4,662)	$(7,065)	$(4,400)
$(11,181)	$(6,819)	$(7,755)	$(7,393)	$(4,790)	$(7,259)	$(4,521)
$(19,356)	$(11,805)	$(13,425)	$(12,797)	$(8,292)	$(12,566)	$(7,826)
$(2,684)	$(1,637)	$(1,861)	$(1,774)	$(1,150)	$(1,742)	$(1,085)
$(51,430)	$(31,365)	$(35,671)	$(34,003)	$(22,032)	$(33,388)	$(20,795)
$(182,017)	$(132,388)	$(144,561)	$(133,174)	$(100,020)	$(131,457)	$(96,381)

continued on next page

Exhibit 13.26 – Example R-1 continued

		Total	Allocation	Smith	Johnson
Step 4	**Determine ancillary services profits pool.**				
	Revenues				
	Ancillary – Technical Component	$315,951	Direct Ancillary Pool		
	Expenses				
	Ancillary Technicians	$(112,085)	Direct Ancillary Pool		
	Ancillary Supplies	$(13,872)	Direct Ancillary Pool		
	Ancillary Net Profit (Revenue – Expense)	$189,994	% of Total Encounters	$10,212	$19,958
Step 5	**Determine amount available for physician compensation and direct expenses.**				
	(Revenue – Operating Expenses + Ancillary Profits)	$3,597,040		$322,076	$533,564
Step 6	**Determine physician-specific direct expenses.**				
	Auto Expense	$(28,023)	Direct to Physician by Utilization		$(2,419)
	Books and Periodicals	$(3,305)	Direct to Physician by Utilization		
	Cellular Phones – Physicians	$(8,124)	Direct to Physician by Utilization	$(780)	$(1,980)
	Computer Expense – Physicians	$(1,819)	Direct to Physician by Utilization		
	Dues and Licenses	$(16,194)	Direct to Physician by Utilization	$(462)	$(1,964)
	Entertainment and Meals	$(30)	Direct to Physician by Utilization		
	Gifts	$(446)	Direct to Physician by Utilization	$(133)	$(133)
	Health Insurance	$(99,257)	Direct to Physician by Utilization	$(10,099)	$(5,579)
	Surgical Instruments	$(326)	Direct to Physician by Utilization		
	Insurance – Long-Term Care	$(5,045)	Direct to Physician by Utilization		
	Insurance – Malpractice	$(303,093)	Direct to Physician by Utilization	$(33,677)	$(33,677)
	Insurance – Term Life	$(3,354)	Direct to Physician by Utilization		
	Meetings and Conventions	$(14,132)	Direct to Physician by Utilization	$(2,324)	
	Nonphysician Provider Comp. and Benefits	$(185,000)	Direct to Physician by Utilization	$(10,000)	$(30,000)
	Office Expense – Specialized	$(32)	Direct to Physician by Utilization		
	Payroll Taxes – Physicians	$(81,593)	Direct to Physician by Utilization	$(8,344)	$(8,657)
	Profit Sharing Contribution	$(75,600)	Direct to Physician by Utilization	$(3,600)	$(4,800)
	Pension Contribution	$(140,940)	Direct to Physician by Utilization	$(15,660)	$(15,660)
	Transcription Service	$(20,003)	Direct to Physician by Utilization	$(685)	$(2,132)
	Total Direct Physician Expenses	$(986,317)		$(85,764)	$(107,002)
Step 7	**Determine physician income after direct expenses (W-2).**	$2,610,724		$236,312	$426,561

* Hypothetical numbers presented for illustrative purposes only. Numbers may not total in all cases due to rounding.
† Actual claim volume not reflected in the example; numbers shown are for illustrative purposes.

Wilson	Einstein	Bornsten	Porter	Mathews	Patel	Kant
$35,693	$28,668	$34,759	$20,269	$12,130	$19,725	$8,579
$256,428	$291,081	$343,674	$556,536	$397,095	$467,735	$428,851
$(587)	$(6,378)		$(2,382)	$(4,981)	$(5,774)	$(5,504)
$(436)	$(143)	$(297)			$(1,833)	$(596)
$(840)	$(780)	$(816)	$(744)	$(804)	$(780)	$(600)
	$(1,275)					$(544)
$(3,642)	$(1,202)	$(1,008)	$(3,046)	$(1,020)	$(2,642)	$(1,206)
						$(30)
		$(180)				
$(10,099)	$(13,580)	$(13,580)	$(13,580)	$(5,579)	$(13,580)	$(13,580)
					$(326)	
$(5,045)						
$(33,677)	$(33,677)	$(33,677)	$(33,677)	$(33,677)	$(33,677)	$(33,677)
$(3,354)						
$(4,310)	$(1,231)	$(877)	$(5,068)		$(164)	$(159)
$(18,000)	$(12,000)	$(25,000)	$(30,000)	$(15,000)	$(25,000)	$(20,000)
			$(8)		$(1)	$(23)
$(7,857)	$(7,906)	$(7,966)	$(10,474)	$(9,603)	$(10,472)	$(10,314)
$(9,600)	$(9,600)	$(9,600)	$(9,600)	$(9,600)	$(9,600)	$(9,600)
$(15,660)	$(15,660)	$(15,660)	$(15,660)	$(15,660)	$(15,660)	$(15,660)
$(5,506)	$(5,506)	$(5,506)	$(74)	$(224)	$(147)	$(222)
$(118,613)	$(108,939)	$(114,168)	$(124,314)	$(96,147)	$(119,656)	$(111,714)
$137,815	$182,143	$229,507	$432,222	$300,948	$348,078	$317,136

EXHIBIT 13.27 Example of Revenue Allocation Method – Strict Cost Accounting

Revenue Category	Allocation Methodology
Net Professional Revenue	Direct to physician producing the revenue.
Ancillary – Technical Component	Allocated to ancillary profit or loss center.
Ancillary – Professional Component	Direct to personally performing physician.
Nonphysician Provider Revenue	Direct to physician supervising the provider producing the revenue based on actual service.
Interest Income	Equal share per physician FTE.
Other Income	Direct to physician producing the income.

EXHIBIT 13.28

Example of Expense Allocation Methods – General Operating Expense Items – Strict Cost Accounting

Accounting	Equal per physician.
Advertising	Equal per physician.
Ancillary Supplies	Direct to ancillary profit or loss center.
Bank Charges	Each physician's percent to total net collections from professional services.
Biomedical Waste	Each physician's percentage of ambulatory encounters.
Business Promotion	Equal per physician.
Cell Phones (administrative)	Equal per physician.
Computer Hardware (administrative)	Equal per physician.
Computer Software	Equal per physician.
Contract Services	Equal per physician.
Drugs & Medical Supplies	Each physician's percentage of ambulatory encounters.
Dues & Licenses (administrative)	Equal per physician.
Food & Entertainment	Equal per physician.
Insurance – General Liability	Equal per physician.
Insurance – Malpractice (corporate)	Equal per physician.
Interest, Penalties, Fees	Equal per physician.
Laundry & Uniforms	Equal per physician.
Lease Equipment	Equal per physician.
Legal Expense	Equal per physician.
Medical Expense Benefits – Flex	Equal per physician.
Mileage Reimbursement (administrative)	Equal per physician.
Miscellaneous Expense	Equal per physician.
Office Supplies	Equal per physician.
Pagers & Answering Service	Equal per physician.
Postage	Equal per physician.
Rent (common)	50% equal share; 50% based on percentage of total encounters.
Rent (division-specific)	Direct to division where possible based on actual per square foot assignment; then based on clinic utilization and time in office.
Repairs & Maintenance	Equal per physician.
Subscriptions & Books	Equal per physician.
Taxes	Equal per physician.
Telephones	Equal per physician.

EXHIBIT 13.29 Example of Expense Allocation Method –
Personnel and Other General Expense Items – Strict Cost Accounting

Employee Salaries

Administrative Staff	Equal per physician.
Billing Staff	50% equal share; 50% based on claims volume.
Clinical Staff	Direct to physician and/or based on % of total encounters.
Nonclinical Staff	Direct to division based on % of total encounters.
Nonclinical Staff (other than direct)	50% equal share; 50% based on % of total encounters.
Scheduling Staff	Direct to division; then based on % of total encounters.
Technicians	Direct to division; then based on % of total encounters.
Ancillary Laboratory Technicians	Direct to ancillary services profit or loss center.
Temporary Employees	Direct to division; then based on % of encounters.

Employee Expenses

Education – Employees	% of allocated salary; consistent with employee-specific allocation.
Insurance, Disability – Employees	% of allocated salary; consistent with employee-specific allocation.
Insurance, Health – Employees	% of allocated salary; consistent with employee-specific allocation.
Payroll Taxes – Employees	% of allocated salary; consistent with employee-specific allocation.
Profit Sharing Contributions	% of allocated salary; consistent with employee-specific allocation.
Worker's Comp – Employees	% of allocated salary; consistent with employee-specific allocation.
Employee Bonuses	% of allocated salary; consistent with employee-specific allocation.

EXHIBIT 13.30

Example of Expense Allocation Method – Direct Expenses – Strict Cost Accounting

Auto Expense	Direct to physician based on utilization.
Books & Periodicals	Direct to physician based on utilization.
Cell Phones	Direct to physician based on utilization.
Computer Expense – Physician	Direct to physician based on utilization.
Dues & Licenses	Direct to physician based on utilization.
Entertainment & Meals	Direct to physician based on utilization.
Gifts	Direct to physician based on utilization.
Health Insurance – Physicians	Direct to physician based on utilization.
Surgical Instruments	Direct to physician based on utilization.
Insurance – Long-Term Care	Direct to physician based on utilization.
Insurance – Malpractice	Direct to physician based on utilization.
Insurance – Term Life	Direct to physician based on utilization.
Meetings & Conventions	Direct to physician based on utilization.
Nonphysician Provider Compensation & Benefits	Direct to physician based on utilization.
Office Expense – Specialized	Direct to physician based on utilization.
Payroll Taxes – Physicians	Direct to physician based on utilization.
Profit Sharing Contribution	Direct to physician based on utilization.
Pension Contribution	Direct to physician based on utilization.
Transcription Service	Direct to physician based on utilization.

EXHIBIT 13.31 Assessment of Group Practice Architecture R –
Strict Cost Accounting Plans

Dimension	Strengths	Weaknesses
Measure	Rewards professional services production.	May result in "cherry-picking" based on reimbursement.
Productivity	Individualistic plan incorporates strong incentives for personal productivity. Promotes personal accountability for work levels.	May lead to competition.
Financial	Allocates practice expenses on perceived "fair" methodology based on utilization.	Cost accounting methodology may create cost allocation disputes. Expense allocation methods are likely to create unrealistic "illusions of precision" related to expenses.
Simplicity		Complex cost allocation formula. Potentially significant administrative burden and challenges in plan administration.
Alignment	Strong emphasis on individual physician performance. Provides clarity of responsibility for share of practice overhead costs.	Productivity orientation may undermine group cohesion. Focus on cost of practice may lead to inappropriate efforts to shift costs. Excessive focus on cost and expense savings may undermine attention to revenue generation as essential to practice success.
"Fairness"	Group physicians may view cost and productivity focus as inherently fair.	May be viewed as promoting culture of co-located individual practices, rather than true "group practice" culture. Use of cost accounting method frequently introduces an unrealistic "illusion of precision" regarding the allocation and responsibility for practice costs.

► GROUP PRACTICE ARCHITECTURE Q – PURE PRODUCTION WITH "MODIFIED" COST ACCOUNTING PLANS
Revenue Element 4 and Expense Element 8

Overview

The perceived weaknesses of strict cost accounting methods – namely, the level of attention and detail to the allocation of both revenues and expenses, and the inherent opportunities for conflict associated with that activity – have led many Group Practices to forego the previous architecture (Architecture R) and adopt "modified" cost accounting plans, such as those illustrated in Architecture Q. Modified cost accounting expense allocation systems allocate a portion of expenses on a shared (e.g., equal share) basis, with a remaining portion allocated on the basis of actual or estimated utilization, as consistent with Expense Element 8.

Application

This plan type is commonly used by single specialty groups, be they primary care, medical specialties, or surgical specialties. It is also used in smaller multispecialty practices. An example of Group Practice Architecture Q is provided in Exhibit 13.32 at the end of this section.

Methodology

Compensation plans using modified cost accounting use agreed upon cost allocation methods to allocate different components of practice expenditures. However, instead of attempting to track each expense item based on actual or perceived resource utilization, these plans tend to recognize that the precision of cost allocation in strict cost accounting is more typically based on illusion than fact. That is, rather than developing a complex infrastructure to measure and track each expenditure item to individual physician utilization, these Group Practices elect to allocate expenses on a reasonable basis – one that balances the objective of allocation based on responsibility with simplicity, understandability, and transparency in expense allocation.

The mathematical steps in these plans are the same as in strict cost accounting models (e.g., Group Practice Example A), but the details of expense allocation differ. Those steps are:

Step 1. Allocate revenues;

Step 2. Allocate expenditures utilizing modified cost accounting;

Step 3. Allocate ancillary services income and profits; and

Step 4. Determine physician-specific compensation.

Modified cost accounting plans typically categorize expenditures into three broad categories: (1) fixed expenditures; (2) variable expenditures; and (3) physician-specific "direct" expenditures, as further defined below.

Fixed Expenditures

A portion of the total expenses for every medical practice is viewed as "fixed" – meaning that the expense will remain largely constant regardless of utilization or productivity. Common "fixed" expenses include building occupancy and rent, furniture, equipment, the majority of support staff costs, legal and accounting, and similar costs. The portion that will be truly fixed will vary somewhat from one practice to another, but the fixed portion of expenses is generally viewed to be in the range of 60 to 85 percent of the total overhead expenses in most practices. The fixed portion is generally allocated on a per capita or equal share per FTE basis.

Variable Expenditures

The portion of practice expenditures that is not fixed, and which does not directly benefit an individual physician (discussed below), will commonly be referred to as the practice's "variable" expenses. Unlike fixed expenses, these expenses typically do vary or change, at least at the margins, based on different levels of physician work, production, or utilization. Such expenses will commonly include medical supplies, laboratory supplies, laundry and linen, and some administrative supplies. The variable portion of expenditures is typically allocated on the basis of actual or estimated utilization.

Physician-Specific "Direct" Expenditures

Physicians in virtually every medical practice have different levels of utilization and costs for physician-specific direct expenses – generally defined as expenses that benefit the individual physician personally. Common physician-specific direct expenses include auto expenses, cell phones, insurance (health, life, malpractice), and others. These expenses are also allocated based on the direct use by individual physicians.

Many compensation plans hold each physician responsible for and "charge" each physician for the physician-specific direct expenses associated with his or her practice on the grounds that the approach promotes individual physician accountability and responsibility. This allows for some level of choice in certain expenses. For example, in some single or multispecialty practices (e.g., cardiology, orthopedics, or divisions in a multispecialty practice), a physician may require special staffing, such as a physician assistant (PA) or surgical PA. In these settings, the nonphysician provider is commonly used to truly extend and support the physician's services, and to enhance the physician's efficiency (rather than billing independently and functioning as an independent provider for revenue generation and other purposes). Accordingly, the additional cost associated with the dedicated nonphysician provider may also constitute a direct expense to the physician benefiting from the provider's services.

Direct allocation of physician-specific direct expenses also allows physicians who do not need a particular expense item (e.g., health or life insurance provided through the practice) to receive benefits (in the form of additional cash) from their nonutilization.

Although three broad categories of expenses are outlined here – fixed, variable, and physician-specific direct – a fourth category termed "fixed/variable" expenses might also be identified. These include expense items that are deemed to contain both fixed and variable components.

As with strict cost accounting methods, the precise means by which a particular expense item is allocated will be subject to discussion and, ultimately, some level of negotiation. Nonetheless, examples of the types of broad categorizations are provided below using the same expense categories referenced in connection with the strict cost accounting example provided in Architecture R.

In Architecture Q, we assume the same professional fee revenue and ancillary revenue treatment as in Architecture R; namely, individual net collections are credited to the physician along with a share of ancillary services income or profits based on a percentage of total ambulatory encounters. The key difference in this example is the modified cost accounting method employed to allocate practice expenses at Step 3 of the calculation. In Architecture R, each individual expense item was allocated as directly as possible to the physician who purchased or consumed the expense. In contrast, with modified cost accounting, the expenditures are generally considered "fixed," "variable," or "direct," with different methods used to allocate these three expenditure categories (as demonstrated in Exhibits 13.33, 13.34, and 13.35).

An assessment of the strengths and weaknesses of Architecture Q is provided in Exhibit 13.36.

EXHIBIT 13.32

Example Q-1 – Group Practice Architecture Q – Modified Cost Accounting Plan*
Revenue Element 4 and Expense Element 8

					Smith	Johnson
Step 1	**Assemble production information.**					
	Physicians	9.00			1.00	1.00
	Physician FTE	8.75			1.00	1.00
	Ambulatory Encounters	5,158			206	504
	Physician % to Total Ambulatory Encounters				4%	10%

		Total	Allocation		Smith	Johnson
Step 2	**Determine revenue.**					
	Net Collections from Professional Services	$4,127,816	Direct		$378,545	$524,376
	Ancillary Net Collections – Professional Component	$155,864	Direct to Reading Physician		$13,342	$62,145
	Other Revenues/Income	$46,897	Equal per Physician		$5,211	$5,211
	Total Revenue	$4,330,577			$397,098	$591,731

		Total	Allocation		Smith	Johnson
Step 3	**Determine operating expenses.**					
	GENERAL OPERATING EXPENSES					
	Accounting	$(18,636)	Fixed (Equal per Physician)		$(2,071)	$(2,071)
	Advertising	$(4,525)	Fixed (Equal per Physician)		$(503)	$(503)
	Bank Charges	$(2,618)	Variable (% of Encounters)		$(105)	$(256)
	Biomedical Waste	$(2,763)	Variable (% of Encounters)		$(110)	$(270)
	Business Promotion	$(2,618)	Fixed (Equal per Physician)		$(291)	$(291)
	Cell Phones (admin)	$(2,400)	Fixed (Equal per Physician)		$(267)	$(267)
	Computer (admin)	$(87,036)	Fixed (Equal per Physician)		$(9,671)	$(9,671)
	Contract Services	$(2,618)	Fixed (Equal per Physician)		$(291)	$(291)
	Drugs and Medical Supplies	$(6,150)	Variable (% of Encounters)		$(246)	$(601)
	Dues and Licenses	$(10,794)	Fixed (Equal per Physician)		$(1,199)	$(1,199)
	Food/Entertainment	$(596)	Fixed (Equal per Physician)		$(66)	$(66)
	Insurance – General Liability	$(1,837)	Fixed (Equal per Physician)		$(204)	$(204)
	Insurance – Malpractice (corp)	$(11,299)	Fixed (Equal per Physician)		$(1,255)	$(1,255)
	Interest/Penalties/Fees	$(742)	Fixed (Equal per Physician)		$(82)	$(82)
	Laundry and Uniforms	$(450)	Variable (% of Encounters)		$(18)	$(44)
	Lease Equipment	$(1,996)	Fixed (Equal per Physician)		$(222)	$(222)
	Legal Expense	$(2,618)	Fixed (Equal per Physician)		$(291)	$(291)
	Medical Expense Benefits – Flex	$(1,430)	Fixed (Equal per Physician)		$(159)	$(159)
	Mileage Reimbursement (admin)	$(220)	Fixed (Equal per Physician)		$(24)	$(24)
	Miscellaneous Expense	$(126)	Fixed (Equal per Physician)		$(14)	$(14)
	Office Supplies	$(16,070)	Fixed (Equal per Physician)		$(1,786)	$(1,786)
	Pagers and Answering Service	$(13,520)	Fixed (Equal per Physician)		$(1,502)	$(1,502)
	Postage	$(8,467)	Fixed (Equal per Physician)		$(941)	$(941)
	Repairs and Maintenance	$(35,782)	Fixed (Equal per Physician)		$(3,976)	$(3,976)
	Subscriptions and Books	$(1,232)	Fixed (Equal per Physician)		$(137)	$(137)
	Taxes	$(3,519)	Fixed (Equal per Physician)		$(391)	$(391)
	Telephone	$(17,520)	Fixed (Equal per Physician)		$(1,947)	$(1,947)

Wilson	Einstein	Bornsten	Porter	Mathews	Patel	Kant
1.00	1.00	1.00	1.00	1.00	1.00	1.00
1.00	1.00	1.00	1.00	0.75	1.00	1.00
1,149	813	1,032	509	300	490	155
22%	16%	20%	10%	6%	9%	3%
$376,499	$356,821	$413,753	$637,903	$434,281	$532,153	$473,486
$13,645	$32,121	$24,512	$1,024	$3,212	$4,512	$1,351
$5,211	$5,211	$5,211	$5,211	$5,211	$5,211	$5,211
$395,355	$394,153	$443,475	$644,137	$442,704	$541,876	$480,048
$(2,071)	$(2,071)	$(2,071)	$(2,071)	$(2,071)	$(2,071)	$(2,071)
$(503)	$(503)	$(503)	$(503)	$(503)	$(503)	$(503)
$(583)	$(413)	$(524)	$(258)	$(152)	$(249)	$(79)
$(616)	$(436)	$(553)	$(273)	$(161)	$(263)	$(83)
$(291)	$(291)	$(291)	$(291)	$(291)	$(291)	$(291)
$(267)	$(267)	$(267)	$(267)	$(267)	$(267)	$(267)
$(9,671)	$(9,671)	$(9,671)	$(9,671)	$(9,671)	$(9,671)	$(9,671)
$(291)	$(291)	$(291)	$(291)	$(291)	$(291)	$(291)
$(1,370)	$(969)	$(1,231)	$(607)	$(358)	$(584)	$(185)
$(1,199)	$(1,199)	$(1,199)	$(1,199)	$(1,199)	$(1,199)	$(1,199)
$(66)	$(66)	$(66)	$(66)	$(66)	$(66)	$(66)
$(204)	$(204)	$(204)	$(204)	$(204)	$(204)	$(204)
$(1,255)	$(1,255)	$(1,255)	$(1,255)	$(1,255)	$(1,255)	$(1,255)
$(82)	$(82)	$(82)	$(82)	$(82)	$(82)	$(82)
$(100)	$(71)	$(90)	$(44)	$(26)	$(43)	$(14)
$(222)	$(222)	$(222)	$(222)	$(222)	$(222)	$(222)
$(291)	$(291)	$(291)	$(291)	$(291)	$(291)	$(291)
$(159)	$(159)	$(159)	$(159)	$(159)	$(159)	$(159)
$(24)	$(24)	$(24)	$(24)	$(24)	$(24)	$(24)
$(14)	$(14)	$(14)	$(14)	$(14)	$(14)	$(14)
$(1,786)	$(1,786)	$(1,786)	$(1,786)	$(1,786)	$(1,786)	$(1,786)
$(1,502)	$(1,502)	$(1,502)	$(1,502)	$(1,502)	$(1,502)	$(1,502)
$(941)	$(941)	$(941)	$(941)	$(941)	$(941)	$(941)
$(3,976)	$(3,976)	$(3,976)	$(3,976)	$(3,976)	$(3,976)	$(3,976)
$(137)	$(137)	$(137)	$(137)	$(137)	$(137)	$(137)
$(391)	$(391)	$(391)	$(391)	$(391)	$(391)	$(391)
$(1,947)	$(1,947)	$(1,947)	$(1,947)	$(1,947)	$(1,947)	$(1,947)

continued on next page

Exhibit 13.32 – Example Q-1 continued

	Total	Allocation	Smith	Johnson
Subtotal General Operating Expenses	$(234,424)		$(25,194)	$(25,887)
RENT – TOTAL	$(115,100)	50% Fixed/50% Variable % Ambulatory Encounters		
Fixed (equal per physician) Portion 50%	$(57,550)	50%	$(6,394)	$(6,394)
Variable (% of ambulatory encounters) Portion 50%	$(57,550)	50%	$(2,298)	$(5,623)
Subtotal – Rent Expense	$(115,100)		$(8,693)	$(12,018)
SUPPORT STAFF EXPENSES				
Administrative Staff	$(123,523)	Fixed (Equal per Physician)	$(13,725)	$(13,725)
Billing, Clinical, Scheduling and Other Staff	$(585,750)	50% Fixed/50% Variable % Ambulatory Encounters		
Fixed (equal per physician) Portion 50%	$(292,875)	50%	$(32,542)	$(32,542)
Variable (% of ambulatory encounters) Portion 50%	$(292,875)	50%	$(11,697)	$(28,617)
Subtotal – Nonphysician Employee Allocated Salary	$(709,273)		$(57,963)	$(74,884)
Total Operating Expenses	$(1,058,797)		$(91,851)	$(112,788)

Step 4 **Determine ancillary services profits pool.**

	Total	Allocation	Smith	Johnson
Revenues				
Technical Component Revenues	$415,424	Ancillary Pool		
Expenses				
Ancillary Technicians	$(211,754)	Direct Ancillary Pool		
Ancillary Net Profit (Revenue – Expense)	$203,670	% of Total Ambulatory Encounters	$10,947	$21,395

Step 5 **Determine amount available for physician compensation and direct expenses.**

	Total	Allocation	Smith	Johnson
(Revenue – Operating Expenses + Ancillary Profits)	$3,475,450		$316,194	$500,338

Step 6 **Determine physician-specific direct expenses.**

	Total	Allocation	Smith	Johnson
Auto Expense	$(28,023)	Direct to Physician		$(2,419)
Books and Periodicals	$(3,305)	Direct to Physician		
Cellular Phones – Physicians	$(8,124)	Direct to Physician	$(780)	$(1,980)
Computer Expense – Physicians	$(1,819)	Direct to Physician		
Dues and Licenses	$(16,194)	Direct to Physician	$(462)	$(1,964)

Wilson	Einstein	Bornsten	Porter	Mathews	Patel	Kant
$(27,385)	$(26,604)	$(27,113)	$(25,898)	$(25,413)	$(25,854)	$(25,076)
$(6,394)	$(6,394)	$(6,394)	$(6,394)	$(6,394)	$(6,394)	$(6,394)
$(12,820)	$(9,071)	$(11,514)	$(5,679)	$(3,347)	$(5,467)	$(1,729)
$(19,214)	$(15,465)	$(17,909)	$(12,074)	$(9,742)	$(11,862)	$(8,124)
$(13,725)	$(13,725)	$(13,725)	$(13,725)	$(13,725)	$(13,725)	$(13,725)
$(32,542)	$(32,542)	$(32,542)	$(32,542)	$(32,542)	$(32,542)	$(32,542)
$(65,241)	$(46,163)	$(58,598)	$(28,901)	$(17,034)	$(27,823)	$(8,801)
$(111,508)	$(92,429)	$(104,864)	$(75,168)	$(63,301)	$(74,089)	$(55,067)
$(158,107)	$(134,499)	$(149,886)	$(113,140)	$(98,455)	$(111,805)	$(88,267)
$38,262	$30,731	$37,261	$21,728	$13,004	$21,145	$9,197
$275,510	$290,385	$330,850	$552,726	$357,253	$451,216	$400,978
$(587)	$(6,378)		$(2,382)	$(4,981)	$(5,774)	$(5,504)
$(436)	$(143)	$(297)			$(1,833)	$(596)
$(840)	$(780)	$(816)	$(744)	$(804)	$(780)	$(600)
	$(1,275)					$(544)
$(3,642)	$(1,202)	$(1,008)	$(3,046)	$(1,020)	$(2,642)	$(1,206)

continued on next page

Exhibit 13.32 – Example Q-1 continued

	Total	Allocation	Smith	Johnson
Entertainment and Meals	$(30)	Direct to Physician		
Gifts	$(446)	Direct to Physician	$(133)	$(133)
Health Insurance	$(99,257)	Direct to Physician	$(10,099)	$(5,580)
Surgical Instruments	$(326)	Direct to Physician		
Insurance – Long-Term Care	$(5,045)	Direct to Physician		
Insurance – Malpractice	$(303,093)	Direct to Physician	$(33,677)	$(33,677)
Insurance – Term Life	$(3,354)	Direct to Physician		
Meetings and Conventions	$(14,132)	Direct to Physician	$(2,324)	
Nonphysician Provider Comp. and Benefits	$(185,000)	Direct to Physician	$(10,000)	$(30,000)
Office Expense – Specialized	$(32)			
Payroll Taxes – Physicians	$(81,593)	Direct to Physician	$(8,344)	$(8,657)
Profit Sharing Contribution	$(75,600)	Direct to Physician	$(3,600)	$(4,800)
Pension Contribution	$(140,940)	Direct to Physician	$(15,660)	$(15,660)
Transcription Service	$(20,003)	Direct to Physician	$(685)	$(2,132)
Total Direct Physician Expenses	$(986,316)	Direct to Physician	$(85,764)	$(107,002)
Step 7 **Determine physician income after direct expenses (W-2).**	$2,489,133		$230,431	$393,336

* Hypothetical numbers presented for illustrative purposes only. Numbers may not total in all cases due to rounding.

Wilson	Einstein	Bornsten	Porter	Mathews	Patel	Kant
						$(30)
		$(180)				
$(10,099)	$(13,580)	$(13,580)	$(13,580)	$(5,579)	$(13,580)	$(13,580)
					$(326)	
$(5,045)						
$(33,677)	$(33,677)	$(33,677)	$(33,677)	$(33,677)	$(33,677)	$(33,677)
$(3,354)						
$(4,310)	$(1,231)	$(877)	$(5,068)		$(164)	$(159)
$(18,000)	$(12,000)	$(25,000)	$(30,000)	$(15,000)	$(25,000)	$(20,000)
			(8)		$(1)	$(23)
$(7,857)	$(7,906)	$(7,966)	$(10,474)	$(9,603)	$(10,472)	$(10,314)
$(9,600)	(9,600)	$(9,600)	$(9,600)	$(9,600)	$(9,600)	$(9,600)
$(15,660)	$(15,660)	$(15,660)	$(15,660)	$(15,660)	$(15,660)	$(15,660)
$(5,506)	$(5,506)	$(5,506)	$(74)	$(224)	$(147)	$(222)
$(118,613)	$(108,939)	$(114,168)	$(124,313)	$(96,147)	$(119,656)	$(111,715)
$156,897	$181,446	$216,683	$428,413	$261,105	$331,559	$289,263

EXHIBIT 13.33   Example of Expense Allocation Method –
General Operating Expense Items – Modified Cost Accounting

Bank Charges	Variable. Based on % of encounters.
Biomedical Waste	Variable. Based on % of encounters.
Drugs & Medical Supplies	Variable. Based on % of encounters.
Laundry & Uniforms	Variable. Based on % of encounters.
Ancillary Supplies	Direct to ancillary profit-and-loss center.
Accounting	Fixed. Equal per physician.
Advertising	Fixed. Equal per physician.
Cell Phones (administrative)	Fixed. Equal per physician.
Computer (administrative)	Fixed. Equal per physician.
Contract Services	Fixed. Equal per physician.
Dues & Licenses (administrative)	Fixed. Equal per physician.
Food & Entertainment	Fixed. Equal per physician.
Insurance – General Liability	Fixed. Equal per physician.
Insurance – Malpractice (corporate)	Fixed. Equal per physician.
Interest, Penalties, Fees	Fixed. Equal per physician.
Lease Equipment	Fixed. Equal per physician.
Legal Expense	Fixed. Equal per physician.
Medical Expense Benefits – Flex	Fixed. Equal per physician.
Mileage Reimbursement (administrative)	Fixed. Equal per physician.
Miscellaneous	Fixed. Equal per physician.
Office Supplies	Fixed. Equal per physician.
Pagers & Answering Service	Fixed. Equal per physician.
Postage	Fixed. Equal per physician.
Repairs & Maintenance	Fixed. Equal per physician.
Subscriptions & Books	Fixed. Equal per physician.
Taxes	Fixed. Equal per physician.
Telephones	Fixed. Equal per physician.
Rent (division-specific and common)	50% Fixed. Equal per physician. 50% Variable. Based on % of encounters.

EXHIBIT 13.34 Example of Expense Allocation Method –
Staffing Expense Items – Modified Cost Accounting

EMPLOYEE SALARIES AND EXPENSES

Administrative Staff	Fixed. Equal per physician.
Billing Staff	50% Fixed. Equal per physician. 50% Variable. Percentage of encounters or claims processed.
Clinical Staff	50% Fixed. Equal per physician 50% Variable. Percentage of encounters
Nonclinical Staff	50% Fixed. Equal per physician. 50% Variable. Percentage of encounters.
Nonclinical Staff (other than direct)	50% Fixed. Equal per physician. 50% Variable. Percentage of encounters.
Scheduling Staff	50% Fixed. Equal per physician. 50% Variable. Percentage of encounters.
Technicians	50% Fixed. Equal per physician. 50% Variable. Percentage of encounters.
Ancillary Laboratory Technician	Direct to ancillary services profit-and-loss pool.
Temporary Employees	50% Fixed. Equal per physician. 50% Variable. Percentage of encounters.
Employee Expenses (education, benefits, bonuses)	50% Fixed. Equal per physician. 50% Variable. Percentage of encounters.

EXHIBIT 13.35

Example of Expense Allocation Method –
Physician-Specific Direct Expenses – Modified Cost Accounting

Auto Expense	Direct to physician based on utilization.
Books & Periodicals	Direct to physician based on utilization.
Cellular Phones	Direct to physician based on utilization.
Computer Expense – Physician	Direct to physician based on utilization.
Dues & Licenses	Direct to physician based on utilization.
Entertainment & Meals	Direct to physician based on utilization.
Gifts	Direct to physician based on utilization.
Health Insurance – Physicians	Direct to physician based on utilization.
Surgical Instruments	Direct to physician based on utilization.
Insurance – Long-Term Care	Direct to physician based on utilization.
Insurance – Malpractice	Direct to physician based on utilization.
Insurance – Term Life	Direct to physician based on utilization.
Meetings & Conventions	Direct to physician based on utilization.
Nonphysician Provider Compensation & Benefits	Direct to physician based on utilization.
Office Expense – Specialized	Direct to physician based on utilization.
Payroll Taxes – Physicians	Direct to physician based on utilization.
Profit Sharing Contribution	Direct to physician based on utilization.
Pension Contribution	Direct to physician based on utilization.
Transcription Service	Direct to physician based on utilization.

EXHIBIT 13.36 Assessment of Group Practice Architecture Q – Modified Cost Accounting

Dimension	Strengths	Weaknesses
Measure	Allows for direct individual production credit.	May lead to "cherry-picking" based on reimbursement.
Productivity	Can use any number of measures for production. Incorporates strong incentives for productivity.	Pure production may lead to internal competition.
Financial	Allocation of expenses promotes accountability for costs. Because strict cost accounting may create cost allocation disputes within a group, modified cost accounting takes the position that costs do not need to be tracked with certainty, but it still uses agreed upon (and "reasonable") allocation method.	Cost categories must still be determined and negotiated.
Simplicity	Reduces cost allocation methods from potentially numerous approaches designed to track actual utilization by using three to four "reasonable" approaches to cost allocation.	Requires judgment to allocate expenses into categories. Still involves complexity and focus on expenses as well as revenues.
Alignment	No need for express performance expectations for productivity due to productivity orientation.	Productivity orientation may undermine group cohesiveness. Productivity orientation may not permit a high enough level of attention to other activities (e.g., quality, efficiency, or service).
"Fairness"	Group physicians may view cost and productivity focus as reasonably "fair."	Physicians may perceive plan as inequitable, given a large proportion of expenditures deemed "fixed" and allocated on an equal share per physician basis. May encourage a practice culture of co-located individual practices rather than a "group practice" orientation.

© 2006 Johnson & Walker Keegan

► GROUP PRACTICE ARCHITECTURE P — PURE PRODUCTION WITH NEGOTIATED EXPENSE ALLOCATION PLANS
Revenue Element 4 and Expense Element 7

Overview

This plan provides individual physicians with direct production credit for professional services, but this example allocates operating expenses based on a negotiated methodology. This method of expenditure treatment effectively further simplifies the cost allocation method from earlier strict cost accounting and modified cost accounting methods. It uses an approach to expense allocation that is acknowledged to be negotiated in a manner that physicians generally perceive to be "fair." This architecture combines Revenue Element 4 (pure production) with Expense Element 7 (negotiated expense allocation).

Application

This plan type is commonly used by single specialty practices, where practice expenses are generally relatively consistent among physicians. The plan architecture is also used in some smaller multispecialty group practices involving similar or complementary practice subspecialties, and in divisions or departments of large multispecialty groups and faculty practice plans.

Methodology

The basic steps in a pure production with negotiated expense allocation plan are presented in Example P-1 below (and illustrated in Exhibit 13.37). We then present a variation on this basic plan in Example P-2 (illustrated in Exhibit 13.38) at the end of this section.

Example P-1 — Basic Example of Architecture P: Pure Production with Negotiated Expense Allocation on a Basis of 70 Percent Equal Share/30 Percent Based on Professional Services Net Collections

Step 1. Determine Individual Production Levels for Physicians
In this example, physician production is measured by net collections from professional services.

Step 2. Allocate Revenue to Individual Physicians
Revenue is allocated to physicians on an individual basis. In this example, net collections from professional services and the professional component of ancillary services are allocated directly to the physician who performed the service. Other revenues are allocated on an equal share per physician basis. Ancillary services are treated as a separate profit-and-loss center in Step 4 below.

Step 3. Negotiate a Method to Allocate Total Operating Expenses to Physicians
In this example, a simple 70 percent equal share (per FTE physician) and 30 percent variable (based on individual physician net collections from professional services as a percentage of total net collections from professional services) is used to allocate cost of

practice or overhead. The use of net collections in this example will mean that physicians who have the highest levels of production will bear the largest portion of operating costs.

Step 4. Determine Ancillary Services Profit-and-Loss Pool, and Allocate Portion of Pool to Individual Physicians

Similar to earlier plan architectures, ancillary services revenues and expenses are used to create an ancillary services profit-and-loss pool. The profits from the ancillary services profits pool are allocated based on each physician's percentage to total of net collections from professional services. Other methods could also be used, including those referenced in other examples and those described in Chapter 9, "The Legal Element."

Step 5. Determine Amount Available for Physician Compensation and Direct Expense

The calculation for this step is:

>   Allocated Revenues
> − Allocated Operating Expense
> + Share of Ancillary Services Profits
>   ———————————————————————————
>   Amount Available for Physician Compensation and Direct Expense

Step 6. Determine Physician-Specific Direct Expenditures

Physician-specific expenditures are directly allocated to physicians based on utilization.

Step 7. Calculate Physician Income after Direct Expenses

Subtract the direct expenses identified in Step 6 from the revenues available for physician compensation and direct expenses (Step 5) to arrive at the earnings for the physician.

Example P-2

This variation of the basic plan architecture demonstrates a different method of negotiating the allocation of total operating expenses in the Group Practice (Step 3).

In this example (illustrated in Exhibit 13.38), while the allocation method involves a combination of fixed and variable methods (consistent with Example P-1), the specific measures and percentages differ. In this example, 60 percent of the total operating expenditures are allocated on a fixed per physician basis (regardless of FTE level, generally reflecting the recognition of the high level of fixed costs in a medical practice), and 40 percent are based on an individual physician's ambulatory encounters as a percentage of total ambulatory encounters. Ambulatory encounters are used as a surrogate for office utilization such that the physicians with the most ambulatory encounters will bear the largest share of practice overhead. This example also involves an equal share or "per capita" allocation of ancillary services profits without regard to physician FTE.

An assessment of the strengths and weaknesses of Architecture P is provided in Exhibit 13.39.

EXHIBIT 13.37

Example P-1 – Group Practice Architecture P –
Pure Production with Negotiated Expense Allocation Plan*
Operating Expenses Allocated 70% Equal Share (per FTE)/30%
Based on Professional Services Net Collections
Revenue Element 4 and Expense Element 7

Step 1	Assemble production information.			Dr. A Gen Ortho	Dr. B Gen Ortho
	Physicians	9.00		1.00	1.00
	Physician FTE	8.75		1.00	0.75
	Ambulatory Encounters	28,523		3,141	2,985
	Physician % to Total Ambulatory Encounters			11%	10%
	Net Collections from Professional Services	$7,874,962		$750,003	$689,542
	Physician % to Total Net Collections	100%		9.52%	8.76%

Step 2	Determine revenue.	Total	Allocation	Dr. A	Dr. B
	Net Collections from Professional Services	$7,874,962	Direct	$750,003	$689,542
	Ancillary Net Collections – Professional Component	$155,864	Direct to Reading Physician	$13,342	$62,145
	Other Revenues/Income	$46,897	Equal per Physician	$5,211	$5,211
	Total Revenue	$8,077,723		$768,556	$756,898

Step 3	Determine operating expenses (negotiated allocation).				
	Total Operating Expenses†	$(3,715,753)			
	Fixed Portion 70%	$(2,601,027)	Equal per FTE	$(297,260)	$(222,945)
	Variable Portion 30%	$(1,114,726)	Physician % to Total Net Collections	$(106,165)	$(97,607)
	Total Operating Expenses	$(3,715,753)		$(403,426)	$(320,552)

Step 4	Determine ancillary services profits pool (e.g., X-ray and MRI).				
	Revenues				
	(excluding personally performed professional component)	$1,074,545	Ancillary Pool		
	Expenses				
	Equipment Rental	$(104,521)			
	Staff	$(245,120)			
	Other Ancillary Expense (supplies, etc.)	$(54,712)	Direct Ancillary Pool		
		$(404,353)			
	Ancillary Net Profit (Revenue – Expense)	$670,192	Distribution: Physician % of Professional Services Net Collections (from above)	$63,828	$58,683

Dr. C Gen Ortho	Dr. D Gen Ortho	Dr. E Sports	Dr. F Sports	Dr. G Foot	Dr. H Spine	Dr. I Spine
1.00	1.00	1.00	1.00	1.00	1.00	1.00
1.00	1.00	1.00	1.00	1.00	1.00	1.00
3,562	3,020	3,500	3,621	3,309	2,501	2,884
12%	11%	12%	13%	12%	9%	10%
$852,141	$798,568	$932,564	$1,021,451	$784,021	$936,458	$1,110,214
10.82%	10.14%	11.84%	12.97%	9.96%	11.89%	14.10%
Dr. C	Dr. D	Dr. E	Dr. F	Dr. G	Dr. H	Dr. I
$852,141	$798,568	$932,564	$1,021,451	$784,021	$936,458	$1,110,214
$13,645	$32,121	$24,512	$1,024	$3,212	$4,512	$1,351
$5,211	$5,211	$5,211	$5,211	$5,211	$5,211	$5,211
$870,997	$835,900	$962,287	$1,027,686	$792,444	$946,181	$1,116,776
$(297,260)	$(297,260)	$(297,260)	$(297,260)	$(297,260)	$(297,260)	$(297,260)
$(120,623)	$(113,040)	$(132,007)	$(144,590)	$(110,981)	$(132,559)	$(157,154)
$(417,883)	$(410,300)	$(429,268)	$(441,850)	$(408,241)	$(429,819)	$(454,415)
$72,521	$67,961	$79,365	$86,930	$66,723	$79,696	$94,484

continued on next page

Exhibit 13.37 – Example P-1 continued

		Total	Allocation	Dr. A Gen Ortho	Dr. B Gen Ortho
Step 5	**Determine amount available for physician compensation and direct expense.**				
	(Revenue – Operating Expenses + Ancillary Profits)	$5,032,162		$428,959	$495,029
Step 6	**Determine physician-specific direct expenses.**				
	Total Direct Physician Expenses	$(815,685)	Direct to Physician	$(75,989)	$(77,172)
Step 7	**Determine physician income after direct expenses (W-2).**	$4,216,477		$352,970	$417,857

* Hypothetical numbers presented for illustrative purposes only. Numbers may not total in all cases due to rounding.
† Operating expenses include rent, nonphysician staff, and other general operating expenses.

Key:
Gen Ortho = General Orthopedic Surgery

© 2006 Johnson & Walker Keegan

Dr. C Gen Ortho	Dr. D Gen Ortho	Dr. E Sports	Dr. F Sports	Dr. G Foot	Dr. H Spine	Dr. I Spine
$525,634	$493,561	$612,384	$672,766	$450,926	$596,058	$756,845
$(101,025)	$(97,190)	$(90,797)	$(94,314)	$(81,788)	$(95,004)	$(102,406)
$424,609	$396,372	$521,587	$578,452	$369,138	$501,054	$654,439

EXHIBIT 13.38

Example P-2 – Group Practice Architecture P –
Pure Production with Negotiated Expense Allocation Plan*
Operating Expenses Allocated 60% Equal Share (per Physician)/40%
Based on Ambulatory Encounters
Revenue Element 4 and Expense Element 7

Step 1	Assemble production information.			Dr. A Gen Ortho	Dr. B Gen Ortho
	Physicians	9.00		1.00	1.00
	Physician FTE	8.75		1.00	0.75
	Ambulatory Encounters	28,523		3,141	2,985
	Physician % to Total Ambulatory Encounters			11%	10%
	Professional Services Net Collections	$7,874,962		$750,003	$689,542
	Physician % to Total Net Collections	100%		10%	9%

Step 2	Determine revenue.	Total	Allocation	Dr. A	Dr. B
	Net Collections from Professional Services	$7,874,962	Direct	$750,003	$689,542
	Ancillary Net Collections- Professional Component	$155,864	Direct to Performing Physician	$13,342	$62,145
	Other Revenues/Income	$46,897	Equal per FTE	$5,360	$4,020
	Total Revenue	$8,077,723		$768,705	$755,707

Step 3	Determine operating expenses (negotiated allocation).				
	Total Operating Expenses[†]	$(3,715,753)			
	Fixed Portion 60%	$(2,229,452)	Equal per Physician	$(247,717)	$(247,717)
	Variable Portion 40%	$(1,486,301)	Physician % to Total Ambulatory Encounters	$(163,674)	$(155,545)
	Total Operating Expenses	$(3,715,753)		$(411,391)	$(403,262)

Step 4	Determine ancillary services profits pool.				
	Revenues				
	(excluding personally performed professional component)	$1,074,545	Direct Ancillary Pool		
	Expenses				
	Equipment Rental	$(104,521)	Direct Ancillary Pool		
	Staff	$(245,120)	Direct Ancillary Pool		
	Other Ancillary Expense (supplies, etc.)	$(54,712)	Direct Ancillary Pool		
	Ancillary Net Profit (Revenue – Expense)	$670,192	Equal per Physician	$74,466	$74,466

Dr. C Gen Ortho	Dr. D Gen Ortho	Dr. E Sports	Dr. F Sports	Dr. G Foot	Dr. H Spine	Dr. I Spine
1.00	1.00	1.00	1.00	1.00	1.00	1.00
1.00	1.00	1.00	1.00	1.00	1.00	1.00
3,562	3,020	3,500	3,621	3,309	2,501	2,884
12%	11%	12%	13%	12%	9%	10%
$852,141	$798,568	$932,564	$1,021,451	$784,021	$936,458	$1,110,214
11%	10%	12%	13%	10%	12%	14%
Dr. C	Dr. D	Dr. E	Dr. F	Dr. G	Dr. H	Dr. I
$852,141	$798,568	$932,564	$1,021,451	$784,021	$936,458	$1,110,214
$13,645	$32,121	$24,512	$1,024	$3,212	$4,512	$1,351
$5,360	$5,360	$5,360	$5,360	$5,360	$5,360	$5,360
$871,146	$836,049	$962,436	$1,027,835	$792,593	$946,330	$1,116,925
$(247,717)	$(247,717)	$(247,717)	$(247,717)	$(247,717)	$(247,717)	$(247,717)
$(185,612)	$(157,369)	$(182,381)	$(188,686)	$(172,428)	$(130,324)	$(150,282)
$(433,329)	$(405,086)	$(430,098)	$(436,403)	$(420,145)	$(378,041)	$(397,999)
$74,466	$74,466	$74,466	$74,466	$74,466	$74,466	$74,466

continued on next page

Exhibit 13.38 – Example P-2 continued

		Total	Allocation	Dr. A Gen Ortho	Dr. B Gen Ortho
Step 5	Determine amount available for physician compensation and direct expense.				
	(Revenue – Operating Expenses + Ancillary Profits)	$5,032,162		$431,780	$426,911
Step 6	Determine physician-specific direct expenses.				
	Total Direct Physician Expenses	$(815,685)	Direct	$(75,989)	$(77,172)
Step 7	Determine physician income after direct expenses (W-2).	$4,216,477		$355,791	$349,739

* Hypothetical numbers presented for illustrative purposes only. Numbers may not total in all cases due to rounding.

† Operating expenses include rent, nonphysician staff, and other general operating expenses.

Key:
Gen Ortho = General Orthopedic Surgery

Dr. C Gen Ortho	Dr. D Gen Ortho	Dr. E Sports	Dr. F Sports	Dr. G Foot	Dr. H Spine	Dr. I Spine
$512,283	$505,429	$606,804	$665,897	$446,913	$642,754	$793,392
$(101,025)	$(97,190)	$(90,797)	$(94,314)	$(81,788)	$(95,004)	$(102,406)
$411,257	$408,239	$516,006	$571,584	$365,125	$547,750	$690,986

EXHIBIT 13.39 Assessment of Group Practice Architecture P –
Pure Production and Negotiated Expense Plans

Dimension	Strengths	Weaknesses
Measure	Encourages individual productivity. Holds physicians accountable for cost of practice but without excessive micromanagement of costs.	Measures tend to focus heavily on clinical production, although additional performance measures may also be employed.
Productivity	Directly recognizes individual production levels.	The focus on production may not permit the level of attention to other key performance indices (e.g., cost of practice, patient access, and patient satisfaction).
Financial	Promotes individual responsibility for a defined level of practice costs. The "negotiated" expense allocation minimizes the administrative complexity associated with plan administration.	Negotiated cost allocation may mitigate individual physician attention to cost management.
Simplicity	Ease of administration.	Equal share and production portions must still be negotiated and set.
Alignment	Encourages individual production, but has a group practice orientation in connection with expenditures.	
"Fairness"	Directly recognizes and rewards physician work and effort.	Physicians may perceive they are being held responsible for expenditures beyond their control.

© 2006 Johnson & Walker Keegan

➤ GROUP PRACTICE ARCHITECTURE O – PURE PRODUCTION WITH EQUAL SHARE EXPENSE ALLOCATION PLANS
Revenue Element 4 and Expense Element 6

Overview

This plan recognizes individual physician work and effort via production measures, but also recognizes the "group" nature of a medical practice and treats expense allocation on an equal share basis. This method combines Revenue Element 4 (pure production) with Expense Element 6 (equal share expense allocation).

Application

This plan architecture is commonly used by single specialty practices, where practice expenses and resource needs are largely consistent among physicians. The plan architecture is also used in some smaller multispecialty group practices involving similar or complementary practice subspecialties, and in divisions or departments of large multispecialty groups and faculty practice plans.

Methodology

The basic steps in a pure production with equal share expense allocation plan are presented in Example O-1 below (and illustrated in Exhibit 13.40). A variation on this basic plan is provided in Example O-2 (and illustrated in Exhibit 13.41) shown at the end of this section.

Example O-1 – Basic Example of Architecture O: Pure Production with Expense Allocation on an Equal Share per Physician Basis

Step 1. Allocate Revenue to Individual Physicians

Revenue is allocated to physicians on an individual basis. In this example (illustrated in Exhibit 13.40), net collections from professional services and the professional component of ancillary services are allocated directly to the physician who performed the service. Other revenues are allocated on an equal share per physician FTE basis.

Step 2. Determine Total Operating Expense and Allocate on an Equal Share Basis to Physicians

Total operating expenditures are then allocated on a per FTE physician basis, meaning that a part-time physician is allocated a lower share of practice expenses than his or her full-time counterpart.

Step 3. Determine Ancillary Services Profit-and-Loss Pool, and Allocate Portion of Pool to Individual Physicians

Similar to earlier plan architectures, ancillary services revenues and expenses are used to create an ancillary services profit-and-loss pool. The allocation method for the ancillary services profit pool is consistent with the treatment of total operating expenses: the ancillary profits are distributed to each physician on a per FTE physician basis. Other allocation methods could also be used, as illustrated in other plan examples and discussed in Chapter 9, "The Legal Element."

Step 4. Determine Amount Available for Physician Compensation and Direct Expense

The calculation for this step is:

> Revenue
> − Operating Expense (equal share per FTE)
> + Ancillary Profits Share
> _____
> Amount Available for Physician Compensation and Direct Expense

Step 5. Determine Physician-Specific Direct Expenditures

Physician-specific expenditures are directly allocated to physicians based on utilization.

Step 6. Calculate Physician Income after Direct Expenses

Subtract the direct expenses identified in Step 5 from the revenue available for physician compensation and direct expenses (Step 4) to arrive at the earnings for the physician.

Example O-2

This variation (illustrated in Exhibit 13.41) of the basic plan architecture allocates total operating expense and ancillary services profits on a per physician basis (as opposed to a per physician FTE basis), recognizing the significant fixed costs in a medical practice, regardless of work levels performed.

An assessment of the strengths and weaknesses of Architecture O is provided in Exhibit 13.42.

EXHIBIT 13.40

Example O-1 – Group Practice Architecture O –
Pure Production with Equal Share Expense Allocation Plan*
Expense Allocation Based on Physician FTE
Revenue Element 4 and Expense Element 6

		Total	Allocation	Dr. A Gen Ortho	Dr. B Gen Ortho
Step 1	Determine revenue.				
	Physician FTE	8.75		1.00	0.75
	Net Collections from Professional Services	$7,874,962	Direct	$750,003	$689,542
	Ancillary Net Collections – Professional Component	$155,864	Direct to Performing Physician	$13,342	$62,145
	Other Revenue/Income	$46,897	Equal per FTE	$5,360	$4,020
	Total Revenue	$8,077,723		$768,705	$755,707
Step 2	**Determine operating expenses (equal share per FTE).**				
	Total Operating Expenses†	$(3,715,753)			
	Fixed Portion 100%	$(3,715,753)	Equal per FTE	$(424,657)	$(318,493)
Step 3	**Determine ancillary services profits pool.**				
	Revenues (excluding personally performed professional component)	$1,074,545	Direct Ancillary Pool		
	Expenses				
	Equipment Rental	$(104,521)	Direct Ancillary Pool		
	Staff	$(245,120)	Direct Ancillary Pool		
	Other Ancillary Expense (supplies, etc.)	$(54,712)	Direct Ancillary Pool		
	Ancillary Net Profit (Revenue – Expense)	$670,192	Equal per FTE	$76,593	$57,445
Step 4	**Determine amount available for physician compensation and direct expense.**				
	(Revenue – Operating Expenses + Ancillary Profits)	$5,032,162		$420,641	$494,659
Step 5	**Determine physician-specific direct expenses.**				
	Total Direct Physician Expenses	$(815,685)	Direct	$(75,989)	$(77,172)
Step 6	**Determine physician income after direct expenses (W-2).**	$4,216,477		$344,652	$417,487

* Hypothetical numbers presented for illustrative purposes only. Numbers may not total in all cases due to rounding.

† Operating expenses include rent, nonphysician staff, and other general operating expenses.

Key:
Gen Ortho = General Orthopedic Surgery

Dr. C Gen Ortho	Dr. D Gen Ortho	Dr. E Sports	Dr. F Sports	Dr. G Foot	Dr. H Spine	Dr. I Spine
1.00	1.00	1.00	1.00	1.00	1.00	1.00
$852,141	$798,568	$932,564	$1,021,451	$784,021	$936,458	$1,110,214
$13,645	$32,121	$24,512	$1,024	$3,212	$4,512	$1,351
$5,360	$5,360	$5,360	$5,360	$5,360	$5,360	$5,360
$871,146	$836,049	$962,436	$1,027,835	$792,593	$946,330	$1,116,925
$(424,657)	$(424,657)	$(424,657)	$(424,657)	$(424,657)	$(424,657)	$(424,657)
$76,593	$76,593	$76,593	$76,593	$76,593	$76,593	$76,593
$523,082	$487,985	$614,372	$679,771	$444,529	$598,266	$768,861
$(101,025)	$(97,190)	$(90,797)	$(94,314)	$(81,788)	$(95,004)	$(102,406)
$422,056	$390,795	$523,574	$585,457	$362,740	$503,261	$666,455

EXHIBIT 13.41

Example O-2 – Group Practice Architecture O –
Pure Production with Equal Share Expense Allocation Plan*
Equal Expense Allocation per Physician (Without Regard to FTE)
Revenue Element 4 and Expense Element 6

		Total	Allocation	Dr. A Gen Ortho	Dr. B Gen Ortho
Step 1	**Determine revenue.**				
	Physician FTE	8.75		1.00	0.75
	Net Collections from Professional Services	$7,874,962	Direct	$750,003	$689,542
	Ancillary Net Collections – Professional Component	$155,864	Direct to Performing Physician	$13,342	$62,145
	Other Revenues/Income	$46,897	Equal per FTE	$5,360	$4,020
	Total Revenue	$8,077,723		$768,705	$755,707
Step 2	**Determine operating expenses (equal share per physician).**				
	Total Operating Expenses†	$(3,715,753)			
	Fixed Portion 100%	$(3,715,753)	Equal per FTE	$(412,861)	$(412,861)
Step 3	**Determine ancillary services profits pool.**				
	Revenues (excluding personally performed professional component)	$1,074,545	Direct Ancillary Pool		
	Expenses				
	Equipment Rental	$(104,521)	Direct Ancillary Pool		
	Staff	$(245,120)	Direct Ancillary Pool		
	Other Ancillary Expense (supplies, etc.)	$(54,712)	Direct Ancillary Pool		
	Ancillary Net Profit (Revenue – Expense)	$670,192	Equal per Physician	$74,466	$74,466
Step 4	**Determine amount available for physician compensation and direct expense.**				
	(Revenue – Operating Expenses + Ancillary Profits)	$5,032,162		$430,309	$417,311
Step 5	**Determine physician-specific direct expenses.**				
	Total Direct Physician Expenses	$(815,685)	Direct	$(75,989)	$(77,172)
Step 6	**Determine physician income after direct expenses(W-2).**	$4,216,477		$354,320	$340,139

* Hypothetical numbers presented for illustrative purposes only. Numbers may not total in all cases due to rounding.

† Operating expenses include rent, nonphysician staff, and other general operating expenses.

Key:
Gen Ortho = General Orthopedic Surgery

© 2006 Johnson & Walker Keegan

Dr. C Gen Ortho	Dr. D Gen Ortho	Dr. E Sports	Dr. F Sports	Dr. G Foot	Dr. H Spine	Dr. I Spine
1.00	1.00	1.00	1.00	1.00	1.00	1.00
$852,141	$798,568	$932,564	$1,021,451	$784,021	$936,458	$1,110,214
$13,645	$32,121	$24,512	$1,024	$3,212	$4,512	$1,351
$5,360	$5,360	$5,360	$5,360	$5,360	$5,360	$5,360
$871,146	$836,049	$962,436	$1,027,835	$792,593	$946,330	$1,116,925
$(412,861)	$(412,861)	$(412,861)	$(412,861)	$(412,861)	$(412,861)	$(412,861)
$74,466	$74,466	$74,466	$74,466	$74,466	$74,466	$74,466
$532,750	$497,653	$624,040	$689,439	$454,197	$607,934	$778,529
$(101,025)	$(97,190)	$(90,797)	$(94,314)	$(81,788)	$(95,004)	$(102,406)
$431,725	$400,463	$533,243	$595,125	$372,409	$512,930	$676,123

EXHIBIT 13.42 Assessment of Group Practice Architecture O –
Pure Production with Equal Share Expense Allocation Plans

Dimension	Strengths	Weaknesses
Measure	Promotes individual physician clinical autonomy and encourages individual productivity. Holds physicians accountable in a direct way for cost of practice due to responsibility for equal share (per physician or share adjusted for FTE) portion of practice operating costs.	Measures tend to focus heavily on clinical production, although additional performance measures may also be employed.
Productivity	Recognizes individual production levels in a direct way.	The focus on production may not permit the level of attention to other key performance indices (e.g., cost of practice, patient access, and patient satisfaction).
Financial	The "equal share" approach to cost of practice minimizes administrative complexity associated with plan implementation and clearly requires physician responsibility for a defined "share" of practice costs.	The "equal share" cost allocation may not promote attention to individual physician cost variances.
Simplicity	Ease of administration.	
Alignment	Encourages not only individual production, but also a group practice orientation toward expenditures.	
"Fairness"	Directly recognizes and rewards physician work and effort.	Physicians may perceive they are being held responsible for expenditures beyond their control.

© 2006 Johnson & Walker Keegan

► GROUP PRACTICE ARCHITECTURE N – PURE PRODUCTION WITH GRADUATED OR NEGOTIATED EXPENSE ALLOCATION PLANS
Revenue Element 4 and Expense Element 5

Overview

Physician perceptions of "fairness" often differ in a medical practice, making the determination of cost allocation methods one of the more challenging tasks of the compensation planning committee. Architecture N uses Element 5; however, unlike Architecture E, which was discussed earlier and focused on *revenues*, this architecture involves a graduated or negotiated approach to *expense allocation* or cost of practice issues. Under this plan architecture, the overhead assessments are negotiated and recognized as the product of such a negotiation process, rather than being based on the "illusion" that overhead can and should be assessed on a precise basis linked to service utilization or otherwise.

In Group Practice Example N-1 (illustrated in Exhibit 13.43 at the end of this section), the overhead assessment is informed by and linked to benchmark costs of practice or overhead rates as measured by market data. Other approaches can also be used, however, including those that assign differing levels of "taxation" to practice revenues based on practice specialty or otherwise, including those illustrated in Architecture E, discussed earlier.

Application

Practices that index their expenditures to published benchmark levels are typically single specialty practices that have significant variation in physician production levels, as well as some multispecialty practices that elect to use differential market-specific overhead rates based on specialty.

Methodology

This architecture is similar to Group Practice Architectures O, P, Q, and R in that it uses a pure production approach to revenue allocation (Revenue Element 4); however, it differs in how cost of practice issues are addressed.

Example N-1 – Pure Productivity with Expenses Linked to Market by Specialty

Step 1. Determine Production Levels of Physician in Comparison to Benchmark Levels

Identify individual physician production levels. In this example, production is measured by net collections from professional services. Determine the production range of the individual physician in comparison to benchmarks, 25th percentile to median, median to 75th percentile, or other range. Overhead rates are then established based on specialty and production. When market data are used, close attention and linkage to median values, potential use of multiple measures that are averaged, and other approaches are recommended to help reduce variation from period to period. Thus, instead of linking to the 25th, median, and 75th percentiles, a practice might link to defined percentages of median values (e.g., 80 percent, 100 percent, 120 percent, etc.) as a means to provide stability from year to year. See Chapter 16 for a more detailed discussion of these concepts.

As demonstrated in this example, if an internist performs below the 25th percentile, he or she is assessed an overhead rate of 64 percent, while an internist reaching production levels greater than the 75th percentile is assessed an overhead rate of 52 percent. In comparison, a physician specializing in gastroenterology performing below the 25th percentile is assessed a 52 percent overhead rate, with the overhead decreasing to 32 percent if his or her production exceeds the 75th percentile.

Step 2. Allocate Revenues to Individual Physicians

In this example, net collections from professional services are allocated to individual physicians who generated the revenue. Other revenue is allocated on an equal share per FTE physician basis.

Step 3. Allocate Ancillary Services Profits Pool

The ancillary services profits pool is allocated to a subset of physicians only. In this example – and consistent with the Stark law – a pool of five physicians is used to allocate the profits pool. The profits pool is allocated based on a percentage to total of net collections from professional services based on the net collections generated by the five physicians. Allocated revenue is then determined for each physician as the sum of the revenue determined in Step 2 (net collections from professional services plus other revenues), plus the portion of the ancillary profits allocated to the physician (in this case, only allocated to a "pod" of five physicians).

Step 4. Allocate Expenditures – Indexed to Market for Specialty, and Tiered

Expense of practice is allocated based on a flat rate up to an established level of allocated revenue. Above this revenue level, the overhead rate determined in Step 1 above (linked to individual physician production and market) applies. As an example, Dr. A will be assessed 60 percent overhead on his or her first $300,000 of allocated revenue. For Dr. A's allocated revenue above $300,000, an overhead rate of 56 percent is assessed. At the end of Step 4, allocated revenues minus negotiated overhead is determined for each physician. These "overhead" rates are informed by market data, as discussed above.

Step 5. Determine Allocated Revenues Minus Negotiated Overhead

The allocated share of practice revenues minus the negotiated overhead amount is calculated for each physician, and each physician's percent of total allocated revenues minus negotiated overhead allocation is determined. This percentage is used in Step 7 below.

Step 6. Compute Actual Practice Net Income (Excluding Physician Compensation), and Determine Revenue Available for Compensation and Direct Expenses

In Step 6, the actual practice net income is determined via the following formula:

$$
\begin{array}{l}
 \text{Revenues from Professional Services (Excluding Ancillary)} \\
+\ \text{Revenues from Ancillary Profits Pool (Pod of Five)} \\
-\ \text{Expenses (Excluding Physician Compensation, Benefits, and Ancillary Expenses)} \\
\hline
 \text{Total Amount Available for Physician-Specific Compensation and Direct Expense}
\end{array}
$$

Step 7. Determine Physician Share of Total Amount Available for Compensation

Although this example shows an amount that would be paid to the physician, the practice may have more (or less) income available to actually pay that amount. In this example, the actual amount available for compensation and direct expenses is greater than the amount allocated through the basic plan. The practice therefore allocates the remaining amount (overage) based on each physician's total allocated income as a percentage of total income previously determined under the model.

Step 8. Determine Physician-Specific Direct Expenses

Consistent with other plan architectures, certain physician-specific direct expenses (retirement contribution) are identified and deducted from the amount otherwise available to pay compensation to each physician. In this example, only select expenses are treated in this manner.

Step 9. Determine Physician Income

In this final step, physician-specific direct expenses (Step 8) are subtracted from revenue available for compensation and direct expenses (Step 7) to determine individual physician income.

The benchmark that is used in Architecture N is the reported specialty-specific "total operating cost as a percentage of total medical revenue" figure, commonly referred to as "overhead." Total operating expense includes support staff salaries and benefits and general operating expenditures, such as building and lease costs, equipment, supplies, information technology, malpractice insurance, etc. In fact, all expenditures except physician and nonphysician provider salary and benefit costs are included in the published "overhead" benchmark rates.

In this model, the physician-specific direct expenses can either be allocated specifically to the physician or be included in the "overhead" that is indexed to the benchmark. This decision typically rests with the physicians' perceptions of equity associated with these types of direct physician expenditures.

Other variations of this basic plan architecture are reported under Architecture E presented earlier.

An assessment of the strengths and weaknesses of Architecture N is provided in Exhibit 13.44.

EXHIBIT 13.43

Example N-1 – Group Practice Architecture N – Pure Production with Negotiated Expense Allocation Plan* Expense Linked to Market by Specialty
Revenue Element 4 and Expense Element 5

Step 1 — Assemble production information.

	Total	Allocation	Dr. A IM	Dr. B IM	Dr. C IM	Dr. D IM	Dr. E IM	Dr. F GI	Dr. G GI
Physician FTE			1.00	0.75	1.00	1.00	1.00	1.00	1.00
Professional Services Production Range by Specialty Based on MGMA Benchmarks†			Median–75th	25th–Median	Over 75th	Median–75th	Median–75th	Median–75th	Over 75th
Overhead Percentage by Specialty and Production‡									
Under 25th			64%	64%	64%	64%	64%	52%	52%
25th–Median			60%	60%	60%	60%	60%	45%	45%
Median–75th			56%	56%	56%	56%	56%	39%	39%
Over 75th			52%	52%	52%	52%	52%	32%	32%

Step 2 — Determine revenue.

	Total	Allocation	Dr. A	Dr. B	Dr. C	Dr. D	Dr. E	Dr. F	Dr. G
Net Collections from Professional Services	$3,449,878	Direct	$320,758	$286,321	$456,231	$425,632	$365,875	$692,761	$902,300
Other Revenues/Income	$46,897	Equal per FTE	$6,948	$5,211	$6,948	$6,948	$6,948	$6,948	$6,948
Total Revenue	$3,496,775		$327,706	$291,532	$463,179	$432,580	$372,823	$699,709	$909,248

Step 3 — Determine ancillary services profits pool allocated using productivity bonus to "pod" of 5 physicians.**

	Total		Dr. A	Dr. B	Dr. C	Dr. D	Dr. E		
Revenues (ancillary services only)	$459,094								
Expenses (ancillary services only)	$(345,124)								
Physician % to Total Professional Services Collections (IM only as pod of 5)			17.29%	15.44%	24.60%	22.95%	19.73%		

	Total							
Allocated Based on % of Professional Services Collections	$113,970	$19,709	$17,593	$28,033	$26,153	$22,481	$—	$—
Allocated Revenues (total revenue + ancillary)		$347,415	$309,125	$491,212	$458,733	$395,304	$699,709	$909,248
Step 4 — Determine negotiated overhead expense allocation based on production.								
Overhead % and Amounts on First $300,000 of Allocated Revenue	60%	$(180,000)	$(180,000)	$(180,000)	$(180,000)	$(180,000)	$(180,000)	$(180,000)
Overhead % Applicable to Amounts over $300,000 (based on benchmark)		56%	60%	52%	56%	56%	39%	32%
Overhead Applicable to Amount over $300,000		$(26,552)	$(5,475)	$(99,430)	$(88,890)	$(53,370)	$(155,886)	$(194,959)
Step 5 — Determine allocated revenues minus negotiated overhead.	$1,726,181††	$140,863	$123,650	$211,782	$189,842	$161,934	$363,822	$534,288
Individual Allocated Revenues Minus Overhead as % of Total		8%	7%	12%	11%	9%	21%	31%

continued on next page

Exhibit 13.43 – Example N-1 continued

	Total	Allocation	Dr. A IM	Dr. B IM	Dr. C IM	Dr. D IM	Dr. E IM	Dr. F GI	Dr. G GI
Step 6 **Determine actual practice net income (excluding physician compensation).**									
Net Collections from Professional Services	$3,496,775								
Expenses (excluding physician compensation, benefits, and ancillaries)	$(1,748,388)								
Total Available for Compensation and Direct Expense	$1,748,388								
Step 7 **Determine amount available for compensation and direct expense.††**	$1,748,388		$142,675	$125,241	$214,506	$192,285	$164,017	$368,503	$541,162
Individual Available for Compensation and Direct Expense as % of Total			8%	7%	12%	11%	9%	21%	31%
Step 8 **Determine direct expenses (retirement contribution only).**			$20,000	$20,000	$25,000	$28,000	$25,000	$40,000	$42,050
Step 9 **Determine physician income after direct expense (W-2).**			$122,675	$105,241	$189,506	$164,285	$139,017	$328,503	$499,112

* Hypothetical numbers presented for illustrative purposes only. Numbers may not total in all cases due to rounding.

† Production ranking using average of multiple benchmark tables (e.g., professional services net collections, WRVUs, etc.).

‡ Negotiated (agreed-to) overhead rates applicable to allocated production based on benchmarks for practice specialty.

** Ancillary services profits allocated to overall profits pool or pod of five or more physicians as allowed by Stark law; then allocated within pod on indirect basis.

†† Actual compensation pool (Step 6) exceeds allocated revenues minus expenses (Step 4). Accordingly, Step 5 amount allocated is based on Step 4 values on percent to total basis.

Key:
IM = Internal Medicine
GI = Gastroenterology

© 2006 Johnson & Walker Keegan

EXHIBIT 13.44 Assessment of Group Practice Architecture N – Pure Production with Negotiated Expense Allocation Plan Linked to Market by Specialty Plans

Dimension	Strengths	Weaknesses
Measure	Rewards professional services production.	Requires use of benchmark or similar expense surrogates.
Productivity	Incorporates strong incentives for productivity through direct production credit for work.	Decreases in production by one physician will impact compensation earned by others.
Financial	Cost categories and allocation methods do not need to be determined. Recognizes a relationship between production and compensation levels based on market data. Allows for multispecialty approach to cost of practice up to an initial level, then specialty-specific variations thereafter.	Sound financial management is required to ensure cost of practice is covered by amounts held back via plan. Less focus on cost issues, since a "flat" rate is assessed on portion of revenues.
Simplicity		Market data may not be viewed as representative. Complex, and requires close attention to reduce year-to-year variation and changes in market data over time.
Alignment	Reduced need for express performance expectations due to productivity orientation.	Productivity orientation may undermine group cohesiveness.
"Fairness"	Linkage of overhead assessment to market may allow for blending of multispecialty and single specialty perspectives, thus promoting potentially greater perception of "fairness" in multispecialty practices.	Linkage to market may be viewed as inappropriate, because "our practice is different."

© 2006 Johnson & Walker Keegan

"MIDDLE GROUND" ARCHITECTURES AND EXAMPLES

Having reviewed the basic plan architectures on both the "team-oriented" and "individualistic" ends of the array of architectures summarized in Exhibit 13.2 (Architectures A through E, and Architectures N through R, respectively), we will now turn to the vast middle ground to review basic architectures that combine different approaches to revenue and expense treatment. The basic elements of the compensation plan matrix can be combined into eight additional architectures (Middle Ground Architectures F through M), with each falling at different points on the array in terms of how the plan approaches revenues and expenses, promotes team or individualistic perspectives, and in other ways.

We illustrate some of the more common approaches by presenting examples (Exhibits 13.45 through 13.52) of the following architectures:

► Architecture F (Exhibit 13.45), guaranteed share (base salary plus incentive), with equal share expense allocation plan (Revenue Element 2 with Expense Element 6);

► Architecture G (Exhibit 13.46), combined equal share and production revenue allocation, with equal share expense allocation plan (Revenue Element 3 with Expense Element 6);

► Architecture H (Exhibit 13.47), guaranteed share (base salary plus incentive), with negotiated expense allocation, and with an equal share and production-based expense component plan (Revenue Element 2 with Expense Element 7);

► Architecture I (Exhibit 13.48), combined equal share and production revenue allocation with negotiated expense allocation, and with an equal share and production-based expense component plan (Revenue Element 3 with Expense Element 7);

► Architecture J (Exhibit 13.49), guaranteed share (base salary plus incentive), with modified cost accounting expense allocation plan (Revenue Element 2 with Expense Element 8);

► Architecture K (Exhibit 13.50), combined equal share and production revenue allocation, with modified cost accounting expense allocation plan (Revenue Element 3 with Expense Element 8);

► Architecture L (Exhibit 13.51), guaranteed share (base salary plus incentive), with strict cost accounting plan (Revenue Element 2 with Expense Element 9); and

► Architecture M (Exhibit 13.52), equal share and production revenue allocation, with strict cost accounting plan (Revenue Element 3 with Expense Element 9).

These architectures are illustrated in the separate exhibits listed above. These "middle ground" architectures generally combine matrix Revenue Elements 2 and 3 with Expense Elements 6, 7, 8, and 9 in different combinations. These examples illustrate the combinations with additional variations, such as different portions of sharing at the revenue or expense levels, or in other ways. Because the examples effectively combine the building blocks illustrated in other examples relating to other architectures, a discussion of the specific steps, strengths, and weaknesses of each is not repeated here.

As noted above, these middle ground examples represent only some of the numerous combinations that are possible. Indeed, the basic plan variations that are illustrated in the examples can be modified in any number of ways by:

► Changing the portion of revenues and/or expenses that are allocated on an equal share basis (e.g., change to smaller or larger equal share portions);

► Changing the method of measuring work, effort, production, or utilization (e.g., by using net collections from professional services, WRVUs, gross charges from professional services, number of encounters, or combinations of one or more of these);

► Modifying the level of guaranteed or "base salary" levels in plans using a guaranteed salary component;

► Changing the measure of market compensation, production, "overhead" percentages, or "tax levels" in models using market data or other norms as part of the compensation methodology;

► Using alternative approaches to the distribution of ancillary services income, expenses, and profits in a legally compliant manner; and

► Introducing quality, practice efficiency, patient satisfaction, and other measures to the compensation plan equation, including measures directed at P4P issues.

EXHIBIT 13.45

Example F-1 – Group Practice Architecture F – Guaranteed Share (Base Salary Plus Incentive) with Equal Share Expense Allocation Plan*
Revenue Element 2 and Expense Element 6

		Total	Dr. A Gen IM	Dr. B Gen IM	Dr. C† Gen IM	Dr. D Gen IM	Dr. E FP w/OB	Dr. F FP w/OB	Dr. G Pulm	Dr. H Rheum	Dr. I Gen Surg
Step 1	**Assemble production information.**										
	FTE Level	9.00	1.00	1.00	1.00	1.00	1.00	1.00	1.00	1.00	1.00
	Median (MGMA) by Specialty		$160,000	$160,000	$160,000	$160,000	$155,000	$155,000	$225,000	$190,000	$280,000
	% of Market for Base	70%									
	Base Salary (% of market)	$1,151,500	$112,000	$112,000	$112,000	$112,000	$108,500	$108,500	$157,500	$133,000	$196,000
	Net Collections from Professional Services	$3,983,012	$480,000	$425,000	$345,000	$400,000	$385,012	$410,200	$458,900	$438,000	$640,900
	Physician % to Total Net Collections		12.05%	10.67%	8.66%	10.04%	9.67%	10.30%	11.52%	11.00%	16.09%
Step 2	**Determine quality incentive pool per physician.**										
	Number of Physicians	$10,000									
		9									
	Total Quality Incentive Pool	$90,000									
Step 3	**Determine physician-specific bonus.**										
	Net Collections from Professional Services	$3,983,012	$480,000	$425,000	$345,000	$400,000	$385,012	$410,200	$458,900	$438,000	$640,900
	Expenses										
	Nonphysician Overhead and Physician-Specific Direct Expenses (equal share)‡	$(2,190,657)	$(243,406)	$(243,406)	$(243,406)	$(243,406)	$(243,406)	$(243,406)	$(243,406)	$(243,406)	$(243,406)
	Base Salaries (from above)	$(1,151,500)	$(112,000)	$(112,000)	$(112,000)	$(112,000)	$(108,500)	$(108,500)	$(157,500)	$(133,000)	$(196,000)
	Quality Incentive Pool (from above)	$(90,000)	$(10,000)	$(10,000)	$(10,000)	$(10,000)	$(10,000)	$(10,000)	$(10,000)	$(10,000)	$(10,000)

	Total									
Bonus (revenue − expense [including base salary])	$550,855	$114,594	$59,594	$(20,406)	$34,594	$23,106	$48,294	$47,994	$51,594	$191,494
Step 4 Determine physician-specific compensation.										
Base Salary	$1,151,500	$112,000	$112,000	$112,000	$112,000	$108,500	$108,500	$157,500	$133,000	$196,000
Quality Incentive Pool Award*	$90,000	$9,000	$10,800	$5,400	$16,200	$900	$7,200	$9,000	$27,000	$4,500
Bonus (after expense allocation)	$550,855	$114,594	$59,594	$—	$34,594	$23,106	$48,294	$47,994	$51,594	$191,494
Step 5 Determine total compensation (after physician-specific direct expenses).	$1,812,762	$235,594	$182,394	$117,400	$162,794	$132,506	$163,994	$214,494	$211,594	$391,994

* Hypothetical numbers presented for illustrative purposes only. Numbers may not total in all cases due to rounding.

† Revenues generated by Dr. C insufficient to cover costs, so no bonus earned for performance during year.

‡ Physician benefit costs included in general overhead for purposes of example.

Key:
FP w/OB = Family Practice with Obstetrics
FP w/o OB = Family Practice without Obstetrics
Gen IM = General Internal Medicine
Gen Surg = General Surgery
Pulm = Pulmonary Medicine
Rheum = Rheumatology

© 2006 Johnson & Walker Keegan

EXHIBIT 13.46

**Example G-1 – Group Practice Architecture G –
Combined Equal Share (25%) and Production (75%) Revenue Allocation with Equal Share Expense Allocation Plan***
Revenue Element 3 and Expense Element 6

		Total	Dr. A Gen Ortho	Dr. B Gen Ortho	Dr. C Gen Ortho	Dr. D Foot/Ankle	Dr. E Hand	Dr. F Sports	Dr. G Sports	Dr. H Spine
Step 1	**Assemble production information.**									
	FTE Level	7.80	1.00	1.00	0.80	1.00	1.00	1	1.00	1.00
	Net Collections from Professional Services	$6,907,387	$750,000	$825,000	$700,350	$815,000	$856,004	$958,000	$1,025,012	$978,021
	Physician % to Total Production		11%	12%	10%	12%	12%	14%	15%	14%
Step 2	**Allocate practice revenues (25% equal/ 75% production).**									
	Net Collections from Professional Services	$6,907,387								
	Equal Share Component (25%)	$1,726,847								
	Equal Share (adjusted by FTE)		$221,391	$221,391	$177,112	$221,391	$221,391	$221,391	$221,391	$221,391
	Production Share Component (75%)									
	% of Total Production (from above)		11%	12%	10%	12%	12%	14%	15%	14%
	Production Share	$5,180,540	$562,500	$618,750	$525,263	$611,250	$642,003	$718,500	$768,759	$733,516
	Total Allocated Share of Production	$6,907,387	$783,891	$840,141	$702,375	$832,641	$863,394	$939,891	$990,150	$954,906
Step 3	**Allocate practice expenses (75% equal/ 25% production).**									
	Expenses									
	Nonphysician Overhead	$(3,108,324)								

		1	2	3	4	5	6	7	8
Equal Share (adjusted by FTE)	$(3,108,324)								
Total Allocated Share of Expenses		$(398,503)	$(398,503)	$(318,802)	$(398,503)	$(398,503)	$(398,503)	$(398,503)	$(398,503)
Step 4	**Determine physician-specific compensation.**								
Total Allocated Share of Revenues		$783,891	$840,141	$702,375	$832,641	$863,394	$939,891	$990,150	$954,906
Total Allocated Share of Expenses		$(398,503)	$(398,503)	$(318,802)	$(398,503)	$(398,503)	$(398,503)	$(398,503)	$(398,503)
		$385,388	$441,638	$383,573	$434,138	$464,891	$541,388	$591,647	$556,403
Step 5	**Determine total compensation (before physician-specific direct expenses).**								
Direct Expenses		$(50,400)	$(52,390)	$(48,983)	$(54,000)	$(40,000)	$(43,000)	$(48,981)	$(50,940)
W-2 Compensation Earned		$334,988	$389,248	$334,590	$380,138	$424,891	$498,388	$542,666	$505,463
Step 6	**Determine year-end bonus.**								
Advance/Draw		$300,000	$300,000	$300,000	$300,000	$300,000	$300,000	$300,000	$300,000
Bonus (end of year)		$34,988	$89,248	$34,590	$80,138	$124,891	$198,388	$242,666	$205,463

* Hypothetical numbers presented for illustrative purposes only. Numbers may not total in all cases due to rounding.

Key:
Gen Ortho = General Orthopedics

© 2006 Johnson & Walker Keegan

EXHIBIT 13.47

Example H-1 – Group Practice Architecture H –
Guaranteed Share (Base Salary Plus Incentive) with Negotiated Expense Allocation with
Production-Based Component (60% Equal/40% Production) Plan*
Revenue Element 2 and Expense Element 7

		Total	Dr. A Gen IM	Dr. B Gen IM	Dr. C† Gen IM	Dr. D Gen IM	Dr. E FP w/OB	Dr. F FP w/OB	Dr. G Pulm	Dr. H Rheum	Dr. I Gen Surg
Step 1	**Assemble production information.**										
	FTE Level	8.75	1.00	1.00	0.75	100	1.00	1.00	1.00	1.00	1.00
	Median (MGMA) by Specialty		$160,000	$160,000	$160,000	$160,000	$155,000	$155,000	$225,000	$190,000	$280,000
	% of Market for Base	70%									
	Base Salary (% of market)	$1,151,500	$112,000	$112,000	$112,000	$112,000	$108,500	$108,500	$157,500	$133,000	$196,000
	Net Collections from Professional Services	$3,983,012	$480,000	$425,000	$345,000	$400,000	$385,012	$410,200	$458,900	$438,000	$640,900
	Physician % to Total Net Collections		12.05%	10.67%	8.66%	10.04%	9.67%	10.30%	11.52%	11.00%	16.09%
Step 2	**Determine quality incentive pool per physician.**	$10,000									
	Number of Physicians	9									
	Total Quality Incentive Pool	$90,000									
Step 3	**Determine physician-specific bonus.**										
	Net Collections from Professional Services	$3,983,012	$480,000	$425,000	$345,000	$400,000	$385,012	$410,200	$458,900	$438,000	$640,900
	Expenses Nonphysician Overhead and Physician Benefits (total)	$(2,190,657)									
	Equal Share (adjusted by FTE) 60%	$(1,314,394)	$(150,216)	$(150,216)	$(112,662)	$(150,216)	$(150,216)	$(150,216)	$(150,216)	$(150,216)	$(150,216)

	Total								
Production Portion (% of net professional services collections) 40%	$(876,263)	$(105,600)	$(93,500)	$(75,900)	$(88,000)	$(84,703)	$(90,244)	$(100,958)	$(96,360)	$(140,998)
Base Salaries (from above)	$(1,151,500)	$(112,000)	$(112,000)	$(112,000)	$(112,000)	$(108,500)	$(108,500)	$(157,500)	$(133,000)	$(196,000)
Quality Incentive Pool (from above)	$(90,000)	$(10,000)	$(10,000)	$(10,000)	$(10,000)	$(10,000)	$(10,000)	$(10,000)	$(10,000)	$(10,000)
Bonus (Revenue – Expense [including base salary]).	$550,855	$102,184	$59,284	$34,438	$39,784	$31,593	$51,240	$40,226	$48,424	$143,686
Step 4 Determine physician-specific compensation.										
Base Salary	$1,151,500	$112,000	$112,000	$112,000	$112,000	$108,500	$108,500	$157,500	$133,000	$196,000
Quality Incentive Pool Award‡	$90,000	$9,000	$10,800	$5,400	$16,200	$900	$7,200	$9,000	$27,000	$4,500
Bonus (after expense allocation)	$550,855	$102,184	$59,284	$34,438	$39,784	$31,593	$51,240	$40,226	$48,424	$143,686
Step 5 Determine total compensation (before physician-specific direct expenses).	$1,792,355	$223,184	$182,084	$151,838	$167,984	$140,993	$166,940	$206,726	$208,424	$344,186

* Hypothetical numbers presented for illustrative purposes only. Numbers may not total in all cases due to rounding.

† Compared to Group Example F-1, Dr. C receives bonus due to different expense allocation method.

‡ Quality incentive pool awarded using point scales or other means. See Chapter 10, "Special Issues in Physician Compensation," and Chapter 15, "Compensation Plans in Academic Practice," for examples.

Key:
FP w/OB = Family Practice with Obstetrics
FP w/o OB = Family Practice without Obstetrics
Gen IM = General Internal Medicine
Gen Surg = General Surgery
Pulm = Pulmonary Medicine
Rheum = Rheumatology

EXHIBIT 13.48

Example I-1 – Group Practice Architecture I – Combined Equal Share (25%) and Production (75%) Revenue Allocation, with Negotiated Expense Allocation with Production-Based Component (50% Equal/50% Production) Plan*
Revenue Element 3 and Expense Element 7

		Total	Dr. A Gen Ortho	Dr. B Gen Ortho	Dr. C Gen Ortho	Dr. D Foot/Ankle	Dr. E Hand	Dr. F Sports	Dr. G Sports	Dr. H Spine
Step 1	**Assemble production information.**									
	FTE Level	7.80	1.00	1.00	0.80	1.00	1.00	1.00	1.00	1.00
	Net Collections from Professional Services	$6,907,387	$750,000	$825,000	$700,350	$815,000	$856,004	$958,000	$1,025,012	$978,021
	Physician % to Total Net Collections		11%	12%	10%	12%	12%	14%	15%	14%
Step 2	**Allocate practice revenues (25% equal/ 75% production).**									
	Total Net collections (professional services + ancillary services)	$7,928,708								
	Equal Share Component (25%)	$1,982,177								
	Equal Share (adjusted by FTE)		$254,125	$254,125	$203,300	$254,125	$254,125	$254,125	$254,125	$254,125
	Professional Services Production Share Component (75%)									
	Physician % to Total Net Collections (from above)		11%	12%	10%	12%	12%	14%	15%	14%
	Production Share	$5,946,531	$645,671	$710,238	$602,927	$701,629	$736,929	$824,737	$882,427	$841,973
	Total Allocated Share of Production	$7,928,708	$899,796	$964,363	$806,228	$955,754	$991,054	$1,078,862	$1,136,552	$1,096,098
Step 3	**Allocate practice expenses (50% equal/ 50% production).**									
	Expenses									
	Nonphysician Overhead	$(3,567,919)								

	Total								
Equal Share Component (50%) (adjusted by FTE)	$(1,783,959)	$(228,713)	$(228,713)	$(228,713)	$(228,713)	$(228,713)	$(228,713)	$(228,713)	$(228,713)
Production Component (50%)									
Physician % to Total Net Collections (from above)		11%	12%	10%	12%	12%	14%	15%	14%
Production Share	$(1,783,959)	$(193,701)	$(213,071)	$(180,878)	$(210,489)	$(221,079)	$(247,421)	$(264,728)	$(252,592)
Total Allocated Share of Expenses	$(3,567,919)	$(422,414)	$(441,784)	$(363,848)	$(439,201)	$(449,791)	$(476,134)	$(493,441)	$(481,305)
Step 4 Determine physician-specific compensation.									
Total Allocated Share of Revenues		$899,796	$964,363	$806,228	$955,754	$991,054	$1,078,862	$1,136,552	$1,096,098
Total Allocated Share of Expenses		$(422,414)	$(441,784)	$(363,848)	$(439,201)	$(449,791)	$(476,134)	$(493,441)	$(481,305)
		$477,382	$522,579	$442,379	$516,553	$541,263	$602,728	$643,112	$614,794
Step 5 Determine total compensation (before physician-specific direct expenses).		$477,382	$522,579	$442,379	$516,553	$541,263	$602,728	$643,112	$614,794
Direct Expenses		$(50,400)	$(52,390)	$(48,983)	$(54,000)	$(40,000)	$(43,000)	$(48,981)	$(50,940)
W-2 Compensation Earned		$426,982	$470,189	$393,396	$462,553	$501,263	$559,728	$594,131	$563,854
Step 6 Determine end-of-year bonus.									
Advance/Draw		$300,000	$300,000	$300,000	$300,000	$300,000	$300,000	$300,000	$300,000
Bonus (end of year)		$126,982	$170,189	$93,396	$162,553	$201,263	$259,728	$294,131	$263,854

* Hypothetical numbers presented for illustrative purposes only. Numbers may not total in all cases due to rounding.

Key:
Gen Ortho = General Orthopedics

© 2006 Johnson & Walker Keegan

EXHIBIT 13.49

Example J-1 – Group Practice Architecture J – Guaranteed Share (Base Salary Plus Incentive) with Modified Cost Accounting Expense Allocation Plan*
Revenue Element 2 and Expense Element 8

		Total	Dr. A Gen IM	Dr. B Gen IM	Dr. C Gen IM	Dr. D Gen IM	Dr. E FP w/OB	Dr. F FP w/OB	Dr. G Pulm	Dr. H Rheum	Dr. I Gen Surg
Step 1	**Assemble production information.**										
	FTE Level	8.90	1.00	1.00	0.90	1.00	1.00	1.00	1.00	1.00	1.00
	Ambulatory Encounters	33,052	4,310	3,895	3,504	3,654	4,185	4,235	4,521	3,185	1,563
	Physician % to Total Ambulatory Encounters		13.04%	11.78%	10.60%	11.06%	12.66%	12.81%	13.68%	9.64%	4.73%
	Median Compensation by Specialty		$160,000	$160,000	$160,000	$160,000	$155,000	$155,000	$225,000	$190,000	$280,000
	% of Market for Base	50%									
	Base Salary (% of market)	$822,500	$80,000	$80,000	$80,000	$80,000	$77,500	$77,500	$112,500	$95,000	$140,000
	Net Collections from Professional Services	$4,014,012	$480,000	$425,000	$376,000	$400,000	$385,012	$410,200	$458,900	$438,000	$640,900
	Physician % to Total Net Collections		11.96%	10.59%	9.37%	9.97%	9.59%	10.22%	11.43%	10.91%	15.97%
Step 2	**Determine ancillary services profits pool.**										
	Ancillary Services Revenues	$498,754									
	Ancillary Services Expenses	$(378,956)									
	Total Ancillary Services Profits (Loss)	$119,798									
Step 3	**Determine physician-specific bonus.**										
	Net Collections from Professional Services	$4,014,012	$480,000	$425,000	$376,000	$400,000	$385,012	$410,200	$458,900	$438,000	$640,900
	Expenses Nonphysician Overhead (modified cost accounting)*	$(2,007,006)									

Fixed Overhead Component (equal share per physician)*	$(1,264,414)	$(142,069)	$(142,069)	$(142,069)	$(142,069)	$(142,069)	$(142,069)	$(142,069)	$(142,069)	$(142,069)
Variable Overhead (% of encounters)*	$(742,592)	$(96,834)	$(87,510)	$(78,726)	$(82,096)	$(94,026)	$(95,149)	$(101,575)	$(71,559)	$(35,117)
Direct Overhead (base salary and direct benefits)										
Base Salaries (from above)	$(822,500)	$(80,000)	$(80,000)	$(80,000)	$(80,000)	$(77,500)	$(77,500)	$(112,500)	$(95,000)	$(140,000)
Direct Benefits	$(313,703)	$(40,400)	$(42,390)	$(28,983)	$(24,000)	$(25,000)	$(33,000)	$(38,981)	$(40,940)	$(40,009)
(Revenue – Expense [including base salary])	$856,596	$120,697	$73,031	$46,222	$71,835	$46,417	$62,482	$63,775	$88,432	$283,706
Step 4 — Determine physician-specific compensation.										
Base Salary	$822,500	$80,000	$80,000	$80,000	$80,000	$77,500	$77,500	$112,500	$95,000	$140,000
Ancillary Services Profits (% of encounters)†	$119,798	$15,622	$14,118	$12,700	$13,244	$15,169	$15,350	$16,387	$11,544	$5,665
Bonus (after expense allocation)	$856,596	$120,697	$73,031	$46,222	$71,835	$46,417	$62,482	$63,775	$88,432	$283,706
Step 5 — Determine total compensation (before physician-specific direct expenses).	$1,798,894	$216,318	$167,148	$138,923	$165,079	$139,086	$155,332	$192,661	$194,977	$429,371

* Hypothetical numbers presented for illustrative purposes only. Numbers may not total in all cases due to rounding.

† Fixed overhead allocated equal share per physician without reduction for FTE level; therefore, Dr. C pays full share of fixed costs despite 0.9 FTE.

Key:
FP w/OB = Family Practice with Obstetrics
FP w/o OB = Family Practice without Obstetrics
Gen IM = General Internal Medicine
Gen Surg = General Surgery
Pulm = Pulmonary Medicine
Rheum = Rheumatology

EXHIBIT 13.50

Example K-1 – Group Practice Architecture K – Combined Equal Share (35%) and Production (65%) Revenue Allocation with Modified Cost Accounting (63% Equal Share/37% Utilization) Expense Allocation Plan*
Revenue Element 3 and Expense Element 8

	Total Total	Dr. A Gen Ortho	Dr. B Gen Ortho	Dr. C Gen Ortho	Dr. D Foot/Ankle	Dr. E Hand	Dr. F Sports	Dr. G Sports	Dr. H Spine
Step 1 **Assemble production information.**									
FTE Level	7.8	1.00	1.00	0.80	1.00	1.00	1.00	1.00	1.00
Ambulatory Encounters		3,141	3,321	2,968	3,309	3,645	3,500	3,654	2,568
Hospital Encounters		87	93	75	82	68	62	72	118
Surgery Cases		612	635	752	638	745	646	720	375
Total Encounters and Surgeries	31,886	3,840	4,049	3,795	4,029	4,458	4,208	4,446	3,061
Physician % to Total Encounters & Surgeries		12%	13%	12%	13%	14%	13%	14%	10%
Net Collections from Professional Services	$6,907,387	$750,000	$825,000	$700,350	$815,000	$856,004	$958,000	$1,025,012	$978,021
Physician % to Total Net Collections		11%	12%	10%	12%	12%	14%	15%	14%
Step 2 **Allocate practice revenues (35% equal/ 65% production).**									
Revenues	$6,907,387								
Equal Share Component (35%)	$2,417,585								
Equal Share (adjusted by FTE)		$309,947	$309,947	$247,957	$309,947	$309,947	$309,947	$309,947	$309,947
Production Share Component (65%)									
Physician % to Total Net Collections (from above)		11%	12%	10%	12%	12%	14%	15%	14%
Production Share	$4,489,802	$487,500	$536,250	$455,228	$529,750	$556,403	$622,700	$666,258	$635,714
Total Allocated Share of Revenues	$6,907,387	$797,447	$846,197	$703,185	$839,697	$866,349	$932,647	$976,205	$945,661

Step 3 — Allocate practice expenses (63% equal/37% utilization).‡

Expenses	Total								
Overhead	$(3,108,324)								
Fixed Overhead Component (equal share per FTE)†	$(1,958,244)	$(251,057)	$(251,057)	$(200,846)	$(251,057)	$(251,057)	$(251,057)	$(251,057)	$(251,057)
Variable Overhead (physician % to total encounters & surgeries)‡	$(1,150,080)	$(138,503)	$(146,041)	$(136,880)	$(145,320)	$(160,793)	$(151,776)	$(160,361)	$(110,406)
Direct Benefit Costs	$(388,694)	$(50,400)	$(52,390)	$(48,983)	$(54,000)	$(40,000)	$(43,000)	$(48,981)	$(50,940)
Total Allocated Share of Expenses	$(3,497,018)	$(439,960)	$(449,488)	$(386,708)	$(450,377)	$(451,850)	$(445,833)	$(460,398)	$(412,403)

Step 4 — Determine physician-specific compensation.

	Total								
Total Allocated Share of Revenues	$6,907,387	$797,447	$846,197	$703,185	$839,697	$866,349	$932,647	$976,205	$945,661
Total Allocated Share of Expenses	$(3,497,018)	$(439,960)	$(449,488)	$(386,708)	$(450,377)	$(451,850)	$(445,833)	$(460,398)	$(412,403)
W-2 Compensation Earned	$3,410,369	$357,487	$396,709	$316,476	$389,320	$414,499	$486,814	$515,806	$533,258

Step 5 — Determine end-of-year bonus.

	Total								
Advance/Draw		$300,000	$300,000	$300,000	$300,000	$300,000	$300,000	$400,000	$400,000
Bonus (end of year)		$57,487	$96,709	$16,476	$89,320	$114,499	$186,814	$115,806	$133,258

* Hypothetical numbers presented for illustrative purposes only. Numbers may not total in all cases due to rounding.

† Fixed overhead allocated on equal share per FTE basis; therefore, Dr. C is allocated a reduced share of fixed overhead.

‡ Variable overhead allocated on percentage of utilization basis, with combination of ambulatory encounters and surgical cases as the measure of utilization for such purposes. Overhead includes physician-specific direct expenses in this example.

Key:
Gen Ortho = General Orthopedics

EXHIBIT 13.51

Example L-1 – Group Practice Architecture L –
Guaranteed Share (Base Salary Plus Incentive) with Strict Cost Accounting Plan*
Revenue Element 2 and Expense Element 9

Step 1	Assemble production information.	Total			Smith	Johnson
	Physician	9.00			1.00	1.00
	Physician FTE	8.75			1.00	1.00
	Base Salary (% of historic compensation)				$140,000	$300,000
	Ambulatory Encounters	5,158			206	504
	Physician % to Total Ambulatory Encounters				4%	10%
	Surgeries	2,172			188	266
	Total Ambulatory and Surgical Encounters	7,331			394	770
	Physician % to Total Encounters – All Divisions	100%			5%	11%
	Physician % to Total Encounters – South Division	100%			11%	21%
	Physician % to Total Encounters – East Division	100%				
	Net Collections from Professional Services	$4,127,816			$378,545	$524,376
	Physician % to Total Net Collections	100%			9%	13%

Step 2	Determine revenue.	Total	Allocation	Smith	Johnson
	Net Collections from Professional Services	$4,127,816	Direct	$378,545	$524,376
	Nonphysician Provider Net Collections	$173,002	Physician Use	$—	$32,203
	Ancillary Net Collections – Professional Component	$155,864	Direct to Performing Physician	$13,342	$62,145
	Interest Income	$46,897	Equal/FTE	$5,360	$5,360
	Other Income	$34,059	Direct	$10,221	$4,512
	Total Revenue	$4,537,638		$407,468	$628,595

Step 3	Determine operating expenses.				
	GENERAL OPERATING EXPENSES				
	Accounting	$(18,636)	Equal per Physician	$(2,071)	$(2,071)
	Advertising	$(4,525)	Equal per Physician	$(503)	$(503)
	Bank Charges	$(6,325)	Equal per Physician	$(703)	$(703)
	Biomedical Waste	$(2,763)	% Ambulatory Encounters	$(110)	$(270)
	Business Promotion	$(2,618)	Equal per Physician	$(291)	$(291)
	Cell Phones (admin)	$(2,400)	Equal per Physician	$(267)	$(267)
	Computer (admin)	$(87,036)	Equal per Physician	$(9,671)	$(9,671)
	Contract Services	$(2,618)	Equal per Physician	$(291)	$(291)
	Drugs and Medical Supplies	$(6,150)	% Ambulatory Encounters	$(246)	$(601)
	Dues and Licenses	$(10,794)	Equal per Physician	$(1,199)	$(1,199)
	Food/Entertainment	$(596)	Equal per Physician	$(66)	$(66)
	Insurance – General Liability	$(1,837)	Equal per Physician	$(204)	$(204)

Wilson	Einstein	Bornsten	Porter	Mathews	Patel	Kant
1.00	1.00	1.00	1.00	1.00	1.00	1.00
1.00	1.00	1.00	1.00	0.75	1.00	1.00
$140,000	$140,000	$160,000	$300,000	$225,000	$250,000	$225,000
1,149	813	1,032	509	300	490	155
22%	16%	20%	10%	6%	9%	3%
228	293	309	273	168	271	176
1,377	1,106	1,341	782	468	761	331
19%	15%	18%	11%	6%	10%	5%
	31%	37%				
37%			21%	13%	20%	9%
$376,499	$356,821	$413,753	$637,903	$434,281	$532,153	$473,486
9%	9%	10%	15%	11%	13%	0.11

Wilson‡	Einstein	Bornsten	Porter	Mathews	Patel	Kant
$376,499	$356,821	$413,753	$637,903	$434,281	$532,153	$473,486
$7,019	$—	$—	$24,991	$40,893	$32,442	$35,455
$13,645	$32,121	$24,512	$1,024	$3,212	$4,512	$1,351
$5,360	$5,360	$5,360	$5,360	$4,020	$5,360	$5,360
$230	$500	$9,852	$164	$2,580	$5,000	$1,000
$402,752	$394,802	$453,476	$669,441	$484,986	$579,467	$516,652

$(2,071)	$(2,071)	$(2,071)	$(2,071)	$(2,071)	$(2,071)	$(2,071)
$(503)	$(503)	$(503)	$(503)	$(503)	$(503)	$(503)
$(703)	$(703)	$(703)	$(703)	$(703)	$(703)	$(703)
$(616)	$(436)	$(553)	$(273)	$(161)	$(263)	$(83)
$(291)	$(291)	$(291)	$(291)	$(291)	$(291)	$(291)
$(267)	$(267)	$(267)	$(267)	$(267)	$(267)	$(267)
$(9,671)	$(9,671)	$(9,671)	$(9,671)	$(9,671)	$(9,671)	$(9,671)
$(291)	$(291)	$(291)	$(291)	$(291)	$(291)	$(291)
$(1,370)	$(969)	$(1,231)	$(607)	$(358)	$(584)	$(185)
$(1,199)	$(1,199)	$(1,199)	$(1,199)	$(1,199)	$(1,199)	$(1,199)
$(66)	$(66)	$(66)	$(66)	$(66)	$(66)	$(66)
$(204)	$(204)	$(204)	$(204)	$(204)	$(204)	$(204)

continued on next page

Exhibit 13.51 – Example L-1 continued

	Total	Allocation	Smith	Johnson
Insurance – Malpractice (corp)	$(11,299)	Equal per Physician	$(1,255)	$(1,255)
Interest/Penalties/Fees	$(742)	Equal per Physician	$(82)	$(82)
Laundry and Uniforms	$(450)	Equal per Physician	$(50)	$(50)
Lease Equipment	$(1,996)	Equal per Physician	$(222)	$(222)
Legal Expense	$(8,750)	Equal per Physician	$(972)	$(972)
Medical Expense Benefits – Flex	$(1,430)	Equal per Physician	$(159)	$(159)
Mileage Reimbursement (admin)	$(985)	Equal per Physician	$(109)	$(109)
Miscellaneous Expense	$(685)	Equal per Physician	$(76)	$(76)
Office Supplies	$(16,070)	Equal per Physician	$(1,786)	$(1,786)
Pagers and Answering Service	$(16,520)	Equal per Physician	$(1,836)	$(1,836)
Postage	$(8,467)	Equal per Physician	$(941)	$(941)
Rent – Common	$(12,692)	Equal per Physician	$(1,410)	$(1,410)
Rent – Division Specific	$(100,488)	Direct to Division	$(14,451)	$(14,451)
Repairs and Maintenance	$(35,782)	Equal per Physician	$(3,976)	$(3,976)
Subscriptions and Books	$(1,232)	Equal per Physician	$(137)	$(137)
Taxes	$(3,519)	Equal per Physician	$(391)	$(391)
Telephone	$(17,520)	Equal per Physician	$(1,947)	$(1,947)
Subtotal – General Operating Expenses	$(384,927)		$(45,421)	$(45,936)
SUPPORT STAFF EXPENSES				
SALARIES				
Administrative Staff	$(99,272)	Equal per Physician	$(11,345)	$(11,345)
Billing Staff	$(139,349)	50% Equal FTE/50% Claims Volume†		
50% of Total (from above)	$(69,675)	Equal per FTE	$(7,963)	$(7,963)
50% of Total (from above)	$(69,675)	% of Claims Volume	$(3,745)	$(7,319)
Clinical Staff	$(25,471)	% of Encounters	$(1,369)	$(2,676)
Nonclinical Staff – South	$(11,818)	Direct Division/ % of Total Encounters	$(1,289)	$(2,520)
Nonclinical Staff – East	$(15,021)	Direct Division/ % of Total Encounters	$—	$—
Scheduling Staff – South	$(56,380)	Direct Division/ % of Total Encounters	$(6,152)	$(12,022)
Scheduling Staff – East	$(126,142)	Direct Division/ % of Total Encounters	$—	$—
Subtotal – Nonphysician Employee Allocated Salary	$(473,454)		$(31,863)	$(43,845)
BENEFITS AND OTHER EXPENSES				
Education – Employees	$(15,234)	% of Allocated Salary	$(1,025)	$(1,411)
Insurance Disability – Employees	$(23,542)	% of Allocated Salary	$(1,584)	$(2,180)
Insurance Health – Employees	$(57,600)	% of Allocated Salary	$(3,876)	$(5,334)
Payroll Taxes – Employees	$(59,182)	% of Allocated Salary	$(3,983)	$(5,481)
Profit-Sharing Contribution – Employees	$(102,450)	% of Allocated Salary	$(6,895)	$(9,488)
Workers Compensation – Employees	$(14,204)	% of Allocated Salary	$(956)	$(1,315)
Subtotal – Employee Benefits	$(272,211)		$(18,320)	$(25,209)
Total Operating Expenses	$(1,130,592)		$(95,604)	$(114,990)

Wilson[‡]	Einstein	Bornsten	Porter	Mathews	Patel	Kant
$(1,255)	$(1,255)	$(1,255)	$(1,255)	$(1,255)	$(1,255)	$(1,255)
$(82)	$(82)	$(82)	$(82)	$(82)	$(82)	$(82)
$(50)	$(50)	$(50)	$(50)	$(50)	$(50)	$(50)
$(222)	$(222)	$(222)	$(222)	$(222)	$(222)	$(222)
$(972)	$(972)	$(972)	$(972)	$(972)	$(972)	$(972)
$(159)	$(159)	$(159)	$(159)	$(159)	$(159)	$(159)
$(109)	$(109)	$(109)	$(109)	$(109)	$(109)	$(109)
$(76)	$(76)	$(76)	$(76)	$(76)	$(76)	$(76)
$(1,786)	$(1,786)	$(1,786)	$(1,786)	$(1,786)	$(1,786)	$(1,786)
$(1,836)	$(1,836)	$(1,836)	$(1,836)	$(1,836)	$(1,836)	$(1,836)
$(941)	$(941)	$(941)	$(941)	$(941)	$(941)	$(941)
$(1,410)	$(1,410)	$(1,410)	$(1,410)	$(1,410)	$(1,410)	$(1,410)
$(8,537)	$(14,451)	$(14,451)	$(8,537)	$(8,537)	$(8,537)	$(8,537)
$(3,976)	$(3,976)	$(3,976)	$(3,976)	$(3,976)	$(3,976)	$(3,976)
$(137)	$(137)	$(137)	$(137)	$(137)	$(137)	$(137)
$(391)	$(391)	$(391)	$(391)	$(391)	$(391)	$(391)
$(1,947)	$(1,947)	$(1,947)	$(1,947)	$(1,947)	$(1,947)	$(1,947)
$(41,136)	$(46,470)	$(46,848)	$(40,030)	$(39,669)	$(39,997)	$(39,418)
$(11,345)	$(11,345)	$(11,345)	$(11,345)	$(8,509)	$(11,345)	$(11,345)
$(7,963)	$(7,963)	$(7,963)	$(7,963)	$(5,972)	$(7,963)	$(7,963)
$(13,089)	$(10,513)	$(12,747)	$(7,433)	$(4,448)	$(7,234)	$(3,146)
$(4,785)	$(3,843)	$(4,660)	$(2,717)	$(1,626)	$(2,644)	$(1,150)
$—	$(3,620)	$(4,389)	$—	$—	$—	$—
$(5,562)	$—	$—	$(3,159)	$(1,890)	$(3,074)	$(1,337)
$—	$(17,269)	$(20,938)	$—	$—	$—	$—
$(46,707)	$—	$—	$(26,524)	$(15,874)	$(25,812)	$(11,226)
$(89,451)	$(54,553)	$(62,042)	$(59,141)	$(38,320)	$(58,071)	$(36,168)
$(2,878)	$(1,755)	$(1,996)	$(1,903)	$(1,233)	$(1,869)	$(1,164)
$(4,448)	$(2,713)	$(3,085)	$(2,941)	$(1,905)	$(2,888)	$(1,798)
$(10,883)	$(6,637)	$(7,548)	$(7,195)	$(4,662)	$(7,065)	$(4,400)
$(11,181)	$(6,819)	$(7,755)	$(7,393)	$(4,790)	$(7,259)	$(4,521)
$(19,356)	$(11,805)	$(13,425)	$(12,797)	$(8,292)	$(12,566)	$(7,826)
$(2,684)	$(1,637)	$(1,861)	$(1,774)	$(1,150)	$(1,742)	$(1,085)
$(51,430)	$(31,365)	$(35,671)	$(34,003)	$(22,032)	$(33,388)	$(20,795)
$(182,017)	$(132,388)	$(144,561)	$(133,174)	$(100,020)	$(131,457)	$(96,381)

continued on next page

Exhibit 13.51 – Example L-1 continued

		Total	Allocation	Smith	Johnson
Step 4	**Determine ancillary services profits pool.**				
	Revenues				
	Ancillary – Technical Component	$315,951	Direct Ancillary Pool		
	Expenses				
	Ancillary Technicians	$(112,085)	Direct Ancillary Pool		
	Ancillary Supplies	$(13,872)	Direct Ancillary Pool		
	Ancillary Net Profit (Revenue – Expense)	$189,994	% of Total Encounters	$10,212	$19,958
Step 5	**Determine amount available for physician compensation and direct expense.**				
	(Revenue – Operating Expenses + Ancillary Profits)	$3,597,040		$322,076	$533,564
Step 6	**Determine physician-specific direct expenses.**				
	Physician Base Salary (Guaranteed) (from above)	$(1,880,000)		$(140,000)	$(300,000)
	Auto Expense	$(28,023)	Direct to Physician by Utilization		$(2,419)
	Books and Periodicals	$(3,305)	Direct to Physician by Utilization		
	Cellular Phones	$(8,124)	Direct to Physician by Utilization	$(780)	$(1,980)
	Computer Expense – Physicians	$(1,819)	Direct to Physician by Utilization		
	Dues and Licenses	$(16,194)	Direct to Physician by Utilization	$(462)	$(1,964)
	Entertainment and Meals	$(30)	Direct to Physician by Utilization		
	Gifts	$(446)	Direct to Physician by Utilization	$(133)	$(133)
	Health Insurance	$(99,257)	Direct to Physician by Utilization	$(10,099)	$(5,579)
	Surgical Instruments	$(326)	Direct to Physician by Utilization		
	Insurance – Long-Term Care	$(5,045)	Direct to Physician by Utilization		
	Insurance – Malpractice	$(303,093)	Direct to Physician by Utilization	$(33,677)	$(33,677)
	Insurance – Term Life	$(3,354)	Direct to Physician by Utilization		
	Meetings and Conventions	$(14,132)	Direct to Physician by Utilization	$(2,324)	
	Nonphysician Provider Compensation and Benefits	$(185,000)	Direct to Physician by Utilization	$(10,000)	$(30,000)
	Office Expense – Specialized	$(32)	Direct to Physician by Utilization		
	Payroll Taxes Physicians	$(81,593)	Direct to Physician by Utilization	$(8,344)	$(8,657)
	Profit-Sharing Contribution	$(75,600)	Direct to Physician by Utilization	$(3,600)	$(4,800)
	Pension Contribution	$(140,940)	Direct to Physician by Utilization	$(15,660)	$(15,660)
	Transcription Service	$(20,003)	Direct to Physician by Utilization	$(685)	$(2,132)
	Total Direct Physician Expenses	$(2,866,317)		$(225,764)	$(407,002)
Step 7	**Determine physician income after direct expenses.**	$730,724		$96,312	$126,561
Step 8	**Determine physician total W-2 compensation.**				
	Sum of guaranteed base plus incentive (if any)‡			$236,312	$426,561

* Hypothetical numbers presented for illustrative purposes only. Numbers may not total in all cases due to rounding.

† Actual claims volume not reflected in the example; numbers shown are for illustrative purposes.

‡ Dr. Wilson receives full base salary despite operating at slight deficit because base salary is guaranteed. Base may be reduced to prevent future deficits.

Wilson‡	Einstein	Bornsten	Porter	Mathews	Patel	Kant
$35,693	$28,668	$34,759	$20,269	$12,130	$19,725	$8,579
$256,428	$291,081	$343,674	$556,536	$397,095	$467,735	$428,851
$(140,000)	$(140,000)	$(160,000)	$(300,000)	$(225,000)	$(250,000)	$(225,000)
$(587)	$(6,378)		$(2,382)	$(4,981)	$(5,774)	$(5,504)
$(436)	$(143)	$(297)			$(1,833)	$(596)
$(840)	$(780)	$(816)	$(744)	$(804)	$(780)	$(600)
	$(1,275)					$(544)
$(3,642)	$(1,202)	$(1,008)	$(3,046)	$(1,020)	$(2,642)	$(1,206)
						$(30)
		$(180)				
$(10,099)	$(13,580)	$(13,580)	$(13,580)	$(5,579)	$(13,580)	$(13,580)
					$(326)	
$(5,045)						
$(33,677)	$(33,677)	$(33,677)	$(33,677)	$(33,677)	$(33,677)	$(33,677)
$(3,354)						
$(4,310)	$(1,231)	$(877)	$(5,068)		$(164)	$(159)
$(18,000)	$(12,000)	$(25,000)	$(30,000)	$(15,000)	$(25,000)	$(20,000)
			$(8)		$(1)	$(23)
$(7,857)	$(7,906)	$(7,966)	$(10,474)	$(9,603)	$(10,472)	$(10,314)
$(9,600)	$(9,600)	$(9,600)	$(9,600)	$(9,600)	$(9,600)	$(9,600)
$(15,660)	$(15,660)	$(15,660)	$(15,660)	$(15,660)	$(15,660)	$(15,660)
$(5,506)	$(5,506)	$(5,506)	$(74)	$(224)	$(147)	$(222)
$(258,613)	$(248,939)	$(274,168)	$(424,314)	$(321,147)	$(369,656)	$(336,714)
$(2,185)	$42,143	$69,507	$132,222	$75,948	$98,078	$92,136
$140,000	$182,143	$229,507	$432,222	$300,948	$348,078	$317,136

EXHIBIT 13.52

Example M-1 – Group Practice Architecture M –
Equal Share (10%)/Production Revenue Allocation (90%) with Strict Cost Accounting Plan*
Revenue Element 3 and Expense Element 9

		Total		Smith	Johnson
Step 1	**Assemble production information.**				
	Physician	9.00		1.00	1.00
	Physician FTE	8.75		1.00	1.00
	Ambulatory Encounters	5,158		206	504
	Physician % to Total Ambulatory Encounters			4%	10%
	Surgeries	2,172		188	266
	Total Ambulatory and Surgical Encounters	7,331		394	770
	Physician % to Total Encounters – All Divisions	100%		5%	11%
	Physician % to Total Encounters – South Division	100%		11%	21%
	Physician % to Total Encounters – East Division	100%			
	Net Collections from Professional Services	$3,912,914		$378,545	$524,376
	Physician % to Total Net Collections	100%		10%	13%
Step 2	**Determine revenue.**	**Total**		**Smith**	**Johnson**
	Net Collections from Professional Services	$3,912,914	Direct	$378,545	$524,376
	Nonphysician Provider Net Revenue	$173,002	Physician Use	$—	$32,203
	Ancillary Net Collections – Professional Component	$155,864	Direct to Performing Physician	$13,342	$62,145
	Interest Income	$46,897	Equal/FTE	$5,360	$5,360
	Other Income	$34,059	Direct	$10,221	$4,512
	Total Revenue	$4,322,736		$407,468	$628,595
Step 3	**Reallocate revenue.**				
	Equal Share Portion (10%) per FTE	$432,274		$49,403	$49,403
	Production Portion (90%) (% of professional services collections)	$3,890,462		$376,373	$521,367
	Allocated Revenue after Equal Share	$4,322,736		$425,776	$570,770

Wilson[‡]	Einstein[‡]	Bornsten	Porter[‡]	Mathews	Patel	Kant
1.00	1.00	1.00	1.00	1.00	1.00	1.00
1.00	1.00	1.00	1.00	0.75	1.00	1.00
1,149	813	1,032	509	300	490	155
22%	16%	20%	10%	6%	9%	3%
228	293	309	273	168	271	176
1,377	1,106	1,341	782	468	761	331
19%	15%	18%	11%	6%	10%	5%
	31%	37%				
37%			21%	13%	20%	9%
$376,499	$356,821	$413,753	$423,000	$434,281	$532,153	$473,486
10%	9%	11%	11%	11%	14%	12%

Wilson	Einstein	Bornsten	Porter	Mathews	Patel	Kant
$376,499	$356,821	$413,753	$423,000	$434,281	$532,153	$473,486
$7,019	$—	$—	$24,991	$40,893	$32,442	$35,455
$13,645	$32,121	$24,512	$1,024	$3,212	$4,512	$1,351
$5,360	$5,360	$5,360	$5,360	$4,020	$5,360	$5,360
$230	$500	$9,852	$164	$2,580	$5,000	$1,000
$402,752	$394,802	$453,476	$454,538	$484,986	$579,467	$516,652
$49,403	$49,403	$49,403	$49,403	$65,870	$49,403	$49,403
$374,339	$354,774	$411,379	$420,573	$431,789	$529,099	$470,770
$423,741	$404,176	$460,781	$469,976	$497,660	$578,502	$520,172

continued on next page

Exhibit 13.52 – Example M-1 continued

		Total	Allocation	Smith	Johnson
Step 4	**Determine operating expenses.**				
	GENERAL OPERATING EXPENSES				
	Accounting	$(18,636)	Equal per Physician	$(2,071)	$(2,071)
	Advertising	$(4,525)	Equal per Physician	$(503)	$(503)
	Bank Charges	$(6,325)	Equal per Physician	$(703)	$(703)
	Biomedical Waste	$(2,763)	% Ambulatory Encounters	$(110)	$(270)
	Business Promotion	$(2,618)	Equal per Physician	$(291)	$(291)
	Cell Phones (admin)	$(2,400)	Equal per Physician	$(267)	$(267)
	Computer (admin)	$(87,036)	Equal per Physician	$(9,671)	$(9,671)
	Contract Services	$(2,618)	Equal per Physician	$(291)	$(291)
	Drugs and Medical Supplies	$(6,150)	% Ambulatory Encounters	$(246)	$(601)
	Dues and Licenses	$(10,794)	Equal per Physician	$(1,199)	$(1,199)
	Food/Entertainment	$(596)	Equal per Physician	$(66)	$(66)
	Insurance – General Liability	$(1,837)	Equal per Physician	$(204)	$(204)
	Insurance – Malpractice (corp)	$(11,299)	Equal per Physician	$(1,255)	$(1,255)
	Interest/Penalties/Fees	$(742)	Equal per Physician	$(82)	$(82)
	Laundry and Uniforms	$(450)	Equal per Physician	$(50)	$(50)
	Lease Equipment	$(1,996)	Equal per Physician	$(222)	$(222)
	Legal Expense	$(8,750)	Equal per Physician	$(972)	$(972)
	Medical Expense Benefits – Flex	$(1,430)	Equal per Physician	$(159)	$(159)
	Mileage Reimbursement (admin)	$(985)	Equal per Physician	$(109)	$(109)
	Miscellaneous Expense	$(685)	Equal per Physician	$(76)	$(76)
	Office Supplies	$(16,070)	Equal per Physician	$(1,786)	$(1,786)
	Pagers and Answering Service	$(16,520)	Equal per Physician	$(1,836)	$(1,836)
	Postage	$(8,467)	Equal per Physician	$(941)	$(941)
	Rent – Division Specific	$(100,488)	Direct to Division	$(14,451)	$(14,451)
	Rent – Common	$(12,692)	Equal per Physician	$(1,410)	$(1,410)
	Repairs and Maintenance	$(35,782)	Equal per Physician	$(3,976)	$(3,976)
	Subscriptions and Books	$(1,232)	Equal per Physician	$(137)	$(137)
	Taxes	$(3,519)	Equal per Physician	$(391)	$(391)
	Telephone	$(17,520)	Equal per Physician	$(1,947)	$(1,947)
	Subtotal – General Operating Expenses	$(384,927)		$(45,421)	$(45,936)
	SUPPORT STAFF EXPENSES				
	Administrative Staff	$(99,272)	Equal per Physician	$(11,345)	$(11,345)
	Billing Staff	$(139,349)	50% Equal FTE/50% Claims Volume†		
	50% of Total (from above)	$(69,675)	Equal per FTE	$(7,963)	$(7,963)
	50% of Total (from above)	$(69,675)	% of Claims Volume	$(3,745)	$(7,319)
	Clinical Staff	$(25,471)	% of Total Encounters	$(1,369)	$(2,676)
	Nonclinical Staff – South	$(11,818)	Direct Division/ % of Total Encounters	$(1,289)	$(2,520)
	Nonclinical Staff – East	$(15,021)	Direct Division/ % of Total Encounters	$—	$—
	Scheduling Staff – South	$(56,380)	Direct Division/ % of Total Encounters	$(6,152)	$(12,022)
	Scheduling Staff – East	$(126,142)	Direct Division/ % of Total Encounters	$—	$—
	Subtotal – Nonphysician Employee Allocated Salary	$(473,454)		$(31,863)	$(43,845)

Wilson‡	Einstein‡	Bornsten	Porter‡	Mathews	Patel	Kant
$(2,071)	$(2,071)	$(2,071)	$(2,071)	$(2,071)	$(2,071)	$(2,071)
$(503)	$(503)	$(503)	$(503)	$(503)	$(503)	$(503)
$(703)	$(703)	$(703)	$(703)	$(703)	$(703)	$(703)
$(616)	$(436)	$(553)	$(273)	$(161)	$(263)	$(83)
$(291)	$(291)	$(291)	$(291)	$(291)	$(291)	$(291)
$(267)	$(267)	$(267)	$(267)	$(267)	$(267)	$(267)
$(9,671)	$(9,671)	$(9,671)	$(9,671)	$(9,671)	$(9,671)	$(9,671)
$(291)	$(291)	$(291)	$(291)	$(291)	$(291)	$(291)
$(1,370)	$(969)	$(1,231)	$(607)	$(358)	$(584)	$(185)
$(1,199)	$(1,199)	$(1,199)	$(1,199)	$(1,199)	$(1,199)	$(1,199)
$(66)	$(66)	$(66)	$(66)	$(66)	$(66)	$(66)
$(204)	$(204)	$(204)	$(204)	$(204)	$(204)	$(204)
$(1,255)	$(1,255)	$(1,255)	$(1,255)	$(1,255)	$(1,255)	$(1,255)
$(82)	$(82)	$(82)	$(82)	$(82)	$(82)	$(82)
$(50)	$(50)	$(50)	$(50)	$(50)	$(50)	$(50)
$(222)	$(222)	$(222)	$(222)	$(222)	$(222)	$(222)
$(972)	$(972)	$(972)	$(972)	$(972)	$(972)	$(972)
$(159)	$(159)	$(159)	$(159)	$(159)	$(159)	$(159)
$(109)	$(109)	$(109)	$(109)	$(109)	$(109)	$(109)
$(76)	$(76)	$(76)	$(76)	$(76)	$(76)	$(76)
$(1,786)	$(1,786)	$(1,786)	$(1,786)	$(1,786)	$(1,786)	$(1,786)
$(1,836)	$(1,836)	$(1,836)	$(1,836)	$(1,836)	$(1,836)	$(1,836)
$(941)	$(941)	$(941)	$(941)	$(941)	$(941)	$(941)
$(8,537)	$(14,451)	$(14,451)	$(8,537)	$(8,537)	$(8,537)	$(8,537)
$(1,410)	$(1,410)	$(1,410)	$(1,410)	$(1,410)	$(1,410)	$(1,410)
$(3,976)	$(3,976)	$(3,976)	$(3,976)	$(3,976)	$(3,976)	$(3,976)
$(137)	$(137)	$(137)	$(137)	$(137)	$(137)	$(137)
$(391)	$(391)	$(391)	$(391)	$(391)	$(391)	$(391)
$(1,947)	$(1,947)	$(1,947)	$(1,947)	$(1,947)	$(1,947)	$(1,947)
$(41,136)	$(46,470)	$(46,848)	$(40,030)	$(39,669)	$(39,997)	$(39,418)
$(11,345)	$(11,345)	$(11,345)	$(11,345)	$(8,509)	$(11,345)	$(11,345)
$(7,963)	$(7,963)	$(7,963)	$(7,963)	$(5,972)	$(7,963)	$(7,963)
$(13,089)	$(10,513)	$(12,747)	$(7,433)	$(4,448)	$(7,234)	$(3,146)
$(4,785)	$(3,843)	$(4,660)	$(2,717)	$(1,626)	$(2,644)	$(1,150)
$—	$(3,620)	$(4,389)	$—	$—	$—	$—
$(5,562)	$—	$—	$(3,159)	$(1,890)	$(3,074)	$(1,337)
$—	$(17,269)	$(20,938)	$—	$—	$—	$—
$(46,707)	$—	$—	$(26,524)	$(15,874)	$(25,812)	$(11,226)
$(89,451)	$(54,553)	$(62,042)	$(59,141)	$(38,320)	$(58,071)	$(36,168)

continued on next page

Exhibit 13.52 – Example M-1 continued

		Total	Allocation	Smith	Johnson
	Education – Employees	$(15,234)	% of Allocated Salary	$(1,025)	$(1,411)
	Insurance Disability – Employees	$(23,542)	% of Allocated Salary	$(1,584)	$(2,180)
	Insurance Health – Employees	$(57,600)	% of Allocated Salary	$(3,876)	$(5,334)
	Payroll Taxes – Employees	$(59,182)	% of Allocated Salary	$(3,983)	$(5,481)
	Profit-Sharing Contribution – Employees	$(102,450)	% of Allocated Salary	$(6,895)	$(9,488)
	Workers Compensation – Employees	$(14,204)	% of Allocated Salary	$(956)	$(1,315)
	Subtotal – Employee Benefits	$(272,211)		$(18,320)	$(25,209)
	Total Operating Expenses	$(1,130,592)		$(95,604)	$(114,990)
Step 5	**Determine ancillary services profits pool.**				
	Revenues				
	Ancillary – Technical Component	$315,951	Direct Ancillary Pool		
	Expenses				
	Ancillary Technicians	$(112,085)	Direct Ancillary Pool		
	Ancillary Supplies	$(13,872)	Direct Ancillary Pool		
	Ancillary Net Profit (Revenue – Expense)	$189,994	% of Total Encounters	$10,212	$19,958
Step 6	**Determine amount available for physician compensation and direct expense.**				
	(Allocated Revenue – Operating Expense + Ancillary Profits Share)	$3,382,138		$340,384	$475,738
Step 7	**Determine physician-specific direct expenses (excluding base salary).**				
	Auto Expense	$(28,023)	Direct to Physician by Utilization		$(2,419)
	Books and Periodicals	$(3,305)	Direct to Physician by Utilization		
	Cellular Phones	$(8,124)	Direct to Physician by Utilization	$(780)	$(1,980)
	Computer Expense – Physician	$(1,819)	Direct to Physician by Utilization		
	Dues and Licenses	$(16,194)	Direct to Physician by Utilization	$(462)	$(1,964)
	Entertainment and Meals	$(30)	Direct to Physician by Utilization		
	Gifts	$(446)	Direct to Physician by Utilization	$(133)	$(133)
	Health Insurance Physicians	$(99,257)	Direct to Physician by Utilization	$(10,099)	$(5,579)
	Surgical Instruments	$(326)	Direct to Physician by Utilization		
	Insurance – Long-Term Care	$(5,045)	Direct to Physician by Utilization		
	Insurance – Malpractice	$(303,093)	Direct to Physician by Utilization	$(33,677)	$(33,677)
	Insurance – Term Life	$(3,354)	Direct to Physician by Utilization		
	Meetings and Conventions	$(14,132)	Direct to Physician by Utilization	$(2,324)	
	Office Expense – Specialized	$(185,000)	Direct to Physician by Utilization	$(10,000)	$(30,000)
	Payroll Taxes Physicians	$(32)	Direct to Physician by Utilization		
	Profit Share Contribution	$(81,593)	Direct to Physician by Utilization	$(8,344)	$(8,657)
	Pension Contribution	$(75,600)	Direct to Physician by Utilization	$(3,600)	$(4,800)
	Telephone Expense	$(140,940)	Direct to Physician by Utilization	$(15,660)	$(15,660)
	Transcription Service	$(20,003)	Direct to Physician by Utilization	$(685)	$(2,132)
	Total Direct Physician Expenses	$(986,317)		$(85,764)	$(107,002)

Wilson[‡]	Einstein[‡]	Bornsten	Porter[‡]	Mathews	Patel	Kant
$(2,878)	$(1,755)	$(1,996)	$(1,903)	$(1,233)	$(1,869)	$(1,164)
$(4,448)	$(2,713)	$(3,085)	$(2,941)	$(1,905)	$(2,888)	$(1,798)
$(10,883)	$(6,637)	$(7,548)	$(7,195)	$(4,662)	$(7,065)	$(4,400)
$(11,181)	$(6,819)	$(7,755)	$(7,393)	$(4,790)	$(7,259)	$(4,521)
$(19,356)	$(11,805)	$(13,425)	$(12,797)	$(8,292)	$(12,566)	$(7,826)
$(2,684)	$(1,637)	$(1,861)	$(1,774)	$(1,150)	$(1,742)	$(1,085)
$(51,430)	$(31,365)	$(35,671)	$(34,003)	$(22,032)	$(33,388)	$(20,795)
$(182,017)	$(132,388)	$(144,561)	$(133,174)	$(100,020)	$(131,457)	$(96,381)
$35,693	$28,668	$34,759	$20,269	$12,130	$19,725	$8,579
$277,417	$300,456	$350,979	$357,071	$409,770	$466,770	$432,371
$(587)	$(6,378)		$(2,382)	$(4,981)	$(5,774)	$(5,504)
$(436)	$(143)	$(297)			$(1,833)	$(596)
$(840)	$(780)	$(816)	$(744)	$(804)	$(780)	$(600)
	$(1,275)					$(544)
$(3,642)	$(1,202)	$(1,008)	$(3,046)	$(1,020)	$(2,642)	$(1,206)
						$(30)
		$(180)				
$(10,099)	$(13,580)	$(13,580)	$(13,580)	$(5,579)	$(13,580)	$(13,580)
					$(326)	
$(5,045)						
$(33,677)	$(33,677)	$(33,677)	$(33,677)	$(33,677)	$(33,677)	$(33,677)
$(3,354)						
$(4,310)	$(1,231)	$(877)	$(5,068)		$(164)	$(159)
$(18,000)	$(12,000)	$(25,000)	$(30,000)	$(15,000)	$(25,000)	$(20,000)
			$(8)		$(1)	$(23)
$(7,857)	$(7,906)	$(7,966)	$(10,474)	$(9,603)	$(10,472)	$(10,314)
$(9,600)	$(9,600)	$(9,600)	$(9,600)	$(9,600)	$(9,600)	$(9,600)
$(15,660)	$(15,660)	$(15,660)	$(15,660)	$(15,660)	$(15,660)	$(15,660)
$(5,506)	$(5,506)	$(5,506)	$(74)	$(224)	$(147)	$(222)
$(118,613)	$(108,939)	$(114,168)	$(124,314)	$(96,147)	$(119,656)	$(111,714)

continued on next page

Exhibit 13.52 – Example M-1 continued

		Total	Allocation		Smith	Johnson
Step 8	Determine physician income after direct expenses (W-2).	$2,395,821			$254,620	$368,736
Step 9	Determine draw amount (previouisly paid not guaranteed).				$(200,000)	$(200,000)
Step 10	Determine bonus/loss (physician income – draw).				$54,620	$168,736
Step 11	Determine total cash compensation.				$254,620	$368,736

* Hypothetical numbers presented for illustrative purposes only. Numbers may not total in all cases due to rounding.

† Based on actual claim volume.

‡ Physicians in deficit status (expenses including exceed revenues). Subsequent draws to be reduced by deficit amount to remove deficit status.

© 2006 Johnson & Walker Keegan

Wilson[‡]	Einstein[‡]	Bornsten	Porter[‡]	Mathews	Patel	Kant
$158,804	$191,517	$236,812	$232,757	$313,622	$347,114	$320,656
$(200,000)	$(200,000)	$(200,000)	$(250,000)	$(300,000)	$(300,000)	$(300,000)
$(41,196)	$(8,483)	$36,812	$(17,243)	$13,622	$47,114	$20,656
$158,804	$191,517	$236,812	$232,757	$313,622	$347,114	$320,656

Each of the middle ground plans may be evaluated and will therefore have its own relative strengths and weaknesses from financial, cultural, and other perspectives. As noted elsewhere, there are literally hundreds of potential compensation plan alternatives – of which only a few are illustrated here. However, through the consideration of the elements on the matrix and reference to the array of compensation architectures, the reader is equipped with the raw materials and basic framework to:

► Assess the practice's current compensation plan in terms of cultural and financial dimensions;

► Assess the potential direction of changes to the current plan in light of the plan's current position on the array of compensation plan architectures; and

► Have a structured tool to evaluate the range of potential plan methodologies that may be considered.

As noted previously, while these architectures address the key financial and cultural dimensions of compensation, they can be supplemented by incentive measures that specifically consider and address quality, patient satisfaction, and other issues. Thus, each of these basic architectures can be viewed as providing the foundation for various compensation plans, to which additional incentive measures can be incorporated or added to address more specific performance-related objectives.

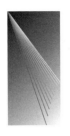

FOURTEEN

Compensation Plans in Hospital-Affiliated Practices
(Direct Employee, Hospital-Affiliated Group and "Contracted" Group)

Compensation plans for physicians who provide services to hospitals via direct employment arrangements or who are employed by a hospital-affiliated medical practice commonly differ somewhat from the plans used in traditional medical groups that are physician-owned and operated. A portion of the variation is due to the unique organizational, political, and cultural factors impacting hospital-affiliated practice arrangements. The most significant reason for methodological differences, however, is due to the legal requirements impacting the physician-hospital relationship.

As discussed in Chapter 9, legal rules that are applicable to compensation arrangements include the Stark and anti-kickback laws, and, in some instances, laws and rules governing tax-exempt organizations. These laws affect the physician compensation methods available in hospital-affiliated physician service and compensation arrangements in several practical ways.

► First, the compensation arrangements commonly rely on exceptions to the Stark law *other than* the law's in-office ancillary services exception, so the physicians generally will not have any ability to benefit financially from their ancillary and other designated health service (DHS) referrals that are subject to the law. The particular Stark law exception being relied upon in the physician-hospital compensation arrangement will dictate the "rules of the road" that will apply to the compensation methodology.

► Second, among its numerous requirements, the anti-kickback law prohibits any payment and/or consideration of referrals from a physician to the hospital (or other entity) in determining compensation.

► Third, where the hospital is a tax-exempt organization, the compensation arrangements must promote the organization's charitable mission, and the compensation paid to physicians must generally not exceed "reasonable" and fair market value (FMV) levels.

As a result of the combination of these laws and rules, the "typical" compensation and incentive system that may be used in a medical group that is physician-owned and operated may not be entirely appropriate in the hospital-affiliated practice setting.

► 401

Of course, even apart from the legal rules governing compensation practices, the underlying organizational features, financial arrangements, culture, and other factors relating to the physician-hospital arrangement will also impact the physician compensation methods that can, or will, be used. For example, many hospital systems have elected to not allow physicians in a captive medical group to receive financial benefit from diagnostic imaging and other ancillary services furnished though the captive medical group's offices – even though such arrangements could be crafted to comply with the Stark law's in-office ancillary services exception. Instead, many hospitals and health systems elect to rely on the Stark law's direct employment exception, which prohibits any direct or indirect consideration of referrals for DHS in determining compensation. In these situations, the hospitals have made business decisions that impact the compensation plans and options that may be used to pay their hospital-affiliated physicians.

The compensation plan development process will also be influenced by the nature of the physician-hospital relationship. In this setting and in others, the *process* of developing a new compensation plan is as critical as the outcome. For that reason, the development of a compensation plan for use with hospital-affiliated physicians is typically conducted by a compensation planning committee that includes both physicians *and* hospital or health system leadership.

The importance of physician participation is no less relevant in this setting in order to promote physician buy-in. However, hospital leadership must also be involved to ensure that the hospital's service and financial goals, business risk-tolerance levels, charitable mission, and/or other objectives are promoted and safeguarded. Moreover, unlike the decision making that occurs in a private practice medical group setting, in a tax-exempt hospital-affiliated practice, the *ultimate* decision regarding compensation methods and levels will generally rest with an independent committee or other decision maker of the hospital – rather than being vested in the physicians who will be the ultimate participants (and recipients) of compensation that is determined and paid under the plan.

Exhibit 14.1 illustrates the common organizational structures and external reimbursement systems that are commonly used in hospital-affiliated practices. As a general matter, when reimbursement is entirely for physician and other health care services under Medicare Part B, and when a bona fide Group Practice is involved, then the plan examples outlined in Chapter 13 may be used.[1]

However, when any portion of the reimbursement is for hospital services, such as when services in a hospital-owned clinic are paid for under the Medicare outpatient prospective payment system (OPPS) (commonly referred to as "provider-based" reimbursement), the compensation methods illustrated in Chapter 13 may not be used in their pure form. This is because, when provider-based reimbursement is used, a portion of the external reimbursement provided from Medicare is in the form of a "facility fee" that is paid because the service is deemed to be provided in a hospital outpatient department. Accordingly, because the Stark law includes inpatient and outpatient hospital services among the DHS to which the Stark law's prohibitions apply, the compen-

Reimbursement Models

Reimbursement for Physician Services Only

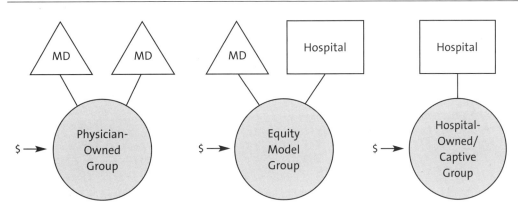

Reimbursement for Physician and Outpatient Hospital Services

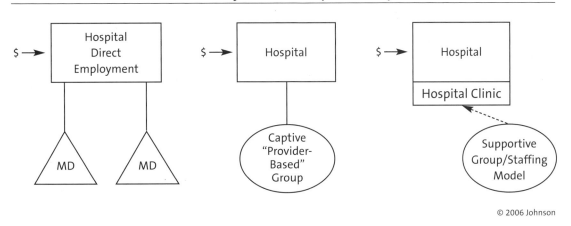

© 2006 Johnson

sation plans for physicians in structures using provider-based reimbursement may not consider the facility fee amount, even if the practice organization otherwise qualifies as a bona fide Group Practice under the Stark law.

The compensation arrangements described in this chapter will generally be structured to comply with Stark law exceptions *other than* the in-office ancillary services exception. The arrangements described here will generally rely upon exceptions to the Stark law governing direct employment arrangements and personal service arrangements, fair market value, indirect compensation arrangements, and potentially others.

Reliance on these exceptions to the Stark law results in a number of practical implications, including:

► Prohibitions on any direct or indirect consideration of referrals in determining physician compensation levels (i.e., referrals for ancillary, inpatient hospital, or other services);

EXHIBIT 14.2   The Compensation Plan Matrix

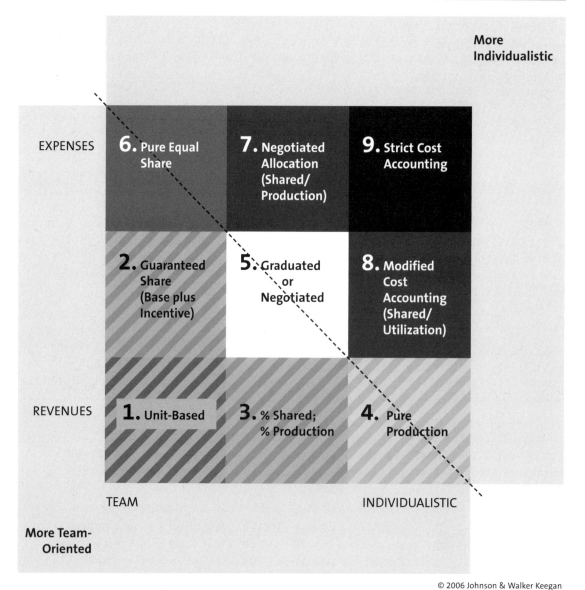

© 2006 Johnson & Walker Keegan

EXHIBIT 14.3 Array of Compensation Plan Architectures

Architecture	A	B	C	D	E	F	G	H	I	J	K	L	M	N	O	P	Q	R
Revenue Element	1	2	3	4	5	2	3	2	3	2	3	2	3	4	4	4	4	4
Expense Element						6	6	7	7	8	8	9	9	5	6	7	8	9
	TEAM					MIDDLE GROUND								INDIVIDUALISTIC				

© 2006 Johnson & Walker Keegan

▶ The imposition of FMV limits on the amount of compensation that may be paid; and

▶ The creation of greater restrictions on the plan methods than are generally applicable to Group Practices.

Thus, the compensation plans in hospital-affiliated groups have a more limited number of methodological options.

The compensation plan examples presented in this chapter *may* also be adapted for use in bona fide Group Practices; therefore, the plan examples in this chapter may be viewed as essentially augmenting the plan examples presented in Chapter 13. However, the plan examples illustrated in Chapter 13 may generally *not* be used in hospital employment arrangements in their pure form (e.g., without modification to take into account the unique rules applicable to the hospital setting).

Nine hospital plan examples are presented. These plans build on different portions of the compensation matrix that were discussed in Chapters 5 and 6 and that are again illustrated in Exhibit 14.2. These plans also build on several of the basic architectures on our array of compensation plan architectures that is again depicted in Exhibit 14.3. The plans can be used in "direct" hospital-physician relationships in which the hospital directly employs the physician, as well as in "indirect" relationships in which: (1) the physician is employed by an entity other than the hospital, such as a hospital-owned medical group, or by a joint venture "equity model" medical group that is owned by physicians and the hospital; or (2) the physicians are legally organized in an entirely separate legal entity that provides services to a hospital-owned clinic on an independent contractor basis.

Exhibit 14.4 illustrates the common types of *direct* compensation relationships involving physicians and hospitals. Examples of direct relationships include:

▶ Employment arrangements in which a hospital employs a physician;

▶ Independent contractor arrangements in which the physician is not an employee, but provides services under a contract that is directly between the physician and the hospital; and

Direct Compensation Arrangement Examples

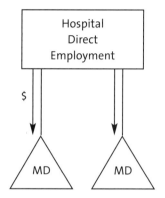

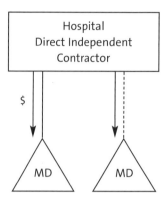

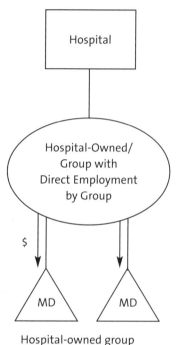

© 2006 Johnson

► Employment (and independent contractor) arrangements between a separately incorporated, hospital-affiliated medical group and individual physicians (in which the direct relationship is with the group, not with the hospital itself).

Plan examples that may be used in *direct* relationships include the following:

► Hospital Example 1 (illustrated in Exhibit 14.6) – Straight Salary Plan (Revenue Element 1, unit-based plan, and Architecture A);

► Hospital Example 2 (illustrated in Exhibits 14.8 through 14.11) – Compensation per WRVU Plan (combining Revenue Element 1, unit-based plans, and Revenue Element 4, pure production plans, and Architectures A and D);

► Hospital Example 3 (illustrated in Exhibits 14.13 and 14.14) – Percentage-based Plan (combining Revenue Elements 1 and 4, unit-based and production, and Architectures A and D);

EXHIBIT 14.5 Indirect Compensation Arrangement Examples

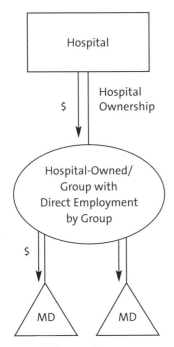

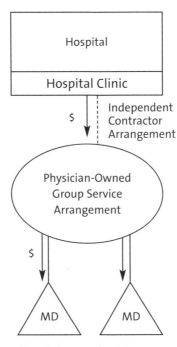

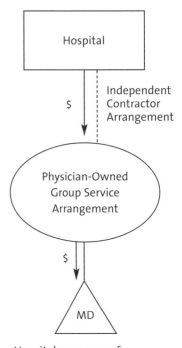

© 2006 Johnson

► Hospital Example 4 (illustrated in Exhibits 14.16 and 14.17) – Base Plus Incentive Plan (Revenue Element 2, guaranteed share, and Architecture C);

► Hospital Example 5 (illustrated in Exhibit 14.19) – Graduated Compensation per WRVU Plan (Revenue Element 5, graduated/negotiated revenues, and Architecture D);

► Hospital Example 6 (illustrated in Exhibit 14.21) – Base Salary with Graduated Compensation per WRVU Plan (Revenue Elements 2 and 5, guaranteed share combined with graduated/negotiated portion of revenues, and Architecture E); and

► Hospital Example 7 (illustrated in Exhibits 14.23 through 14.25) – Hourly Pay Arrangement Plan (using Revenue Element 1, unit-based plan, and Architecture A).

Exhibit 14.5 illustrates the common types of *indirect* compensation relationships involving physicians and hospitals. An indirect relationship is generally present when an intervening legal entity stands in between the hospital (or other organization) that is paying compensation and the organization that has the direct financial relationship with the physician benefiting from that compensation. Examples of indirect relationships include:

► Employment (and independent contractor) arrangements between a separately incorporated, hospital-owned medical group and individual physicians, but the hospital provides funds for compensation; in this case, the physicians may have an indirect compensation arrangement with the hospital;

► Employment arrangements between a physician and a medical practice that provides services to a hospital outpatient department under an independent contractor service arrangement; and

► A contract between a privately owned and operated physician group and a hospital for the delivery of medical director or similar services in which the compensation for such services is paid to the medical group that employs the physician, and not directly to the physician providing the services.

Examples of plans that may be used with *indirect* arrangements include:

► Hospital Example 8 (illustrated in Exhibits 14.27 and 14.28) – Indirect Hospital or Contracted Group with Cost Control Plan (simple) (Revenue Elements 4 and 5, production-based and graduated/negotiated revenues);

► Hospital Example 9 (illustrated in Exhibits 14.30 through 14.33) – Indirect Hospital or Contracted Group Using WRVUs and Cost Control Plan (complex) (Revenue Elements 4 and 5, production-based and graduated/negotiated revenues).

Consistent with the approach we took in the last chapter, we evaluate each of these plans on six separate dimensions that are generally present in better-performing compensation plans, including:

Measure: Selection of a measure(s) that is clear and understandable;

Productivity focus: Strength of the plan's focus on clinical productivity;

Financial: Fiscal viability of the plan;

Simplicity: Level of simplicity represented by the plan;

Alignment: Alignment of the plan with the medical practice's goals; and

Fairness: Issues of equity that may be of concern to physicians.

As noted previously, the plan examples generally illustrate the basic architecture being described using hypothetical data. The plan examples are intended to illustrate the mathematical calculations. The same basic methods can be adapted for use in other settings and arrangements, and the methodological features illustrated in one example can frequently be incorporated into others. For this reason, each of the plan architectures and examples, along with the various details illustrated in each, can be viewed as building blocks that can be mixed and combined to create alternative plans and models.

➤ HOSPITAL EXAMPLE 1 – STRAIGHT SALARY PLAN
Revenue Element 1 (Unit-Based Plan)

Overview

Straight salary arrangements are used to pay physicians for the services they furnish to a hospital, health plan, or other organization. Straight salary arrangements involve payment of a predefined level of compensation for services. These methods generally use Revenue Element 1 and build on Architecture A in that they are "unit-based" by paying compensation for a unit of service (i.e., compensation in the form of a salary for one year's service). Because they also incorporate a largely "guaranteed" amount of compensation, straight salary plans also build on Revenue Element 2 (involving a guaranteed income).

Application

Straight salary compensation plans are commonly paid by hospitals or medical groups to physicians under full- or part-time employment arrangements. Such systems are commonly used with primary care physicians and with medical and surgical specialists. Straight salary arrangements are also commonly used in many large, multispecialty medical groups, and will frequently be used when physicians are in their early years of practice.

When a compensation arrangement relies on the Stark law's employment exception, as is common in many hospital-physician relationships, an essential legal requirement is that the compensation may not exceed fair market value for the physician's services. When a tax-exempt organization is involved, compensation must also be "reasonable." Chapter 9 provides more information on these legal issues.

Methodology

The steps in any straight salary plan generally involve the following:

Step 1. Identify physician specialties and services;

Step 2. Establish performance expectations for receipt of salary;

Step 3. Establish salary levels; and

Step 4. Determine and pay compensation.

Steps 2 and 3 are further detailed below.

Step 2: Establish Performance Expectations for Receipt of Salary

Although straight salary plans effectively involve the agreed upon payment of compensation for a defined unit of service (e.g., a salary for a full year of service), an essential element for successful salary plans is the establishment of *minimum* performance expectations for receipt of the salary amount. Such performance expectations will commonly consider any number of work-related factors that are defined in advance of setting the salary, and that constitute *minimum* levels of performance that are deemed to be acceptable for receipt of the full salary.

Minimum performance expectations may be distinguished from targets defined in connection with incentive compensation. Performance expectations constitute the bare minimum expected performance levels, and physicians who fail to perform at such levels will typically be subject to reduced compensation, financial and/or other sanctions for nonperformance, and potentially termination of the underlying service and compensation relationship. Conversely, targets and goals that are defined for incentive compensation are established so that, if they are achieved, they typically result in additional compensation. Physicians who fail to meet or exceed the incentive targets will not receive additional compensation, but neither will they generally be at risk of additional sanctions as long as their performance conforms with the minimum performance expectations.

Performance expectations are further discussed in Chapter 10 and are generally defined in any number of objective and more subjective areas of physician performance, including:

- ► Weeks worked per year (e.g., 46 or 47 weeks of service per year);

- ► Scheduled days of clinical service (clinic, hospital, and/or surgical services) per week, typically requiring some defined level (e.g., four and one-half days or five days per week) for "full-time" employment, with reduced levels for part-time employment status;

- ► Clinical productivity defined by charges, WRVUs, or other measures (e.g., production from professional services no less than 80 percent of the median or other production percentiles as reported in published survey data);

- ► Professional service hours including clinic operating hours and time devoted to hospital care/rounds within benchmarks (e.g., no less than 36 hours of scheduled clinic time per week and four and one-half day week for primary care physicians);

- ► Maintenance of a clinic scheduling template to maximize patient access and to provide next available appointment times within benchmarks for routine, urgent, and acute care (new and return patients), and consistent with third-party contract requirements;

- ► Starting the scheduled clinic on time (without chronic tardiness);

- ► Participating in clinic or site and specialty-specific planning and budgeting activities directed at enhancing clinic efficiency and meeting fiscal and other goals;

➤ Submission of charge tickets and medical record documentation in accordance with completion and accuracy standards (e.g., within 48 hours of encounter; coding levels to accurately match documentation of services performed); and

➤ Use of electronic health records.

Other performance expectations can also be defined to establish minimum performance requirements. Achievement of the minimum performance expectations should be well within every physician's capabilities such that a physician's failure to meet the minimum expectations should generally constitute the exception rather than the rule.

The performance expectations also should consider both the goals and desires of the physicians, as well as the requirements of the hospital or other organization from financial, business, service, and other perspectives. This reality commonly leads to changes in performance expectations and requirements in the hospital practice setting over those that may have been imposed in private practice or elsewhere in the past.

For example, although many practices that are physician-owned and operated may be willing to allow physicians to maintain a "typical" work schedule of four or four and one-half days per week, the combination of declining reimbursement, increased operating costs, and increased patient demand is requiring many practices and hospitals to assess whether the continuation of such practices is viable or appropriate. As a result, many practice organizations, including those that are hospital-affiliated, are defining minimum work requirements that generally expand upon the typical work week or scheduling practices that may have been used in the past. In addition to the inherent challenges with instituting any change in work requirements, hospital-affiliated practices arguably have an additional hurdle in instituting such a change, because the physicians who work for the hospital-affiliated practice may develop a level of "insulation" from external market forces and realities, given their position.

Because performance expectations are, by definition, standards of *minimum* performance for receipt of the salary, the compensation plan (and underlying contractual documents and/or policies governing the compensation relationship) should also address what happens when such performance requirements are not met.

In most instances, the failure to meet performance minimums will yield predefined reductions in salary levels, while still providing a reasonable level of compensation. Thus, a physician's failure to achieve minimum production or other service levels may allow for a "midterm" adjustment of the salary amount being paid up to a predefined reduction (e.g., 20 percent). The reduction may be allowed for a short time or for the remainder of the term and be linked to performance that rises to minimum performance standards, the achievement of which will allow the salary to return to previous levels. In some cases, the failure to meet minimum performance requirements results in reductions in compensation, counseling, and "probationary" plans to improve performance, and, in more extreme (or chronic) instances, termination of employment.

Performance standards and expectations should optimally include objective measures that can be achieved. In addition to the specific standards themselves, organizations that define performance expectations should also consider and address such issues as:

► What type of hospital or other system support should be provided to help ensure that all physicians can and do perform at expected levels (e.g., physician mentoring programs, formal training, schedule management, etc.)?

► How will physicians be informed via reports and face-to-face interaction regarding their performance in relation to the minimum standards?

► Who will be responsible for monitoring and implementing corrective adjustments when minimum performance expectations are not received?

► What actions or sanctions will be imposed for nonperformance in accordance with the minimum expectations?

► What procedural and other safeguards are available to the physician to ensure that the performance standards are developed and administered in a "fair" manner?

► At what point will the failure to meet the minimum requirements trigger specific actions, including reduction in salary or compensation levels and potential termination?

See Chapter 10 for more information on developing and implementing performance expectations.

Step 3. Establish Salary Levels

Certainly one of the key issues under any straight salary plan is the appropriate means to establish the salary arrangement. Salaries generally will be linked to a defined benchmark (e.g., Medical Group Management Association [MGMA] median by specialty) or to some estimated measure of performance or production per physician in relation to the defined benchmark.

The approach involving a set salary level that is directly linked to a published benchmark was commonly used in the 1990s in connection with many hospital-affiliated practices and integrated delivery systems. Such a method was generally deemed to be problematic as a long-term strategy, because the methodology divorced any measure of work from compensation. As a result, the use of set salaries without any express consideration of work levels was viewed to be at least partially responsible for significant operating losses for hospital-affiliated physician practices.

As a result of these experiences, variations of straight salary plans have been used to incorporate different measures of productivity. The basic methodology of paying a straight salary for physician services has remained, but hospitals have used different approaches to link physician production to compensation levels – even under straight salary arrangements. Hospital Example 1 (illustrated in Exhibit 14.6 at the end of this section), shows the use of a tiered grid to determine salary levels, with the various tiers in the grid based on consideration of market and other data.

Other methods involving similar grids linked to production are provided in other hospital examples. In each of these plans, production at the individual physician level is effectively benchmarked against market or other expected performance levels for purposes of determining compensation levels to be paid.

Hospital Example 1 also demonstrates the use of a straight salary plan for new physicians and a different straight salary plan for established physicians in the practice. In this example, the new physician plan is used during the initial year of employment. During year two of employment, the physician is paid the greater of the year-one salary, or the amount that would be earned under the "established physician" plan. In year three, the physician automatically moves to the established physician plan, which uses production levels to determine salary amounts. This general three-year progression mimics the transition from "associate" to "partner" status in most private medical groups, but with appropriate adaptations for a hospital-affiliated arrangement.

This example also illustrates the reality that some physician production levels will exceed the top (or bottom) levels of the preestablished salary ranges. Reaching the upper limit can be used to provide a de facto cap on total salary that will be paid; or, more commonly, the achievement of production that is above defined levels will likely require the salary arrangement to be considered via a separate method. Such separate methods include a review of the appropriateness of compensation levels by a non-physician compensation committee and/or a review as part of a compliance process directed at ensuring that the proposed compensation level is reasonable and consistent with the FMV of the physician's services.

Other methods can also be used to develop salary levels beyond those illustrated in Example 1. By illustration, for a primary care physician, production at a defined percentage of market median production levels (e.g., 85 to 90 percent of MGMA median) might yield a salary level that is benchmarked at 80 to 90 percent of MGMA median salary levels by specialty. See Architecture A in Chapter 13 for additional examples of straight salary plans. (*Note:* Discussion of the survey instruments as they relate to production and salary levels is provided in Chapter 16, "The Special World of Hospital and Academic Practices – Assessing Reasonableness and Promoting Compliance.")

Exhibit 14.7 provides an assessment of the strengths and weaknesses of Hospital Example 1.

EXHIBIT 14.6

Hospital Example 1 – Straight Salary Plan*
Revenue Element 1 (Unit-Based Plan)

Step 1 **Identify physician specialties.**
Note: General surgery illustrated here.

Step 2 **Establish minimum performance expectations.**

Measure	Minimum
Clinical service production (WRVUs) per year	5,500
Average per month	458
Weeks worked per year	46 weeks
Scheduled days per week	4.5 days
On-call obligations	Pro rata night and weekend within department
Service	Quality improvement committee

Step 3 **Establish salary levels.[†]**
Note: Links salary to year of employment and production as follows.

	Salary Level
Employment Year 1	$220,000
Employment Year 2	Greater of $220,000 or amount under established physician grid (see below)
Employment Year 3 and beyond	Established physician grid (see below)

Established Physician Grid

WRVU Level	Salary Level
Over 8,500[‡]	$275,000[‡]
8,001 to 8,500	$263,380
7,501 to 8,000	$247,887
7,001 to 7,500	$232,394
6,501 to 7,000	$216,901
6,001 to 6,500	$201,408
5,501 to 6,000	$185,915
5,001 to 5,500	$170,423
Under 5,000	$154,930

* Hypothetical numbers presented for illustrative purposes only. Numbers may not total in all cases due to rounding.

[†] Salary levels derived from market data to promote consistency with fair market value and reasonableness standards.

[‡] Physicians with high production levels can have variation from salary under grid (within limits) when approved by compliance or other committee.

Assessment of Hospital Example 1 – Straight Salary Plan

EXHIBIT 14.7

Dimension	Strengths	Weaknesses
Measure	Determines salary based on physician specialty. Compensation must not exceed FMV and must be reasonable in a tax-exempt setting.	Infrequently used in pure form other than in initial "start up" and guaranteed periods of new physician practices.
Productivity	Can link fixed salary to prior year production levels (e.g., prior year WRVUs as a percentage of benchmark).	Many straight salary plans have no linkage to actual production.
Financial	Salaried arrangements facilitate budgetary and financial planning.	May result in operating losses due to limited "real time" relationship to production. Performance expectations likely to be essential to successful financial performance. No consideration of revenues generated by physician during work period.
Simplicity	Simple to administer.	
Alignment	Market data can be used to inform salary levels and promote compliance. Coupled with performance expectations and/or strong practice culture, may facilitate "group practice" approach to care.	Generally, only limited application.
"Fairness"	Salary provides income stability.	May allow for relatively low work levels and result in hospital (or other organization) operating losses unless carefully managed.

© 2006 Johnson & Walker Keegan

➤ HOSPITAL EXAMPLE 2-A – COMPENSATION PER WRVU PLAN
Revenue Elements 1 and 4 (Unit-Based and Production)

Overview

In this plan, physicians are paid a set rate of compensation for each WRVU that is personally performed by the physician. This plan uses a unit-based architecture (Architecture A) and Revenue Element 1, but it is also productivity-based using Revenue Element 4 on the compensation matrix. Variations of this plan can incorporate non-clinical production-based bonus criteria, such as those used in pay-for-performance (P4P) reimbursement systems, and other incentive measures linked to quality, patient satisfaction, or other measures.

Application

Examples of relationships in which compensation per WRVU are commonly used include a hospital's direct employment of physicians in virtually all specialties. The methodology may also be adopted for use with indirect payment arrangements from a hospital to a physician group that provides services in a hospital-owned outpatient clinic or urgent care center. These plan types are also used in multispecialty groups and in departments or divisions of such groups, including those that are hospital affiliated, faculty practice plans, or physician-owned groups.

When the employment exception to the Stark law is being relied upon for the compensation arrangement, the compensation per WRVU and the total compensation paid to the physician must not exceed FMV, and compensation must only be paid for personally performed services. When the arrangement is used in a tax-exempt health system, then the compensation must also be reasonable.

Methodology

We will present three variations of a compensation per WRVU plan – Plan 2-A, 2-B, and 2-C; however, there are four basic steps in any compensation per WRVU plan. These steps are described below.

Step 1. Identify Physician Specialties

In a compensation plan that is based on payments per WRVU levels, physicians will receive differential income based on their ability to generate WRVUs. Physicians are able to earn more or less WRVUs due to their specialty and the type of services they perform. For example, a general surgeon can typically earn more WRVUs than a primary care physician. Similarly, an orthopaedic surgeon who performs both inpatient and outpatient services will likely generate more WRVUs than an orthopaedist who has an office-based practice. Thus, the first step in this plan is to identify the specialties of each physician, and if appropriate, the subspecialties of the physicians to be covered by the plan.

Step 2. Establish Performance Expectations

Although compensation per WRVU plans effectively pay an agreed upon level of compensation per unit of work, the definition of *minimum* performance expectations will also be important in such plans. Performance expectations will commonly consider any number of work-related factors that are defined in advance of setting the dollar amount per WRVU, and that will constitute *minimum* levels of performance deemed to be acceptable for receipt of such amounts.

Hospital Example 2-A (illustrated in Exhibit 14.8) and Hospital Example 2-B (illustrated in Exhibit 14.9) presented at the end of this section, both show performance expectations in areas such as minimum production by specialty (measured by WRVUs), weeks worked, scheduled work week, and other activities. Hospital Example 2-A also illustrates the use of a predefined (and automatic) adjustment for a failure to meet minimum performance expectations. In this example, Physician E has WRVU production levels below the minimum for the physician's practice specialty; therefore, the dollar per WRVU amount is automatically adjusted downward by 10 percent, meaning that the physician receives only 90 percent of the expected amount for his or her work. This example also assumes that nonperformance in other areas would result in additional reductions (e.g., reduction of an additional 10 percent for failure to work 47 weeks, or for maintaining a clinic schedule that is less than 4.5 days per week). Note that this example caps the total adjustment at 20 percent of the total amount otherwise due and payable. Performance deficiencies that exceed this 20 percent maximum may require more significant actions.

In compensation plans such as the straight dollar amount per WRVU plan illustrated in Example 2-A, minimum performance expectations are important to assess individual physician performance, as well as for the hospital or other organization's financial performance. This is because a hospital that is expecting (and planning for) a cost structure that is consistent with the minimum standards will be negatively impacted if production and work levels fall short. Accordingly, while performance expectations are required to define minimum performance requirements, they also can be used as an objective means to identify service arrangements that may need intervention and/or adjustment.

Step 3. Establish Compensation per WRVU Levels by Specialty

Market data can be used to determine the compensation per WRVU payment rate. Market data might consist of reported compensation per WRVU, or the compensation per WRVU could be calculated by dividing the median compensation for a particular specialty by the median WRVUs for the same specialty. Importantly, the tables found in benchmark sources do not directly correlate. This means, for example, that the table that reflects median WRVUs and the table that reports median compensation do not necessarily provide data for the same individual physician. Consequently, a compensation system that pays a physician the median level of compensation per WRVUs, as reported in MGMA or other data, will typically *not* yield median levels of compensation in the aggregate, even if the physician's production is at median levels. See Chapter 7 for a discussion of benchmark sources and uses in compensation systems.

Hospital Example 2-A illustrates the use of market data from different tables and sources to derive compensation per WRVU amounts for individual physician practice specialties. In this model, the average of several values as reported by benchmark sources is used for the compensation per WRVU conversion factor for the defined time period (typically one year).

Hospital Example 2-B is similar to Example 2-A, except that it provides a defined level of compensation per WRVU based on the procedures that are performed by physicians in related subspecialties – in this instance, cardiology subspecialties. In Hospital Example 2-B, compensation per WRVU amounts are also informed by market data, plus other factors. In this example, the market data for select cardiology subspecialties are further adjusted by considerations related to the relative recruitment challenges for the particular subspecialty. An "adjustment factor" is assigned to the average of market data to reflect the relative challenge of recruiting and retaining particular subspecialties. In this example, physicians specializing in electrophysiology are more difficult to recruit and retain; thus, an adjustment factor has been implemented. Note that while this assumes a relatively greater difficulty in recruitment and retention, which is translated into an adjustment of the compensation per WRVU, it will not change the underlying compliance requirement that the total compensation must not exceed that which is consistent with FMV. Moreover, the adjustment would likely change over time as recruitment becomes easier and/or compensation levels among practice subspecialties become more similar.

Step 4. Determine and Pay Compensation Based on Production

In Hospital Example 2-A, each physician is paid a defined dollar amount per WRVU, with the amount linked to practice specialty. The use of a set dollar amount per WRVU for each specialty is generally viewed as desirable, because it provides for a relatively straightforward, easily understandable payment method. Moreover, the method can be linked to market data, which means that it can change over time to correspond with changes in the market data.

While such a method provides for a relatively easy and straightforward compensation method, it may not accurately reflect the market realities with respect to reimbursement per WRVU. The rate that is set needs to be realistic based on actual practice revenues, expense levels, and work volumes. In reality, a physician in a practice with low levels of production would typically not earn median levels of compensation per WRVU. This fact is discussed in greater detail with respect to Example 3, below, which uses a graduated level of compensation per WRVU as a surrogate or estimate of true market realities. Likewise, the "market" in a community with extremely low (or high) levels of external reimbursement due to payer mix (e.g., in a poor inner city or rural area, or in an affluent resort community) may not correspond with the market data reflected in benchmark resources. As a result, some special adjustments may be required to align the compensation per WRVU amount with the local market conditions and realities.

► HOSPITAL EXAMPLE 2-B – COMPENSATION PER WRVU PLAN
Revenue Elements 1 and 4 (Unit-Based and Production)

Hospital Example 2-B also illustrates a slightly different approach to how dollar per WRVU amounts can be determined and paid based on individual physician subspecialties, or based on the services that are performed by individual subspecialties. In the case of cardiology, for example, as illustrated in Hospital Example 2-B (Exhibit 14.9), different dollar amounts per WRVU are assigned to individual procedures and current procedural terminology (CPT) codes (e.g., angioplasty, diagnostic catheterization, and other interventional or invasive procedures are assigned one level of reimbursement, while noninvasive procedures, including evaluation and management codes and others, are assigned another, and electrophysiology procedures are assigned still another). This recognizes that in many practices, even though there will be considerable subspecialization, each physician will commonly perform some of the same types of procedures as part of his or her normal work process but with different frequencies.

Of course, while such a system may make sense from the perspective of paying physicians based on the work they actually perform, close monitoring and management may also be required to prevent inappropriate "cherry-picking" of more highly reimbursed procedures or other inappropriate behavior. In this example, the total compensation paid to the physician is based on the combination of the work and dollar amounts per type of work.

Under a direct compensation arrangement that pays a defined level of compensation per WRVU, physicians may generally only be paid for the services that they personally perform. However, the physician may be compensated for supervision of nonphysician providers through a separate supervision stipend or similar means, as long as that compensation is consistent with FMV for the physician's services.

When the compensation arrangement is indirect, such that a separate legal entity stands between the physician and the hospital that serves as the source of compensation, the intervening legal entity may be paid compensation based on the services performed by the physician entity. In this scenario, the intervening entity could, if it desired, pay a portion of the compensation it received from the services of nonphysician providers to physicians who are employed by the intervening entity. In such a circumstance, the physicians (and other providers) in the entity must not be paid in excess of the FMV of the services they personally perform. Exhibit 14.10 illustrates the type of indirect contractual arrangement discussed here and in Hospital Example 2-C.

► HOSPITAL EXAMPLE 2-C – COMPENSATION PER WRVU PLAN – INDIRECT COMPENSATION ARRANGEMENT
Revenue Elements 1 and 4 (Unit-Based and Production)

Hospital Example 2-C (Exhibit 14.11) illustrates an indirect arrangement such as that described above. In this example, a set dollar amount per WRVU is paid from the hospital to the physician practice that is staffing a hospital outpatient clinic. The practice, in turn, reallocates the total received from the hospital among the practice's physician and nonphysician employees. Under this service arrangement the dollar amount per WRVU paid by the hospital to the practice is adjusted upward to reflect the cost of benefits (such that the dollar conversion factor in this example is increased by 20 percent), because the practice must pay the benefit costs. Here, too, while this indirect model allows the practice to reallocate compensation somewhat, it will not change the underlying compliance requirement that the total compensation must not exceed FMV.

A compensation per WRVU model can also incorporate qualitative and other measures in determining and paying physician compensation, such as those being used in the emerging P4P reimbursement environment. In this setting, the compensation per WRVU method will provide the foundation for the majority of total compensation (typically 70 to 80 percent of the total compensation earned by individual physicians), with the qualitative incentive component that is aligned with P4P reimbursement or other objectives comprising the remaining 20 to 30 percent of total compensation. See Chapter 8 for a discussion of P4P and plan examples.

Exhibit 14.12 provides an assessment of the strengths and weaknesses of Hospital Example 2 and its plan variations.

EXHIBIT 14.8

Hospital Example 2-A –
Compensation per WRVU Plan*
Revenue Elements 1 and 4 (Unit-Based and Production)

Step 1 **Identify physician specialties.**
Note: Primary care specialties illustrated here.

Step 2 **Establish minimum performance expectations.**

Measure	Minimum
Clinical service production (WRVUs) per year (for full-time service by subspecialty)	
Family Practice	3,500
General Internal Medicine	3,400
Pediatrics	3,200
OB/GYN	5,200
Weeks worked per year	47 weeks
Scheduled days per week	4.5 days per week
On-call obligations	Pro rata night and weekend within department
Adjustment for nonperformance	10% per measure of nonperformance

Step 3 **Assess market data.†**
(compensation per WRVU)

	All Practices	Single Specialty	Multispecialty	Other Benchmark	Average
Family Practice	$41.20	$37.50	$41.00	$39.65	$39.84
Internal Medicine General	$42.12	$38.80	$42.00	$41.20	$41.03
Pediatrics	$38.45	$38.20	$38.50	$40.00	$38.79
Obstetrics/ Gynecology	$40.39	$39.60	$40.50	$41.25	$40.44

Step 4 **Establish compensation per WRVU by specialty (and/or subspecialty).‡**

Family Practice	$39.84
Internal Medicine General	$41.03
Pediatrics	$38.79
Obstetrics/ Gynecology	$40.44

Step 5 Determine physician-specific compensation.

Example Physicians	Specialty	Actual WRVU	$ per WRVU without Adjustment	Adjustments	Compensation
Dr. A	Pediatrics	4,236	$38.79		$164,304
Dr. B	Pediatrics	4,167	$38.79		$161,628
Dr. C	Family Practice	4,102	$39.84		$163,413
Dr. D	Family Practice	5,301	$39.84		$211,179
Dr. E**	Family Practice	3,142	$39.84	−10%	$112,652
Dr. F	Family Practice	3,952	$39.84		$157,438
Dr. G	Family Practice	3,720	$39.84		$148,196
Dr. H	General Internal Medicine	3,894	$41.03		$159,771
Dr. I	General Internal Medicine	3,720	$41.03		$152,632
Dr. J	General Internal Medicine	4,125	$41.03		$169,249
Dr. K	General Internal Medicine	4,420	$41.03		$181,353
Dr. L	Obstetrics/Gynecology	6,449	$40.44		$260,765
Dr. M	Obstetrics/Gynecology	7,852	$40.44		$317,496
Total					$1,431,212

* Hypothetical numbers presented for illustrative purposes only. Numbers may not total in all cases due to rounding.

† Market data assume combination of numerous benchmarks to develop average of measure for each subspecialty.

‡ Average of market used to determine preset dollar amount per WRVU under compensation plan.

** Physician E fails to meet minimum performance standards; therefore, is subject to reduced dollar per WRVU amount for services as provided under plan.

EXHIBIT 14.9

Hospital Example 2-B –
Compensation per WRVU Plan*
Revenue Elements 1 and 4 (Unit-Based and Production)

Step 1 Identify physician specialties.
Note: Cardiology illustrated here.

Step 2 Establish minimum performance expectations.

Measure	Minimum
Clinical service production (WRVUs) per year (by primary cardiology subspecialty)	
Invasive/Interventional	7,500
Noninvasive	5,000
Electrophysiology	6,700
Weeks worked per year	45 weeks
Scheduled days per week	5 days
On-call obligations	Pro rata night and weekend within department
Outreach activities	Pro rata based on subspecialty
Service	Quality improvement committee
Other	EHR Usage

Step 3 Assess market data.[†]
(compensation per WRVU)
Determine adjustment factor.

	All Practices	Single Specialty	Multi-specialty	Average	Adjustment Factor
Invasive/Interventional	$50.61	$50.60	$50.73	$50.65	1.10
Noninvasive	$49.80	$46.20	$50.81	$48.94	1.00
Electrophysiology	$40.91	$39.13	$50.50	$43.51	1.36

Step 4 Establish compensation per WRVU by specialty (and/or subspecialty)[‡]
(after adjustment applied): average × adjustment factor.

Invasive/Interventional	$55.71
Noninvasive	$48.94
Electrophysiology	$59.18

Step 5 Determine physician-specific compensation.

Dr. X (example physician)	Actual WRVU	$ per WRVU	Compensation
WRVU from interventional procedures	1,765	$55.71	$98,331
WRVU from noninvasive procedures	3,452	$48.94	$168,929
WRVU from electrophysiology procedures	19	$59.18	$1,124
WRVU from other procedures (paid at noninvasive)	3,168	$48.94	$155,031
	8,404		
Total Compensation			$423,416

* Hypothetical numbers presented for illustrative purposes only. Numbers may not total in all cases due to rounding.

† Median values from multiple survey tables used in determining average.

‡ For example, compensation per WRVU for invasive/interventional procedures calculated by multiplying average of $50.65 per WRVU (calculated in Step 3) times 1.10 to yield $55.71 per WRVU.

© 2006 Johnson & Walker Keegan

EXHIBIT 14.10 Indirect Compensation Arrangement in Hospital Example 2-C

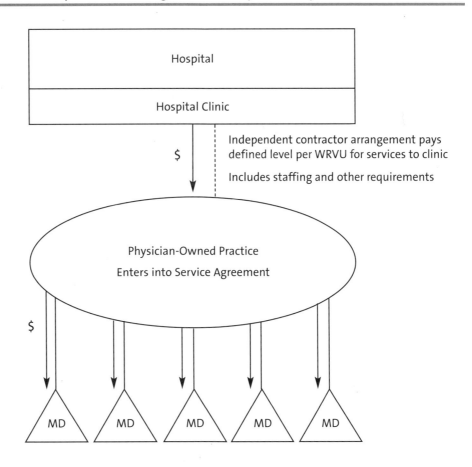

Hospital pays physician group to staff hospital-owned and operated outpatient clinic; group pays physician and other providers it employs for services performed. PA paid at lower rate. Profit from contract allocated among practice owners.

© 2006 Johnson

EXHIBIT 14.11

Hospital Example 2-C –
Compensation per WRVU Plan – Indirect Compensation Arrangement*
Revenue Elements 1 and 4 (Unit-Based and Production)

Note: Model assumes physician staffing of a hospital-based clinic, with hospital paying defined dollar amount per WRVU for services furnished through "provider-based" outpatient clinic. Compensation involves "indirect" compensation arrangement.

Step 1 **Identify hospital-based clinic.**
Note: Primary care specialties illustrated here.

Step 2 **Establish minimum performance requirements under contract.**
Note: Expectations would be established for the hospital clinic as a whole under the contract.

Measure	Requirements
Clinical FTE levels per day	5 providers during weekdays, 2 providers during weekends and holidays
Weeks worked per year	52 weeks
Scheduled days per week	6 days per week
Total provider weekdays (exclude holidays)	1,255
Total provider weekends	208
Total provider days	1,463

Step 3 **Assess market data.†**
(compensation per WRVU)

	All	Single Specialty	Multi-pecialty	Other Benchmark	Average
Family Practice	$41.20	$37.50	$41.00	$39.65	$39.84
Internal Medicine (General)	$42.12	$38.80	$42.00	$41.20	$41.03
Pediatrics	$38.45	$38.20	$38.50	$40.00	$38.79
Average of All (used for contract rate)					$39.89

Step 4 **Establish compensation per WRVU by specialty.‡**

Contract Rate per WRVU	$39.89
Benefit Adjusment (+20%)	$7.98
$ per WRVU under contract	$47.86

Step 5 **Determine compensation from hospital to physician group under service contract.**

Total work WRVU	30,681
$ per WRVU under contract	$47.86
Total Compensation to Practice	$1,468,454

Step 6   Allocate contract compensation within physician group.**
Note: Assumes allocation on dollar per WRVU basis, with adjustment for specialty.

Example Physicians	Specialty	Actual WRVU	$ per WRVU within Practice	Allocated for Compensation & Benefits	Profit among Practice Owners
Dr. B	Pediatrics	4,167	$47.86	$199,433	$7,959
Dr. C	Family Practice	4,102	$47.86	$196,322	$7,959
Dr. D	Family Practice	5,301	$47.86	$253,706	$7,959
Dr. F	Family Practice	3,952	$47.86	$189,143	$7,959
Dr. G	Family Practice	3,720	$47.86	$178,039	$7,959
Dr. H	Internal Medicine (General)	3,894	$47.86	$186,367	$7,959
Dr. J	Internal Medicine (General)	2,125	$47.86	$101,703	$7,959
Dr. K	Physician Assistant	3,420	$31.59	$108,030	
		30,681			
Total				$1,412,741	$55,713
Difference from contract amount (profit to owners)				$55,713	

* Hypothetical numbers presented for illustrative purposes only. Numbers may not total in all cases due to rounding.

† Market data assume combination of numerous benchmarks to develop average of measure for each subspecialty.

‡ Average of market used to determine preset dollar amount per work RVU under contract. Additional amount paid for benefits.

** Assumes practice has physician assistant (PA) providing services, for which payment is received. PA is paid lower dollar per WRVU amount with profit allocated among practice owners (here assumed to be on an equal share basis).

© 2006 Johnson & Walker Keegan

EXHIBIT 14.12 Assessment of Hospital Example 2 – Compensation per WRVU Plan

Dimension	Strengths	Weaknesses
Measure	Can pay physicians a market-based rate per WRVU based on physician specialty.	Physicians may have limited understanding of WRVUs.
Productivity	Encourages direct focus on work or production without consideration of expenses.	Pays same rate of compensation per WRVU regardless of payer mix or production.
Financial	Can be used in hospital and similar employment arrangements. Can also be used in compensation plans used in bona fide Group Practices with some adjustment to promote fiscal solvency.	Divorces actual financial performance from compensation paid. No consideration of revenues or income generated by physician during work period. Does not directly or indirectly consider practice operating costs. May result in operating losses in hospital-affiliated practices when other monitors or measures are not instituted (e.g., performance expectations, cost of practice thresholds).
Simplicity	Easy to understand and administer.	
Alignment	Compensates for personal work.	May require other measures to promote nonphysician provider supervision and other goals.
"Fairness"	Payer-neutral compensation system.	

➤ HOSPITAL EXAMPLE 3 — PERCENTAGE-BASED COMPENSATION PLAN
Revenue Elements 1 and 4 (Unit-Based and Production)

Overview

In this example, physicians are paid compensation based on a set percentage of the gross charges or net collections from their personal services. This plan combines Revenue Elements 1 and 4 (unit-based and pure production).

Application

Percentage-based compensation systems may be used in a number of settings to include employment or personal service arrangements between physicians and hospitals, medical groups, or other organizations. They can also be used in indirect compensation arrangements between a hospital and a physician group for the provision of physician professional services in support of hospital-operated departments, clinics, and urgent care centers.

Under a percentage-based compensation plan used in a direct compensation arrangement that relies on the Stark law's employment exception, physicians may only be paid for services that they personally perform. Moreover, when a tax-exempt organization is involved, the compensation must also be reasonable.

Methodology

There are generally five steps involved in any percentage-based compensation plan.

Step 1. Identify Physician Specialties and Services

Consistent with Hospital Example 2, the first step is to identify the specialty of each physician, along with his or her subspecialty as appropriate. This involves also recognizing the type of services he or she performs. For example, a family practice physician who performs obstetrical services will be categorized separately from a family practice physician who does not maintain an obstetrical practice.

Step 2. Establish Performance Expectations

Although percentage-based plans effectively pay an agreed upon percentage of compensation per unit of production, when production is measured by gross charges or net collections from professional services, the definition of *minimum* performance expectations will also be important. Such performance expectations will commonly consider any number of work-related factors that will constitute minimum performance levels required to be acceptable for receipt of such compensation amounts.

Hospital Examples 3-A and 3-B (illustrated in Exhibits 14.13 and 14.14 at the end of this section) show general performance expectations akin to those illustrated in Hospital Examples 2-A, 2-B, and 2-C.

Step 3. Assess Market and Benchmark to Establish Applicable Percentage

The percentage-based arrangement can be applied either to a percentage of the gross charges for the physicians' professional services or to net collections derived from those professional services. A determination of whether a standard charge master or fee schedule would be used for the arrangement, or whether collections that measure actual reimbursement to the hospital or other organization would be used, will be based on financial modeling, the overall goals of the arrangement, and compliance considerations. The percentage can also be applied to an "adjusted-charges" measure that is calculated by multiplying the total gross charges for professional services by a practice-wide (or other level, e.g., service line, department, division, specialty) collection percentage.

Step 4. Determine Applicable Percentage to Be Applied to Charges or Collections

The exact percentage to be applied to the production measure can be based on actual performance, on a negotiated arrangement, on market data, or on a combination of these means. Hospital Examples 3-A and 3-B (Exhibits 14.13 and 14.14, respectively) use market data and an averaging of several market sources to adjust the percentage levels. The applicable percentage must also be modeled to assess financial and legal feasibility based on historic or anticipated production data. Hospital Example 3-A illustrates the use of market data to determine a compensation to professional gross charges ratio (illustrated using neurosurgery as an example), while Hospital Example 3-B uses net collections from professional services. When charges are used, the method will be payer-neutral. However, the use of net collections from professional services will more directly link to the organization's financial performance.

When the employment exception to the Stark law is relied upon, the total amount of compensation must not be in excess of FMV for the physician's services, and similar standards apply when the hospital is tax-exempt. In a tax-exempt setting, the hospital will also commonly impose a cap on total compensation as an additional compliance safeguard. See Chapter 9, "The Legal Element," and Chapter 16, "The Special World of Hospital and Academic Practices – Assessing Reasonableness and Promoting Compliance," for more information regarding the applicable legal requirements.

Step 5. Determine and Pay Compensation

In the percentage-based arrangement, the predefined percentage is applied to the professional services gross charges or net collections from professional services generated by the physician. In all instances, the number to which the percentage is applied (charges or collections) must be based solely on the physician's professional services charges, and may not include credit for ancillary services, technical components, facility fees, or the like. Because of this, the use of gross charges (which can be assigned and mapped to individual CPT codes) is commonly the preferred method from an administrative perspective because of the difficulty of ensuring that collections data do not include ancillary services, facility fees, or other revenue.

While percentage of professional services gross charges or net collections arrangements are commonly used in direct employment, contractual, and similar arrangements, they can also be used in indirect contractual service arrangements, such as those illustrated in Exhibit 14.10, and as demonstrated in Example 2-C (Exhibit 14.11).

An assessment of the strengths and weaknesses of Hospital Example 3 is provided in Exhibit 14.15.

EXHIBIT 14.13

Hospital Example 3-A – Percentage of Professional Services Charges Plan*
Revenue Elements 1 and 4 (Unit-Based and Production)

Step 1 Identify physician specialties and set fee schedule using standard method.
Note: Neurosurgery illustrated here. Assumes fees set via standard method
(e.g., 150% of Medicare RBRVS).

Step 2 Establish minimum performance expectations.

Measure	Minimum
Clinical service production (gross charges) per year	
Neurosurgery	$1,500,000
Weeks worked per year	47 weeks
Scheduled days per week	4.5 days per week
On-call obligations	Pro rata night and weekend within department

Step 3 Assess the compensation to professional services gross charges ratio from market data.[†]

	Reported Compensation/ Professional Services Charges	Reported Compensation	Reported Charges	Calculated Ratio Compensation/ Professional Services Charges
Neurosurgery				
MGMA				
All Physicians	0.267	$542,000	$2,250,000	0.241
Single Specialty	0.244	$528,000	$2,400,000	0.220
Multispecialty	0.291	$550,000	$1,900,000	0.289
Other Survey Data				
All Physicians	0.287	$495,620	$1,987,546	0.249
Region (same as practice)	0.275	$562,103	$2,054,562	0.274
Average of Measure	0.273			0.255

Step 4 Establish percentage of gross charges for compensation.[‡]

Neurosurgery   0.270

Step 5 Determine physician-specifc compensation.

Example Physicians	Specialty	Actual Professional Services Charges at Fee Schedule	Compensation % of Gross Charges	Compensation
Dr. A	Neurosurgery	$2,750,231	0.270	$742,562
Dr. B	Neurosurgery	$2,462,020	0.270	$664,745
Dr. C	Neurosurgery	$1,875,421	0.270	$506,364
Total				$1,913,671

* Hypothetical numbers presented for illustrative purposes only. Numbers may not total in all cases due to rounding.

† Market data assume combination of numerous benchmarks to develop average of measure. Use calculated and reported values.

‡ Percentage shown here informed by average of calculated measures, but ultimately negotiated within range of market values.

© 2006 Johnson & Walker Keegan

EXHIBIT 14.14

Hospital Example 3-B – Percentage of Net Collections Plan*
Revenue Elements 1 and 4 (Unit-Based and Production)

Step 1 Identify physician specialties and set fee schedule using standard method.
Note: General surgery illustrated here. Assumes fees set via standard method
  (e.g., 150% of Medicare RBRVS).

Step 2 Establish minimum performance expectations.

Measure	Minimum
Clinical service production (net collections) per year	
General Surgery	$400,000
Weeks worked per year	47 weeks
Scheduled days per week	4.5 days per week
On-call obligations	Pro rata night and weekend within department

Step 3 Assess market data for compensation as percentage of net collections from professional services.[†]

General Surgery Survey Data	Reported Compensation/ Collections	Reported Compensation	Reported Collections	Calculated Ratio Compensation/ Collections
All Physicians	0.542	$282,504	$520,215	0.543
Single Specialty		$290,000	$500,000	0.552
Multispecialty		$265,200	$525,000	0.530
Region (same as practice)	0.547	$301,500	$590,700	0.510
Average of Measure	0.545			0.534

Step 4 Establish percentage of professional service net collections for compensation.[‡]

General Surgery   0.539

Step 5 Determine physician-specific compensation.

Example Physicians	Specialty	Actual Collections	Compensation as % of Collections	Compensation
Dr. A	General Surgery	$685,300	0.539	$369,569
Dr. B	General Surgery	$645,020	0.539	$347,847
Dr. C	General Surgery	$452,002	0.539	$243,756
Dr. C	General Surgery	$520,402	0.539	$280,643
Total				$961,171

* Hypothetical numbers presented for illustrative purposes only. Numbers may not total in all cases due to rounding.

† Market data assume combination of numerous benchmarks to develop average of measure. Use calculated and reported values.

‡ Percentage shown here informed by average of calculated measures.

EXHIBIT 14.15 Assessment of Hospital Example 3 — Percentage-Based Compensation Plan

Dimension	Strengths	Weaknesses
Measure	Market data can be used to inform percentage-based compensation level (e.g., gross charges or net collections from professional services) and promote legal compliance.	Gross charges do not reflect payer mix and are subject to potential "gamesmanship" in fee setting. Basing percentage on net collections may be viewed as penalizing physicians with adverse payer mix. Results may be impacted by inconsistencies in fee schedules.
Productivity	Can combine with draw mechanism to provide stability of income while also linking to personal production.	When gross charges from professional services are used, pays same rate of compensation per dollar of charges, regardless of actual reimbursement level.
Financial	Use of charges allows for payer-neutral measures.	Divorces actual financial performance from compensation paid. Does not consider practice operating costs.
Simplicity	Relatively simple and understandable. Can be linked to market data.	
Alignment	Direct arrangements compensate physicians for personal work only. Performance expectations (e.g., hours and weeks worked, etc.) typically recommended.	May result in "cherry-picking" of patients when based on net collections from professional services. May result in seeing large (potentially unsustainable) levels of indigent or uninsured when based on gross charges.
"Fairness"	When percentage is based on gross charges, the compensation system is payer-neutral.	Nonpayer-neutral compensation system when percentage is based on net collections from professional services.

© 2006 Johnson & Walker Keegan

▶ HOSPITAL EXAMPLE 4-A – BASE PLUS INCENTIVE PLAN
Revenue Element 2 (Guaranteed Share)

Overview

Base salary coupled with incentive-based compensation arrangements are frequently used to pay physicians for the services they furnish to hospitals and other organizations. These models generally use Revenue Element 2 from the compensation plan matrix, involving a guaranteed payment, coupled with production and/or nonclinical production incentive measures. Basic base plus incentive plans and variations of such plans (commonly referred to as "XYZ plans") are often used in academic settings; therefore, the additional examples presented in Chapter 15 for academic practices have potential application to hospital-affiliated practices.

Most base salaries are linked to market data (e.g., MGMA median compensation), to the historic or anticipated performance of a physician (e.g., relationship between prior year of production, which establishes a base salary level), or to a negotiated amount. Although the base salary portion of compensation is generally "guaranteed," it is also typically coupled with performance expectations and can frequently be modified (and reduced) for performance that is significantly below those predefined expectations.

Application

Base salary plus incentive compensation systems are used in direct employment arrangements in hospitals, academic practices, and many physician-owned group practice settings. They are used with all types of medical practices (primary care, medical, and surgical specialties).

When the employment exception to the Stark law is relied upon, an essential legal requirement imposed on base plus incentive arrangements is that the compensation may not exceed FMV for the physician's services. By illustration, a physician could be paid a base salary equal to 70 percent of MGMA median compensation levels and be eligible for a productivity bonus based upon work level production in excess of a defined threshold. Close attention to financial planning and modeling would, however, be required in order to evaluate financial solvency under such models and the FMV and reasonableness of the compensation to be paid.

Methodology

The following steps are used in determining a base plus incentive plan.

Step 1. Identify Physician Specialties
The base salary levels are generally tailored to each respective primary care, medical, or surgical specialty based on market or other factors. Consistent with the previous hospital plan examples, the first step is to identify each physician's specialty, subspecialty (as appropriate), and the types of services he or she performs.

Step 2. Establish Performance Expectations for Receipt of Base Salary

In base plus incentive plans, the base salary effectively involves the agreed upon payment of compensation for a defined unit of service (e.g., a base salary for a full year of service). However, as with any arrangements involving guaranteed payments, an essential element for successful salary plans is the establishment of *minimum* performance expectations for receipt of the salary amount. Such performance expectations will commonly consider any number of work-related factors that are defined in advance and that constitute *minimum* performance levels required to receive the full base salary amount.

Because performance expectations are, by definition, standards of *minimum* performance for receipt of the salary, the compensation plan (and underlying contractual documents and/or policies governing the compensation relationship) should also address what happens when such performance requirements are not met. In most instances, the failure to meet performance minimums will yield predefined reductions in salary levels, while still providing a reasonable level of compensation. Thus, a physician's failure to achieve minimum production or other service levels may allow for an adjustment of the salary amount being paid up to a predefined reduction (e.g., 20 percent). The reduction may be allowed for a short time or for the remainder of the term or it can be established that if performance rises to minimum performance standards the salary may return to previous levels. In some cases, the failure to meet minimum performance requirements results in reductions in compensation, counseling, performance-improvement plans, or other actions, with more extreme (or chronic) conditions leading to physician termination. See Chapter 10 for more information on developing and implementing performance expectations.

Step 3. Determine Base Salary Levels by Specialty

As referenced above, determination of base salary can be based upon market data or percentage of market levels of compensation. By illustration, the base salary, which is a guaranteed portion of compensation, might be based upon a defined percentage (e.g., 70 percent) of a relevant market benchmark. Other methods to determine base salary levels are discussed in Chapter 10.

In addition, in order to take into account inherent variations in physician production, different percentages of market median benchmarks may be used to set different base salary levels based upon different relative levels of production. Close attention to market levels and potential consideration of "composite" measures of market are frequently appropriate due to the significant year-to-year variations in such measures, as discussed in Chapter 16. Under such a methodology, composite market median benchmarks could be used as a standard reference point, with different base salary levels linked to different percentages of the market benchmark (e.g., 80 percent of composite market median, composite market median, and 120 percent of composite market median). The applicable base salary percentage (70 percent in this example) would be applied to the reference point to yield base salary compensation levels for physicians with "low," "median," and "high" production levels, as illustrated below:

	Percentage of Median Production	Benchmark	Base as a Percentage of Benchmark	Base Salary
Low Production	80%	$160,000	70%	$112,000
Median Production	100%	$200,000	70%	$140,000
High Production	125%	$250,000	70%	$175,000

A similar type of method is also illustrated in Group Practice Example E-2 in Chapter 13.

Step 4. Determine Incentive Compensation

Incentive compensation in a base salary plus incentive system may be based on any number of measures. In some settings, the incentive is linked solely to physician production, and, as such, is paid based on production in excess of defined production thresholds (e.g., 30 percent of gross charges or net collections from professional services in excess of a defined target level). Likewise, nonclinical production measures are also being used with greater frequency, including those that consider P4P reimbursement criteria.

In some settings, the combination of both revenues and expenses will be used to determine physician compensation levels, with physicians paid a defined percentage of revenues in excess of allocated expenses. This is illustrated in Hospital Example 4-A (Exhibit 14.16 presented at the end of this section), which pays each physician a defined percentage (50 percent) of the surplus remaining after allocated expenses of practice (including physician base salary and benefit costs) are subtracted from the revenues allocated to the physician.

For purposes of Hospital Example 4-A, each physician's "allocated revenues" will include revenues from direct professional services (net collections plus managed care bonuses or deficits), but will not include revenues from ancillary services (e.g. laboratory, radiology) or other services that are classified as DHS under the Stark law. The allocated revenues may also be calculated by multiplying the physician's gross charges times an agreed upon collection percentage for the division or organization as a whole to "even out" an adverse payer mix (or variable revenue cycle performance) among physicians in the division.

The expense allocation methods used in a base plus incentive plan can be based on full cost allocation systems using strict or "modified" cost accounting methods (using Expense Elements 9 and 8 of the compensation plan matrix, respectively). In the context of hospital-affiliated systems, however, consideration is often given to the allocation of only those costs that are "controllable" by the physician, or that are otherwise reasonable and consistent with a more typical physician practice. For example, although a hospital may have purchased an office building in which 16 physicians can practice, if only eight physicians actually work in the facility, the cost allocation system might allocate only one-half of the total lease cost among the physicians actually practicing in the facility, rather than allocating the full cost.

If a surplus is identified, that amount is allocated between the physician and the hospital or employer on an agreed upon basis. Although Hospital Example 4 uses a straight 50 percent of surplus approach – 50 percent of the surplus distributed to physicians and 50 percent retained by the hospital – other methods are also feasible, such as the following:

► First $15,000 of surplus – 100 percent to physician;

► $15,001 to $50,000 of surplus – 50 percent to physician, 50 percent retained by hospital; and

► Surplus in excess of $50,001 – 60 percent to physician, 40 percent retained by hospital.

Each incentive measure and method is subject to its own limits, issues, and business risks. Again, it is important to consider FMV and reasonableness related to compensation levels.

Step 5. Determine Physician Total Compensation

Physician compensation is equal to the sum of base salary plus incentive compensation.

Any number of variations from this basic model is also feasible, including those that allocate the incentive based on other measures, including quality, practice efficiency, patient access, and related measures.

The incentive measure illustrated in Hospital Example 4-A is focused at the individual production level and, as such, treats each individual physician as a solo practitioner. Because of this, individual physicians have no financial incentive to consider approaches to practice that might promote greater levels of clinical efficiency, cost control, or appropriate utilization of nonphysician staff.[2] For this reason, system-wide, specialty, department, or other "group-wide" incentive measures will also commonly be developed and applied. Thus, some hospital systems will, for example, evaluate primary care physicians or each primary care practice in relation to targeted goals for the primary care practices in the aggregate. While many hospital-affiliated primary care practices lose money, efforts to focus attention on overall financial performance are commonly important, and "system-wide" incentives are often directed at the performance of a defined subset of employed physicians.

For example, financial incentives can be provided to primary care practices for performance resulting in an improvement in aggregate clinic operating losses as compared to present levels (e.g., decrease operating losses on a per primary physician FTE basis to $70,000 per year, down from the current losses of $100,000 per FTE). In the event that the primary care physician component achieves this goal, additional compensation may be provided as a means of creating a true incentive to focus attention on practice costs, efficiency, and productivity. Any such model should result in a "win-win" situation in which primary care physician practices have a real opportunity to earn incentive based on improvements in performance, which, in the process, will yield improvements at the overall system level. See Chapter 10 for more examples of such system-wide incentive systems.

In addition, other group-level incentives can use a similar approach to measure and encourage performance in relation to defined targets – for example, growth in charges, revenues, and WRVUs; improvement of net margins; or other appropriate measures. These incentive measures can also result in a win-win scenario for the physicians and the organization as a whole.

➤ HOSPITAL EXAMPLE 4-B – BASE PLUS INCENTIVE PLAN
Revenue Element 2 (Guaranteed Share)

Hospital Example 4-B (Exhibit 14.17) illustrates a base plus incentive plan involving hospitalist physicians. In this example, physicians who have prior experience in functioning as hospitalists are paid a slight premium in total anticipated compensation. Base salary levels are based on 80 percent of the market using specialty and experience level of the physicians as criteria. The remaining 20 percent of expected compensation can be "earned back" by meeting certain performance standards. Given the use of hospitalists in this example, two specific measures are used:

▶ WRVU production; and

▶ Peer evaluations.

WRVU production is a basic measure of work and effort but without regard to payer mix or reimbursement levels. In this example, each physician is expected to have at least 3,000 WRVUs in order to receive the full 5 percent of additional total compensation based on individual production. The amount at risk under this measure is predefined; physicians that exceed (or fall short) of the 3,000 WRVU target will have their award adjusted accordingly.

Of the two measures in Example 4-B, assessment of the hospitalist's performance via peer evaluation involves the greatest amount "at risk," with 15 percent of additional compensation beyond the base determined via this measure. In a hospitalist setting, this may be appropriate, given the role that the hospitalist plays on behalf of the patient's primary treating physician and the hospital itself. Peer evaluations in this example are assessed via a simple 1-to-5 point scale, but physicians who perform below acceptable levels (in this case, below 3.5 on the 5-point scale) receive a reduced portion of the amount at risk. In this example, Dr. D receives only a 30 percent share of the amount at risk because of his 3.0 performance on the peer evaluations.

Hospital Example 4-B also illustrates the payment of a P4P award by the third-party payer and hospital. Full participation in the award is limited to physicians who achieved full WRVU production (therefore, Drs. C and D receive reduced awards, with Dr. D receiving a significantly reduced portion). The P4P award in this example ($65,000) is allocated solely on a percentage of WRVUs basis, with adjustments for Drs. C and D as referenced above. Note that this treatment of the P4P dollars may or may not be aligned with the determination of the P4P award dollars (further discussed in Chapter 8).

In many instances, compensation levels will be linked to a cap or maximum level of compensation. The cap may be linked to market annual levels (e.g., equal to the MGMA 75th percentile [national] for the physician specialty), expressed as a percentage of median values (e.g., equal to 130 percent of the MGMA median value), or it may be determined in other ways. Compensation can frequently be paid in excess of the maximum when it is warranted by physician performance; however, in such circumstances, the total amount of compensation that would be earned under the plan will commonly be subject to review and approval by a compliance committee and verified by an external valuation. Such external validation will generally take into account physician production levels, compensation-to-production ratios (e.g., compensation per WRVU, compensation to professional services net collections, etc.), physician schedules, physician scarcity in the service area, and other factors. Chapter 16, "The Special World of Hospital and Academic Practices," provides more information on these issues.

Exhibit 14.18 provides an assessment of the strengths and weaknesses of Hospital Example 4.

EXHIBIT 14.16

Hospital Example 4-A –
Base Plus Incentive Plan*
Revenue Element 2 (Guaranteed Share)

Step 1 **Identify physician specialties.**
Note: General surgery illustrated here.

Step 2 **Establish minimum performance expectations.**

Measure	Minimum
Clinical service production (WRVUs) per year	5,500
Weeks worked per year	46 weeks
Scheduled days per week	4.5 days
On-call obligations	Pro rata night and weekend within department
Service	Medical staff credentials committee
Other	EHR usage

Step 3 **Establish salary levels.†**

Established Physician Grid

WRVU Level Based on Market	Market-Based Salary Level	Base Salary (70% of Market)
Over 120% of Median	$264,000	$184,800
Median to 120% of Median	$220,000	$154,000
80% of Median to Median	$176,000	$123,200
Under 80% of Median	$143,000	$100,100

Step 4 **Determine incentive compensation.‡**

	Allocated Production (Charges x Collections %)	Overhead Expense	Base Salary Expense	Benefit Expense	Surplus (Deficit)	Incentive (50% of Surplus)
Dr. A	$589,859	(241,050)	(184,800)	(42,150)	$121,859	$60,930
Dr. B	$583,748	(230,120)	(184,800)	(43,612)	$125,216	$62,608
Dr. C	$490,956	(215,212)	(123,200)	(40,221)	$112,323	$56,162
Dr. D	$512,938	(248,502)	(154,000)	(49,562)	$60,874	$30,437
Dr. E	$457,833	(213,225)	(100,100)	(36,542)	$107,966	$53,983

Step 5 **Determine total compensation.**

	Base Salary	Incentive Compensation	Total Compensation
Dr. A	$184,800	$60,930	$245,730
Dr. B	$184,800	$62,608	$247,408
Dr. C	$123,200	$56,162	$179,362
Dr. D	$154,000	$30,437	$184,437
Dr. E	$100,100	$53,983	$154,083

---

* Hypothetical numbers presented for illustrative purposes only. Numbers may not total in all cases due to rounding.

† Salary levels derived from market data to promote consistency with fair market value and reasonableness standards.

‡ Incentive can be based on any number of measures. Example illustrates payment of predefined percentage of "surplus" of revenues over expenses.

EXHIBIT 14.17

Hospital Example 4-B –
Base Plus Incentive (with System-Wide Bonus) Plan*
Revenue Element 2 (Guaranteed Share)

Step 1 **Identify physician specialties.**
Note: Hospitalist physicians (multiple specialties) illustrated here.

Step 2 **Establish minimum performance expectations at individual physician level.**

Measure	Minimum
Clinical service production (WRVUs) per year (minimum)	2,900
Weeks worked per year	46 weeks
Scheduled days per week	4 12-hour shifts

Step 3 **Establish salary levels.†**

	Market-Based Salary Level	Base Salary (80% of Market)
General Internal Medicine	$165,000	$132,000
Hospitalist (with prior experience)	$176,000	$140,800

Step 4 **Determine incentive measures and awards.‡**

		Amount "At Risk"	
Measure	Weight	General Internal Medicine	Hospitalist (Prior Experience)
1. Achieves 3,000 WRVUs	5% of Market	$8,250	$8,800
2. Peer Physician Evaluation/ Ranking	15% of Market	$24,750	$26,400
3. Pay-for-Performance Award† $65,000 to be awarded	Additive (% of WRVUs)	Additive	Additive

Step 5 **Assess performance in relation to incentive measures.**

	Actual WRVU	Measure 1 Achieves 3,000 WRVUs	Measure 2 Peer Eval (1-5 score)	Measure 3 P4P	WRVU for P4P	% for P4P
Dr. A	3,252	108%	4.50	100% WRVU Credit	3,252	24%
Dr. B	3,623	121%	5.00	100% WRVU Credit	3,623	27%
Dr. C	2,985	100%	4.00	75% WRVU Credit	2,239	17%
Dr. D	2,868	96%	3.00	25% WRVU Credit	717	5%
Dr. E	3,452	115%	5.00	100% WRVU Credit	3,452	26%
	16,180				13,283	

Step 6 **Determine incentive compensation – Measure 1.**

	Specialty	Measure 1 Performance	Measure 1 Amount "At Risk"	Measure 1 Award (Performance × "At Risk")
Dr. A	General Internal Medicine	1.08	$8,250	$8,943
Dr. B	General Internal Medicine	1.21	$8,250	$9,963
Dr. C	Hospitalist (prior experience)	1.00	$8,800	$8,756
Dr. D	Hospitalist (prior experience)	0.96	$8,800	$8,413
Dr. E	Hospitalist (prior experience)	1.15	$8,800	$10,126
				$46,201

Step 7 Determine incentive compensation – Measure 2.

	Specialty	Measure 2 Performance	Measure 2 Amount "At Risk"	Measure 2 Award‡
Dr. A	General Internal Medicine	4.50	$24,750	$22,275
Dr. B	General Internal Medicine	5.00	$24,750	$24,750
Dr. C	Hospitalist (prior experience)	4.00	$26,400	$21,120
Dr. D	Hospitalist (prior experience)	3.00	$26,400	$7.920
Dr. E	Hospitalist (prior experience)	5.00	$26,400	$26,400
				$102,465

Step 8 Determine incentive compensation – Measure 3.

	Specialty	Measure 3 Performance (P4P)	Measure 3 WRVU for P4P	% of WRVU	Measure 3 P4P Award (% of WRVU)
Dr. A	General Internal Medicine	100% WRVU Credit	3,252	24%	$15,914
Dr. B	General Internal Medicine	100% WRVU Credit	3,623	22%	$17,729
Dr. C	Hospitalist (prior experience)	75% WRVU Credit	2,239	18%	$10,955
Dr. D	Hospitalist (prior experience)	25% WRVU Credit	717	18%	$3,509
Dr. E	Hospitalist (prior experience)	100% WRVU Credit	3,452	21%	$16,893
					$65,000

Step 9 Determine total compensation.

	Base Salary	Measure 1	Measure 2	Measure 3	Total Compensation
Dr. A	$132,000	$8,943	$22,275	$15,914	$179,132
Dr. B	$132,000	$9,963	$24,750	$17,729	$184,443
Dr. C	$140,800	$8,756	$21,120	$10,955	$181,631
Dr. D	$140,800	$8,413	$7,920	$3,509	$160,641
Dr. E	$140,800	$10,126	$26,400	$16,893	$194,218

* Hypothetical numbers presented for illustrative purposes only. Numbers may not total in all cases due to rounding.

† Salary levels derived from market data to promote consistency with fair market value and reasonableness standards.

‡ Peer evaluation incentive assumes percent of target based on score, but requires minimum 3.5 ranking. Scores below 3.5 subject to 50% penalty. Example: Physician A scored 4.5 out of 5, therefore receives 90% (4.5/5) of award. Physician D achieved 3.0 out of 5, therefore receives 30% ([3/5] x 50% = 30%) of award.

EXHIBIT 14.18   Assessment of Hospital Example 4 – Base Plus Incentive Plan

Dimension	Strengths	Weaknesses
Measure	Market data can be used to inform base salary levels.	
Productivity	Can link base salary to prior year production levels.	Base salary may comprise too large of a component of total compensation, therefore removing productivity incentive.
Financial	Can incorporate cost of practice in incentive awards.	Strong financial management required to prevent operating losses.
Simplicity	Sophisticated, yet reasonably simple.	Potential complexity and subjectivity in incentive component.
Alignment	Production incentive component must be linked to personal services of physicians receiving compensation. Incentive may include consideration of cost of practice, quality, patient satisfaction, and similar measures.	Incentive measures that are linked to quality, patient satisfaction, and other nonclinical production-based factors can be viewed as excessively subjective.
"Fairness"	Incentive may focus on individual production levels and other factors. Base salary provides income stability and guaranteed pay.	Eligibility for incentive may depend upon individual and other factors, which may be viewed as unfair. Depending on performance measure, physicians may be asked to do more than clinical production (e.g., WRVUs), such as hospital committee work for which they are not directly compensated.

➤ ## HOSPITAL EXAMPLE 5 –
GRADUATED COMPENSATION PER WRVU PLAN
Revenue Element 5 (Graduated/Negotiated Revenues)

Overview

Under this plan methodology, physicians receive a set rate of compensation per WRVU, but the rate is graduated based on production levels. In general, the compensation per WRVU increases as physician production levels increase, up to a maximum. This model is intended to approximate the reality that in a private practice setting, physicians will typically not receive the same amount of compensation per unit of work for low levels of production as for high production levels. Therefore, this plan approximates, in a general manner, the relationship between production and compensation in the marketplace. This plan incorporates Element 5, involving a graduated compensation level, along with a heavily production-based system.

Application

Compensation plans based on graduated WRVUs may be used in a variety of relationships, including hospital-physician direct employment relationships with virtually all primary care, medical, and surgical practice specialties. These plans may also be used with faculty practice plans and more traditional group practices.

Methodology

The steps in this model are outlined below and depicted in Hospital Example 5.

Step 1. Identify Practice Specialties
The first step is to identify each physician's specialty and subspecialty, as appropriate. Equally important is to identify the type of services the physician performs (e.g., an obstetrician gynecologist who practices gynecology only, or a hematologist-oncologist who limits his or her practice to hematology only).

Step 2. Establish Performance Expectations
As in other plans, models using graduated payments linked to WRVUs or other types of production will benefit from the establishment of *minimum* performance expectations. Such performance expectations will commonly consider any number of work-related factors that are defined in advance. These expectations constitute *minimum* performance levels.

Because performance expectations are, by definition, standards of *minimum* performance, the compensation plan (and underlying contractual documents and/or policies governing the compensation relationship) should also address what happens when such performance requirements are not met. See Chapter 10 for more information on developing and implementing performance expectations.

Step 3. Establish Composite Data Values Based on the Market

Under this plan, each physician receives a predefined dollar amount per WRVU for the work the respective physician personally performs. The actual dollar amount varies depending upon the physician's specialty and production level. The dollar amount to be paid per WRVU is defined in a "grid" that is constructed through the use of two "composite" measures:

▶ Composite market-based median compensation by practice specialty; and

▶ Composite "median WRVUs" by individual physician specialty.

These "composite" measures are generally developed by averaging median values from various tables in compensation surveys (e.g., MGMA, American Medical Group Association [AMGA] and others). Each "composite" measure is developed by averaging the information contained in several tables reported in such surveys as reported (e.g., all physician respondents, by specific geographic section, multispecialty or single specialty practices, percent capitation, practice size, private/hospital/academic practice, etc.) for the respective specialty. This is to provide for an average and "fair" level of compensation for each specialty and to minimize the influence of wide fluctuations in market survey data from year to year. Separate "grids" are then created for each primary care, medical, and surgical specialty through the use of composite measures of market compensation and production. In this fashion, separate composite median compensation and composite median WRVU levels are determined for each respective specialty. This calculation method is illustrated in Step 3 of Hospital Example 5 (Exhibit 14.19) presented at the end of this section.

Step 4. Use Composite Values to Determine a Grid for Each Specialty

The composite median compensation and WRVU levels are then used to construct a grid that provides for different levels of compensation per WRVU based on differing levels of production. A graduated scale may be more appropriate than use of a standard dollar amount of payment per WRVU for a variety of reasons, including:

▶ As a means to provide a positive incentive for increased levels of work – consistent with the goals of encouraging hard work and rewarding individual physician work levels; and

▶ Because the cost of practice, or "overhead percentage," tends to vary based upon production levels. For example, the physician with a low level of production but average overhead costs will receive a lower amount of compensation per WRVU than his or her colleague with similar overhead costs but a higher level of production, because, in the case of the physician with a low level of production, the fixed costs associated with the overhead are spread across fewer units of service.

The starting point for the grid is the amount determined by dividing the composite median compensation by the composite median WRVUs, by specialty, to determine the composite median dollar per WRVU for the particular specialty. This amount is then used to determine dollar amounts per WRVU that are paid for work that is less than or greater than the composite median levels. These WRVUs and the dollars per WRVU composite medians are then used to construct the grid for the particular specialty. In this example, the lower and upper extremes of the grid are set at 80 percent and 120 percent of the composite median values, respectively.

Step 5. Determine Compensation Based on Performance

Compensation levels are determined by assessing performance in relation to the WRVU production as set forth on the grid, and multiplying actual WRVU production by the corresponding dollars per WRVU amount identified in the grid.

Exhibit 14.20 provides an assessment of the strengths and weaknesses of Hospital Example 5.

EXHIBIT 14.19

Hospital Example 5 –
Graduated Compensation per WRVU Plan*
Revenue Element 5 (Graduated/Negotiated Revenues)

Step 1 Identify physician specialties.

Step 2 Establish minimum performance expectations at individual physician level.

Measure	Minimum
Clinical service production (WRVUs)	3,500
Weeks worked per year	46 weeks
Scheduled days per week	4 12-hour shifts

Step 3 Establish composite data values based on market.†

Specialty: Neurology	Median Compensation	Median WRVU
All Respondents (Survey 1)	$178,937	4,296
Multispecialty (Survey 1)	$185,666	4,973
Western Section (Survey 2)	$176,346	4,219
11–25 FTE Physicians (Survey 2)	$186,946	4,190
Composite (average of above)	$181,974	4,420

Step 4 Use composite values to determine grid by specialty.

% of Median	Composite Median	WRVU for Specialty	$ per WRVU	Compensation (WRVU × $ per WRVU)
80%		3,536	$32.94	$116,463
84%		3,712	$34.59	$128,401
88%		3,889	$36.23	$140,920
92%		4,066	$37.88	$154,023
96%		4,243	$39.53	$167,707
100%	$181,974	4,420	$41.18	$181,974
104%		4,596	$42.82	$196,823
108%		4,773	$44.47	$212,254
112%		4,950	$46.12	$228,268
116%		5,127	$47.76	$244,864
120%		5,303	$49.41	$262,042

Step 5 Determine compensation based on performance.

	Actual WRVU	$ per WRVU at Level	Total Compensation
Dr. A	4,235	$37.88	$160,427
Dr. B	3,623	$32.94	$119,342
Dr. C	4,987	$46.12	$229,982
Dr. D	5,874	$49.41	$290,236
Dr. E	5,102	$46.12	$235,286

* Hypothetical numbers presented for illustrative purposes only. Numbers may not total in all cases due to rounding.

† Data derived from market data to promote consistency with fair market value and reasonableness standards.

EXHIBIT 14.20	Assessment of Hospital Example 5 – Graduated Compensation per WRVU Plan	
Dimension	**Strengths**	**Weaknesses**
Measure	Market data can be used to determine compensation per WRVU. WRVUs provide for payer-neutral system.	Does not consider actual reimbursement.
Productivity	Encourages work and relates physician work to compensation levels. Pays varying level of compensation based on production levels.	Uses negotiated method to approximate cost of practice without direct consideration of actual costs.
Financial	Indirectly considers cost of practice and overhead issues in determining physician compensation (e.g., in setting the WRVU values).	Divorces actual revenues from compensation paid. Does not directly consider practice operating costs. Cap on total compensation commonly required in tax-exempt organizations.
Simplicity	Straightforward once implemented, but requires significant initial education.	Sophisticated plan requiring communication planning to ensure physician understanding and engagement.
Alignment	Rewards personal productivity on a payer-neutral basis. Some indirect consideration of cost of practice.	No direct linkage to actual operating costs.
"Fairness"	System has reasonable flexibility to accommodate part time or reduced time, maternity and family leave, and similar transition arrangements. Can combine with draw mechanism to provide stability of income while also linking to personal production.	

► HOSPITAL EXAMPLE 6 – BASE SALARY WITH GRADUATED COMPENSATION PER WRVU PLAN
Revenue Elements 2 and 5 (Guaranteed Share Combined with Graduated/Negotiated Revenues)

Overview

The previous example involved a "pure productivity" payment method that results in payment of 100 percent of the compensation earned based on the physician's production and the application of the grid. Defined levels of compensation are paid for different WRVU production levels. Under this Hospital Example 6 (Exhibit 14.21) shown at the end of this section, the same concepts are coupled with a guaranteed base salary (therefore combining Elements 2 and 5 of the compensation plan matrix). Specifically, rather than using a pure production method, this example pays a base salary that is combined with a reduced-dollar per WRVU incentive payment.

The base salary constitutes a guaranteed amount of compensation that is paid throughout the year, typically set at a defined percentage (e.g., 60 to 80 percent) of the total anticipated compensation based on a combination of historic performance and expected future performance. Receipt of the base salary is linked to minimum levels of WRVU production and would be reduced for failure to meet minimum performance expectations (e.g., minimum WRVUs, insufficient weeks worked per year, etc.). Because the base salary is guaranteed, the dollar amount per WRVU for the incentive component is set at a reduced level (with all amounts linked to composite medians). The plan can also incorporate nonclinical production performance measures and criteria as discussed in Chapter 10.

Application

This plan can be used in a variety of relationships, including direct employment between a hospital or medical group and physician, and with virtually all specialties.

Methodology

The steps required in a base plus incentive model with a graduated payment per WRVU are similar to those referenced in the previous example. The key steps are presented below.

Step 1. Identify Physician Specialties
As with the other hospital plan examples, the first step is to identify the physicians' specialties, subspecialties (if appropriate), and scope of practices and services they perform.

Step 2. Establish Performance Expectations
Consistent with other examples, the establishment of physician performance expectations related to basic work levels will be important to an effective plan.

Step 3. Define a Dollar Amount for Each WRVU in the Grid

The same basic methodology referenced in Hospital Example 5 above is used to determine the grid as a starting point under this plan example and requires the following substeps:

- ► Defining the composite median compensation and the composite median WRVU levels for each respective specialty; and
- ► Determining the grid.

Step 4. Determine the Base Salary to Be Paid

Rather than making the entire compensation determined through a productivity-based plan, a portion of total anticipated compensation is guaranteed through a base salary component. That base salary could be determined on the basis of any number of factors, including percentage of median compensation by specialty; by historic compensation (e.g., prior year's total compensation); by variations in the market based upon low, medium, and high production levels, as illustrated in Hospital Example 4 (Exhibit 14.16); or by other factors (further described in Chapter 10).

Step 5. Determine Compensation per WRVU at a Reduced Level in the Grid

The base salary portion is guaranteed under this plan; therefore, the incentive compensation per WRVU is reduced from that contained in Hospital Example 5. Accordingly, this model uses the same basic methodology as in Hospital Example 5 (illustrated for neurology), but it reduces the dollar amounts per WRVU in light of the base salary guarantee.

Step 6. Determine and Pay Physician Compensation

Hospital Example 6 illustrates the use of the base salary plus incentive payment plan using graduated dollars per WRVUs. Base salary is calculated at 60 percent of the composite median amount, and the incentive amounts per WRVU have also been decreased by 60 percent.

Under the base plus incentive method using graduated WRVUs, payment of the physician's total compensation is determined based on the sum of the base salary plus the incentive, which is calculated by multiplying the physician's total WRVUs by the applicable dollars per WRVU based on production and specialty.

Exhibit 14.22 provides an assessment of the strengths and weaknesses of Hospital Example 6.

EXHIBIT 14.21

Hospital Example 6 –
Base Salary with Graduated Compensation per WRVU Plan*
Revenue Elements 2 and 5
(Guaranteed Share Combined with Graduated/Negotiated Revenues)

Step 1 Identify physician specialties.

Step 2 Establish minimum performance expectations at individual physician level.

Measure	Minimum
Clinical service production (WRVUs)	3,500
Weeks worked per year	46 weeks
Scheduled days per week	4 12-hour shifts

Step 3 Establish composite data values based on market.†

Specialty: Neurology	Median Compensation	Median WRVU
All Respondents (Survey 1)	$178,937	4,296
Multispecialty (Survey 1)	$185,666	4,973
Western Section (Survey 2)	$176,346	4,219
11–25 FTE Physicians (Survey 2)	$186,946	4,190
Composite (average of above)	$181,974	4,420

Step 4 Determine base salary to be paid.

Composite Median Compensation Target	$181,974
Base Salary as % of Target	60%
Base Salary Portion	$109,184
Incentive as % of Target	40%
Incentive Portion	$72,790

Step 5 Use composite values to determine grid by specialty.

% of Median	40% of Composite Median	WRVU for Specialty	$ per WRVU	Incentive (WRVU × $ per WRVU)	Total Base + Incentive at % of Median
80%		3,536	$13.18	$46,604	$155,770
84%		3,712	$13.83	$51,337	$160,545
88%		3,889	$14.49	$56,352	$165,552
92%		4,066	$15.15	$61,600	$170,793
96%		4,243	$15.81	$67,082	$176,267
100%	$72,790	4,420	$16.47	$72,797	$181,974
104%		4,596	$17.13	$78,729	$187,913
108%		4,773	$17.79	$84,912	$194,086
112%		4,950	$18.45	$91,328	$200,491
116%		5,127	$19.11	$97,977	$207,130
120%		5,303	$19.76	$104,787	$214,001

Step 6 Determine compensation based on performance.

	Base Salary	Actual WRVU	$ per WRVU at Level	Total Compensation
Dr. A	$109,184	4,235	$15.15	$173,355
Dr. B	$109,184	3,623	$13.18	$156,921
Dr. C	$109,184	4,987	$18.45	$201,177
Dr. D	$109,184	5,874	$19.76	$225,279
Dr. E	$109,184	5,102	$18.45	$203,298

* Hypothetical numbers presented for illustrative purposes only. Numbers may not total in all cases due to rounding.
† Data derived from market data to promote consistency with fair market value and reasonableness standards.

EXHIBIT 14.22 Assessment of Hospital Example 6 –
Base Salary Plus Variation of Graduated Payment per WRVU Plan

Dimension	Strengths	Weaknesses
Measure	Base salary is linked to market, with individual credit for WRVU production.	Does not consider actual reimbursement.
Productivity	Encourages clinical productivity. Provides stability in base.	
Financial	Approximates cost of practice, though indirectly.	Does not expressly consider revenue or expenditures.
Simplicity	Relatively straightforward once the grid is determined.	Base salary level and grid must be determined.
Alignment	Individualistic focus with production orientation, while also providing level of income security through base salary component.	Performance expectations are also generally required in connection with base salary component. Incentives can also include non-clinical production measures (e.g., quality, patient satisfaction, etc.)
"Fairness"	Base salary provides greater security and stability, while also encouraging production orientation.	

© 2006 Johnson & Walker Keegan

► HOSPITAL EXAMPLE 7 – HOURLY PAY FOR PHYSICIAN PROFESSIONAL SERVICES PLAN
Revenue Element 1 (Unit-Based)

Overview

Hourly pay arrangements compensate physicians for services based on time. They may be used in direct or indirect compensation arrangements. These arrangements use Revenue Element 1, and they build on Architecture A, presented in Chapter 13, involving unit-based compensation plans.

Application

Examples of common relationships in which hourly rate compensation systems are used include but are not limited to:

- ► Hospital payments to a physician for medical director services;

- ► Payments by a hospital to a physician for trauma or obstetrical call services;

- ► Emergency room staffing services provided by an emergency room staffing company under an indirect arrangement; and

- ► Arrangements between a hospital and a group of physicians for staffing of a hospital outpatient or inpatient department (e.g., critical care) or urgent care clinic under an indirect compensation arrangement.

The essential requirements related to hourly payment methods are that the compensation paid per hour may not exceed FMV, and such compensation may be paid only for services that are actually performed.

The Phase II final rule to the Stark law defined a new safe harbor methodology for determining hourly rates for a physician's personal services. The safe harbor hourly rate methodology can potentially be used to determine rates that would be paid to individual physicians or to a group of physicians in which an indirect relationship between the hospital and the physicians is present. Because of the applicable FMV standards, however, the underlying contract and payment governing the indirect compensation arrangement would need to consider the mix of physician specialties and the actual time devoted by each, as well as potentially other issues.

Methodology

The following are the basic steps in any hourly payment arrangement.

Step 1. Identify Physician Specialties and Services
Identify each physician's specialty, subspecialty (as appropriate), and the types of services that the physician performs.

Step 2. Establish Performance Expectations and Physician Services

Minimum performance expectations are also useful in an hourly rate arrangement, especially when the physician's services are on a full-time or largely full-time basis. In this step, in addition to basic performance expectations, the description of the required services is documented. In the case of urgent care services, the precise services need to be expressed in the contractual documents governing the service arrangement, to include hours of service and documentation requirements. In the case of less than full-time arrangements, such as those used in medical directorships and similar arrangements, time cards and similar verification tools are also commonly used to document the provision of services for which payment is being provided.

Step 3. Establish an Hourly Rate

The Stark law's final rule outlines a specific "safe harbor" approach to determining FMV hourly payment levels. These methods can therefore be used to establish an hourly rate, although there is no requirement that such a method be used.

In Hospital Example 7-A (Exhibit 14.23, involving the staffing of a hospital urgent care center), the basic concepts referenced in the Stark law final rule's hourly payment safe harbor are used as the starting point in that the average of multiple market median compensation measures are divided by 2,000 hours to derive the hourly rate.[3] In this example, given that an urgent care center is being staffed by physicians who generally provide urgent care services and also by family practitioners, two different hourly rates are calculated, with the particular hourly rate assigned based on the practice's specialty or physician's expertise. An alternative to this approach is to establish the hourly rate through the use of bona fide bargaining between the parties.

Step 4. Determine and Pay Compensation

Compensation may only be paid for services that are actually performed. As a result, verification of services via time cards or similar evidence is generally required, and additional monitoring methods may be instituted to verify work levels.

Hourly pay arrangements can also be coupled with limited incentive measures as a means to encourage and reward certain types of performance. Such incentive arrangements will commonly be linked to issues of patient satisfaction, quality, and/or work levels, with the particular type of incentive typically dependent upon the type of services for which hourly payments are being made.

Hospital Example 7-B (Exhibit 14.24) illustrates an incentive payment that considers: (1) patient satisfaction by physician; and (2) patient visit volume by physician FTE in hospital urgent care centers. It pays an incentive payment based on patient visit volume by reference to targets. The hourly rate is set at 95 percent of the expected value, with additions to the hourly rate paid for performance in relation to incentive performance. Incentive is paid in the form of increased hourly rate amounts, with the level of increase linked to patient satisfaction and patient visit volume. Central to such a system is the adoption of a survey or similar instrument to assess patient satisfaction within the organization. When such tools exist and have been used to establish base-line measures, targets and incentive payments can be assigned to improvements in scores with respect to particular measures.

Other measures can also be used to determine incentive payments paid over and above the hourly wage rates. The example below creates a flat dollar incentive payment defined in advance based on two measures: (1) performance in improving the clinic's overall financial condition; and (2) performance based on customer satisfaction survey instruments.

Performance Metric 1: Incentive Payment Based on Financial Performance

Incentive compensation will be paid based upon increases to net patient revenue over the prior fiscal year.

Flat dollar incentives shall be determined and paid as follows:

- ► Three percent (3%) increase in net revenues   = $1,000
- ► Seven percent (7%) increase in net revenues   = $2,000
- ► Ten percent (10%) increase in net revenues   = $3,000

Total cumulative incentive for financial performance = $6,000

Performance Metric 2: Incentive Payment Based on Customer Satisfaction

Customer satisfaction will be tabulated based on results from the health system's exter-nal customer satisfaction survey, to include surveys of employers and patients. The incentive will be paid based on the total cumulative overall score for the program dur-ing the year. Incentives will be determined and paid as follows:

- ► One-half percent (.5%) improvement   = $1,000
- ► One percent (1%) improvement   = $1,000
- ► One and one-half percent (1.5%) improvement   = $1,000
- ► Two percent (2%) improvement   = $1,000

Total cumulative incentive for customer service = $4,000

It should be recognized, however, that in hourly pay arrangements, the hourly rate will typically comprise the majority of the compensation to be earned for professional services, and the hourly rate is generally selected as a means to compensate for work per-formed, but without focusing attention on payer mix or similar issues. Under an hourly pay arrangement, the hourly rate is determined and paid so that physicians can provide necessary services when the services are required, without consideration of whether the reimbursement for such services, if any, is sufficient to cover cost of practice or similar issues. Therefore, in these settings, any incentive compensation will typically comprise only a small portion of the physician's expected compensation (e.g., between 10 and 20 percent), and will generally be based on financial performance and paid as a true additional incentive bonus. Accordingly, the compensation under the straight hourly rate arrangement will generally need to be at an acceptable level to allow the organization to purchase physician services, and any bonus will generally be relatively slight in relation to the full amount of compensation earned through the hourly rate.

Exhibit 14.25 (Hospital Example 7-C) presents a third example of an hourly pay arrangement involving compensation for on-call services.

Exhibit 14.26 provides an assessment of the strengths and weaknesses of Hospital Example 7.

EXHIBIT 14.23

Hospital Example 7-A –
Hourly Pay for Physician Professional Services Plan*
Revenue Element 1 (Unit-Based)

Step 1   **Identify physician specialties.**
Note: Urgent care clinic staffing illustrated here.

Step 2   **Establish minimum performance expectations at individual physician level.**

Measure	Minimum
Hours per urgent care shift	12

Step 3   **Establish composite data values based on market.†**

	Urgent Care Median	Family Practice Median
All Respondents (Survey 1)	$177,113	$165,124
Multispecialty (Survey 1)	$181,079	$168,967
Hospital-Owned (Survey 2)	$192,337	$170,000
Midwest Section (Survey 2)	$184,386	$172,594
Average of Above	$183,729	$169,171
FMV Rate (average/2,000 hours)	$91.86	$84.59
Rate per Contract	$91	$87

Step 4   **Determine and pay compensation.**

	Documented Hours of Service	Practice Specialty	Hourly Rate per Contract	Total Compensation
Dr. A	1,900.0	Urgent Care	$91	$172,900
Dr. B	900.0	Family Practice	$87	$78,300
Dr. C	2,100.0	Urgent Care	$91	$191,100
Dr. D	1,987.5	Urgent Care	$91	$180,863
Dr. E	1,700.0	Urgent Care	$91	$154,700

* Hypothetical numbers presented for illustrative purposes only. Numbers may not total in all cases due to rounding.
† Data derived from market data to promote consistency with fair market value and reasonableness standards.

EXHIBIT 14.24

Hospital Example 7-B – Hourly Pay Arrangement with Incentive Plan*
Revenue Element 1 (Unit-Based)

Step 1 **Identify physician specialties.**

Note: Urgent care clinic staffing illustrated here.

Step 2 **Establish minimum performance expectations at individual physician level.**

Measure	Minimum
Hours per urgent care shift	12

Step 3 **Establish composite data values based on market.†**

	Urgent Care Median
All Respondents (Survey 1)	$177,113
Multispecialty (Survey 1)	$181,079
Hospital-Owned (Survey 2)	$192,337
Midwest Section (Survey 2)	$184,386
Average of Above	$183,729
FMV Rate (average/2,000 hours)	$91.86
Rate per Contract (95% of FMV)	$87

Step 4 **Determine incentive measure(s).**

INDIVIDUAL INCENTIVE – PATIENT SATISFACTION

Satisfaction Score	% of Actual Physician Compensation	Additional Amount per Hour
< 85.99%	0.00%	$ —
86.0–87.49%	0.50%	$0.44
87.5–88.99%	1.00%	$0.87
89.0–90.99%	1.50%	$1.31
91.0–92.99%	2.00%	$1.74
93.0% +	2.50%	$2.18

LOCATION/GROUP INCENTIVE

Patient Visit Volume per FTE	Percent of Physician Compensation	Additional Amount per Hour
< 4,300	0%	$—
4,301–4,600	1%	$0.87
4,601–4,900	2%	$1.74
4,901–5,200	3%	$2.61
5,201–5,500	4%	$3.48
5,501+	5%	$4.35

Location A	Documented Hours of Service	Physician FTE	Base Hourly Rate per Contract	Patient Satisfaction Score	Patient Satisfaction Incentive per Hour	Patient Visits	Patient Visits per FTE	Patient Visit Incentive per Hour	Total Compensation‡
Dr. A	1,900.00	0.95	$87	89.00%	$1.31	3,909	4,115	$0.87	$169,442
Dr. B	900.00	0.45	$87	92.20%	$1.74	2,292	5,093	$2.61	$82,215
Dr. C	2,100.00	1.05	$87	89.20%	$1.31	5,200	4,952	$1.74	$189,105
Dr. D	1,987.50	0.99	$87	90.34%	$1.34	4,787	4,817	$1.74	$179,034
Dr. E	1,700.00	0.85	$87	85.00%	$—	4,562	5,367	$3.48	$153,816

* Hypothetical numbers presented for illustrative purposes only. Numbers may not total in all cases due to rounding.

† Data derived from market data to promote consistency with fair market value and reasonableness standards.

‡ Total compensation = hours of service × (base hourly contract rate + patient satisfaction incentive + patient visit incentive)

Hospital Example 7-C –
Hourly Pay Arrangement for On-Call Services Plan*
Revenue Element 1 (Unit-Based)

EXHIBIT 14.25

Step 1   **Identify physician specialties.**

Note: Neurosurgery illustrated here.

Step 2   **Establish minimum performance expectations at individual physician level.**

Measure	Requirement
On-call services	
Primary on-call nights (physically present)	12-hour shifts
Secondary on-call nights (beeper only)	12-hour shifts

Step 3   **Establish hourly rates based on market values.**

Neurosurgery	Median		Hourly rate
Survey 1	$524,894		
Survey 2	$498,920		
Survey 3	$501,992		
Survey 4	$467,629		
Average	$498,359		
Fair Market Value Hourly (average / 2,000)			$249
Nights (physically present)		33%	$82
Nights (beeper)		10%	$25

Step 4   **Determine on-call compensation.**

Primary On-Call Pay (physically present)

Physician	Shifts	Physically Present Hours per Shift	Rate per Hour	Total Pay
Dr. A	68	12	$82	$66,912
Dr. B	87	12	$82	$85,608
Dr. C	65	12	$82	$63,960
Dr. D	73	12	$82	$71,832
Dr. E	72	12	$82	$70,848
Total	365			$359,160

Secondary On-Call Pay (beeper)

Physician	Shifts	Beeper Hours per Shift	Rate per Hour	Total Pay
Dr. A	88	12	$25	$26,400
Dr. B	45	12	$25	$13,500
Dr. C	67	12	$25	$20,100
Dr. D	56	12	$25	$16,800
Dr. E	109	12	$25	$32,700
Total	365			$109,500

* Hypothetical numbers presented for illustrative purposes only. Numbers may not total in all cases due to rounding.

† Data derived from market data to promote consistency with fair market value and reasonableness standards.

Assessment of Hospital Example 7 – Hourly Rate for Physician Professional Services Plan

EXHIBIT 14.26

Dimension	Strengths	Weaknesses
Measure	Tracks and pays for time (e.g., hours of work) directly to each physician.	
Productivity	Limits compensation to hours actually worked, without regard to production (e.g., professional services) actually furnished.	No linkage to actual production when providing services for which hourly compensation is paid.
Financial		No consideration of revenues generated by physician during work period. No consideration of expense of practice.
Simplicity	Simple to administer, although records to demonstrate services or hours actually worked (as opposed to those contracted for) are required.	
Alignment	Use of FMV safe harbor can promote compliance with legal requirements. Compliance is frequently promoted by application of a cap on total hours and/or payments. When coupled with performance expectations or strong group culture, can encourage and support true "group practice" approach to care.	Generally only limited application. FMV safe harbor pay level may be so low that physicians will not provide services for agreed upon rate.
"Fairness"	Allows physician to receive compensation without regard to patient payer mix.	Unless performance expectations are established and enforced, may allow for low work effort or shirking behaviors.

© 2006 Johnson & Walker Keegan

► HOSPITAL EXAMPLE 8 – INDIRECT HOSPITAL OR CONTRACTED GROUP WITH COST CONTROL PLAN
Revenue Element 4 (Production-Based) and Element 5 (Graduated/Negotiated Revenues)

Background

Many hospital-affiliated medical practices use structures involving either direct employment of physicians by the hospital or employment through a captive medical group that is owned by the hospital. In some settings, however, hospitals will use a structure involving an "indirect" contractual relationship between the hospital and individual physicians who furnish services on the hospital's behalf. As illustrated in Exhibit 14.5, these structures commonly involve ambulatory care clinics that are hospital-owned and operated and that are staffed via contractual arrangements by one or more medical groups. However, the groups remain entirely independent of the hospital and health system, rather than being owned by the hospital.

Under such indirect contractual service arrangements, the hospital obtains the services of various physician specialties (e.g., primary care and frequently many medical and surgical subspecialties) who reassign their right to payment to the hospital, but without direct employment. Such structures allow for physician-hospital collaboration, while enabling the physician group to maintain some enhanced level of governance, decision making, and other autonomy. These indirect contractual structural models can also benefit from provider-based reimbursement and can encompass potentially other desirable structural features and characteristics.

Application

The basic structural setting for such indirect contractual models and associated plans involves the following characteristics:

- ► A hospital that desires to obtain and bill for physician professional services furnished in hospital-affiliated clinics, and potentially in inpatient and other settings;

- ► A separate medical practice that employs physicians and contracts with the hospital to furnish patient care services on the hospital's behalf; and

- ► Physician reassignment of payment for professional fees to the hospital.

When these indirect structures are established, there are effectively two different compensation plans: (1) a plan involving payments from the hospital to the physician practice for services furnished pursuant to a contractual arrangement (referred to here as "Level I" payments); and (2) a plan involving payments from the physician practice to the physicians of amounts received under the contract, which serves as the actual physician compensation plan that is used to distribute contracted dollars to the physician (referred to here as "Level II" payments).

The financial performance of such structural models is commonly a product of numerous factors, including:

▶ Decisions regarding clinical time and service levels required and acquired by the hospital;

▶ Variations in physician production or work levels; and

▶ Other decisions that involve both controllable and uncontrollable costs, such as facility and occupancy costs, personnel costs, and other practice expenses that are commonly more characteristic of a hospital than a physician group.

A successful contractual relationship typically requires a multifaceted approach, including an effective funds flow from the hospital to the physician practice through the Level I payments, and an effective internal physician practice compensation plan through the Level II compensation system. These two compensation structures optimally create incentives for physicians to engage in activities that will benefit them personally, their practices, and the hospital as the ultimate source of compensation. Effective compensation plans directed at such ends create a strong relationship between physician performance and compensation and permit physicians to be held responsible for activities that they perceive are within their control.

Good financial margins in such structures generally require focused attention on both cost control and productivity enhancement; therefore, the compensation plans will frequently be designed to provide the contracted physician practice(s) with the financial incentive to both increase production *and* manage costs. As a result, effective plans will typically include the following core features:

1. A clear definition of desired clinical FTE ("CFTE," or clinical full-time equivalency) levels of physician services being purchased by a hospital from the physician group;

2. Identification of "controllable" costs of practice that are viewed to be within the control of individual physicians and/or the physician practice, and the assessment of practice operating costs by reference to "controllable costs"; and

3. Definition of targets and goals related to both production and cost control as part of the "Level I" compensation plan involving payment from the hospital to the physician practice, and in the context of "Level II" payments to physicians as part of the practice's compensation plan.

Methodology

Two different plans are presented that are commonly used in an indirect, contracted group plan. Hospital Example 8 (Exhibit 14.27), presented at the end of this section, illustrates a basic model. Hospital Example 9 involves a model with significantly greater complexity. The basic steps as illustrated in Hospital Example 8 are described below.

Step 1. Define Physician Specialties and CFTE Time Being Purchased by the Hospital

Under this model, the hospital purchases physician services to staff hospital-owned outpatient clinics and provide other clinical services. The time in which such staffing is being acquired is defined in advance in the aggregate, and therefore defines a minimum controllable performance requirement. The compensation paid from the hospital to the practice at Level I may be adjusted for failure to meet that expectation.

Step 2. Define Performance Expectations

Performance expectations are defined at multiple levels, including:

► Entity, department, or division (e.g., time in the clinic);

► Individual physician (e.g., production per CFTE, medical records or quality requirements, and patient access); and

► Site level (e.g., attention to financial performance and role in cost management).

Step 3. Determine Level I Compensation per CFTE

Under this example, a production-based payment is made by the hospital to the physician practice on a dollars per WRVU basis. However, the dollars paid per WRVU are arrayed along an inverted curve, with fewer dollars per WRVU being paid for performance at each end of the curve. Hospital Example 8 (Exhibit 14.27) illustrates the award measured in the aggregate (for the practice as a whole, based on practice production per CFTE).

In the middle of the curve, the hospital pays dollars per WRVU that would result in a defined level of compensation for a defined or "target" level of production (e.g., median compensation levels for median levels of production). Below this target level, (e.g., below median in this example), the dollars per WRVU decline. For productivity levels that fall between the target level and another higher, or "maximum" level, the dollars per WRVU increase by a fixed percentage. Above the maximum level (e.g., 120 percent of the median percentile in the example above), the dollars per WRVU again decline.

The plan is designed to assure that the hospital pays compensation that bears a close relationship to market expectations for production. By doing so, it provides an incentive to increase the production levels of physicians who fall below target levels, while also rewarding work effort beyond that target level up to a specific maximum level.

Level I payments from the hospital are measured and paid for on an individual physician basis (as illustrated in this example), although they could be measured and paid for at the group level per CFTE. This plan pays defined levels for each increment of production (standardized for CFTE). This means, for example, that the hospital pays X_1 amount per WRVU for the first defined number of units of production per CFTE, X_2 for the next increment of WRVU production, and so on.[4]

Hospital Example 8 uses hypothetical data and assumes payment per WRVU at an increased level over market rates based on the need to provide compensation for benefits and certain other costs (e.g., malpractice insurance) that are paid for by the hospital.

Precise target and maximum values, as well as the payment levels for WRVUs and the number of steps in the grid, are determined as part of the plan design process and informed by financial modeling.

Based on this example, if annual production per 1.0 CFTE for the physician practice as a whole is 4,660 WRVUs (assuming 5.3 CFTE), during a particular time period, the medical practice receives $48.99 per WRVU for the first 3,925 WRVUs (per 1.0 CFTE), $53.25 per WRVU for the next 185 WRVUs between 3,925 and 4,110, etc. The total compensation per 1.0 CFTE is then multiplied by the 5.3 FTE "purchased" by the hospital to determine the total payment to the physician group based on physician production.

Step 4. Determine the Cost of Practice Incentive

A cost of practice incentive is provided under this example based on improvements to financial performance at the local practice site level. Improvements in financial performance due to cost savings are shared between the hospital and the physicians working at the particular practice site. The means to measure the cost-savings incentive can be designed using any number of measures to include:

- ► Current year costs in comparison to prior year costs;
- ► Performance vs. budget (including performance in relation to budgeted deficits);
- ► Improvements in operating margins; and/or
- ► Improvements in total operating cost as a percentage of total medical revenue.

An example of this approach to a cost of practice incentive using improvements in current-year costs as compared to the prior year is provided in Exhibit 14.28.

In this example, it is assumed that if the physicians in practice site "A" achieved their target related to cost control, the hospital would make a Level I payment in an amount equal to 50 percent of that savings through payments to the medical group as an entity. Additional compensation paid for performance in relation to cost-savings targets would typically be limited to no more than a defined percentage of total production payments from the hospital (e.g., 10 percent). Hospital Example 8 illustrates such an incentive payment based on the difference between the practice site's budgeted controllable costs and the actual controllable costs.

Although some incentive can be earned and paid through cost-savings measures, the level of practice efficiency that can be promoted and achieved is likely to be limited. Furthermore, savings can typically be achieved in most cases in a relatively short time period, but such savings will typically be non-reoccurring. Care must always be taken to ensure that the desire to cut and save costs *does not* result in a less efficient (and largely ineffective) clinical practice setting.[5] In addition, close attention to compliance issues is required in arrangements considering costs. In particular, when the services are furnished in a hospital outpatient clinic in which services are reimbursed on a provider-based basis, the use of a direct cost award could potentially raise "gainsharing" and similar concerns. See Chapter 12 for a general discussion of these issues.

Level II Payment (to Individual Physicians via the Compensation Plan)

As a general matter, the means by which individual physicians are compensated by a physician practice in an indirect contracted group plan are determined by local (practice–specific) decision making within the practice. Nonetheless, even these plans must then be structured with the following points in mind:

► The Level I (hospital to medical practice) and Level II (medical practice to individual physicians) plans that are actually used should be evaluated to ensure alignment of incentive. As part of any performance expectations between a hospital and medical practice relating to payment of Level I funds, the Level II payment methods must reasonably promote the same basic goals; and

► At least a minimum defined percentage (e.g., 30 to 50 percent) of dollars that are earned from specific incentive components of the plan should be linked to the individual physician's compensation in order to align Level I and II incentives.

Hospital Example 8 illustrates such a Level II (medical practice to physician) compensation plan. As noted above, a portion of the amount paid by the hospital should also optimally be allocated to the physicians responsible for generating the original payment based on their performance in the Level II plan. In addition, the ultimate levels of compensation received by practice physicians may not exceed FMV and, when a tax-exempt organization is involved, must be reasonable.

Hospital Example 8 illustrates a within-practice allocation method after payment of physician benefits, malpractice, and other costs (Step 6), involving a combined equal share and percentage of production methodology within the physician practice (Step 7). In this model, the entire pool available for compensation is allocated to individual practice physicians on a 50 percent equal share basis (based on CFTE) and 50 percent on a percent to total basis (measured by WRVUs). Other methods, including many of those described in Chapter 13, could be used in such an internal compensation plan model.

An assessment of the strengths and weaknesses of Hospital Plan 8 is provided in Exhibit 14.29.

EXHIBIT 14.27

Hospital Example 8 –
Indirect Hospital or Contracted Group with Cost Control Plan*
Revenue Element 4 (Production-Based) and Element 5 (Graduated/Negotiated Revenues)

LEVEL I – PAYMENT FROM HOSPITAL TO PHYSICIAN PRACTICE

Step 1 **Define physician specialties and clinical full time equivalency (CFTE) being purchased by hospital.**

Note: Family practice and general internal medicine illustrated here.

Family Practice 7.5 CFTE
Internal Medicine 5.3 CFTE

Step 2 **Define performance expectations.**

Requirements for 1.0 CFTE by Specialty

	Scheduled Clinic Hours per Week	Weeks per Year	Hospital Rounds	On-Call
Family Practice	36	47	No	Yes
Internal Medicine	34	47	Yes	No

Step 3 **Establish compensation per WRVU (based on CFTE).**

	WRVU	Compensation per WRVU
Benchmark Median	3,925	$42.60

Production Range	WRVU per 1.0 CFTE	$ per WRVU‡	% of Target Value
Maximum (120% of median)	Over 4,851	$48.99	92%
	4,666 – 4,851	$57.51	108%
	4,481 – 4,665	$56.45	106%
	4,296 – 4,480	$55.38	104%
	4,111 – 4,296	$54.32	102%
Target (e.g., median)	3,926 – 4,110	$53.25	100%
	First 3,925	$48.99	92%

continued on next page

Exhibit 14.27 – Hospital Example 8 continued

Step 4 **Establish cost of practice incentive.**

Measure:

50% of difference between budgeted controllable costs and actual controllable costs at site level.

Note: Controllable costs predefined to include personnel costs, supplies, and other costs deemed to be within the control of physicians at the local practice level.

Difference between budget and actual to be allocated 50% to physicians at site/50% to hospital.

Step 5 **Determine compensation based on production per CFTE and cost of practice.**

Production-Based Payment

Internal Medicine Only	WRVU Total
Actual Production	24,700
CFTE	5.30
Production Adjusted for 1.0 CFTE	4,660

Compensation per WRVU Thresholds	Rate	Per 1.0 CFTE	Total per 5.3 CFTE
First 3,925	$48.99	$192,237	$1,018,855
3,926 – 4,110	$53.25	$9,851	$52,212
4,111 – 4,295	$54.32	$9,994	$52,968
4,296 – 4,480	$55.38	$10,190	$54,007
4,481 – 4,665	$56.45	$10,104	$53,549
4,666 – 4,851	$57.51		
Over 4,851	$48.99		
Production-Based Compensation		$232,376	$1,231,590
Total Production Compensation to Physician Practice (for Internal Medicine physicians only)			$1,231,590

Cost of Practice Incentive

	Controllable Operating Cost per Physician FTE	Total
Budget	$258,956	$1,372,467
Actual	$237,654	$1,259,566
Difference	$21,302	$112,901
Physician Practice Share	50%	$56,450

Total Cost of Practice Incentive to Physician Practice (for Internal Medicine physicians only)	$56,450
Total Level I (Hospital to Physician Practice) Payment (sum of production payment plus cost of practice incentive)	$1,288,041

LEVEL II – PAYMENT FROM PHYSICIAN PRACTICE TO INDIVIDUAL PHYSICIANS

Step 6 **Determine amount available for physician compensation (net of expenses).**

Total Payment from Hospital	$1,288,041
Physician Benefit Cost	$(231,847)
Malpractice Insurance Cost	$(58,300)
Available for Physician Compensation	$997,893

Step 7 **Determine physician-specific compensation (within physician practice).**

Internal Medicine Only	Total	Dr. A	Dr. B	Dr. C	Dr. E	Dr. F	Dr. G
Actual Production (WRVU)	24,700	2,988	4,129	5,628	3,392	4,401	4,162
% of Actual Production	100%	12%	17%	23%	14%	18%	17%
CFTE	5.30	0.60	1.00	1.00	0.90	1.00	0.80
Equal Share per CFTE (50%)	$498,947	$56,485	$94,141	$94,141	$84,727	$94,141	$75,313
% of WRVU Production (50%)	$498,947	$60,358	$83,407	$113,687	$68,519	$88,901	$84,074
Total W-2 Compensation	$997,893	$116,843	$177,548	$207,828	$153,246	$183,042	$159,386

* Hypothetical numbers presented for illustrative purposes only. Numbers may not total in all cases due to rounding.

† Data derived from market data to promote consistency with fair market value and reasonableness standards.

‡ Level I payment increased 25% from straight market rate per WRVU to provide compensation for physician benefits, malpractice, and other costs incurred by group.

© 2006 Johnson & Walker Keegan

EXHIBIT 14.28 Cost of Practice Incentive Grid – Example

Practice Site	Prior Year Cost	Current Year Cost	Difference	Split 50% Hospital 50% Physicians
A	$250,000	$225,000	$25,000	$12,500 Hospital $12,500 Physicians
B	$350,000	$375,000	-$25,000	No incentive

EXHIBIT 14.29

Assessment of Hospital Example 8 – Indirect Hospital or Contracted Group with Cost Control Plan

Dimension	Strengths	Weaknesses
Measure	Links market compensation to market levels of work. Uses WRVUs to measure and determine compensation.	
Productivity	Encourages enhanced focus on productivity at individual physician level.	Individual physician production focus may not carry through to practice Level II plan, resulting in potential misalignment of incentives.
Financial	Focuses group physicians and leadership on cost of practice issues at local practice site level. Production orientation promoted at physician and practice level.	Focuses on practice-wide production per CFTE, which may allow individual physicians to maintain low production levels with the expectations that others will make up the difference (e.g., shirking or "free rider" behaviors). Relatively limited focus on cost of practice. Additional plan administration costs (though not high). Once cost of practice goals have been reached, creating additional incentives for cost reduction may be detrimental to practice efficiency.
Simplicity	Relative ease of administration once developed. Allows hospital to purchase necessary services, while also allowing greater physician practice autonomy and control over practice-physician compensation system, internal group management, and in other areas.	Indirect contractual relationship creates additional complexity.
Alignment	Provides foundation for stronger "group practice" plan of service delivery. Promotes higher level of physician group autonomy than is found in many more typical hospital-affiliated group models.	Performance expectations are required to ensure that physicians are engaged in activities beyond productivity and cost issues. Continued emphasis on individual physician productivity; only small "group" emphasis by virtue of practice site cost measures.
"Fairness"	Pays for work performed and creates limited cost-savings incentives.	

► HOSPITAL EXAMPLE 9 – INDIRECT HOSPITAL OR CONTRACTED GROUP USING WRVUS AND COST CONTROL PLAN

Overview

This second option of a plan for an indirect hospital or contracted group uses more complex but arguably more objective measures to make Level I payments from a hospital to the physician practice while also varying those payments based upon production and cost management at the regional and "local" group levels.

This plan is generally only available in systems with extensive hospital-affiliated group infrastructure system support. Nonetheless, the model involves significantly greater objective measures and potentially greater understandability, once implemented.

The steps with respect to Level I payments from the hospital to physician practice involve the following.

Step 1. Define Time Being Purchased by Hospital for Service in Hospital Ambulatory Clinics

Similar to Hospital Example 8, this variation of a hospital-contracted plan involves the purchase of physician services to staff hospital-owned clinics. The time in which such staffing is being acquired is defined for each practice site and in the aggregate. This amount of time constitutes a minimum performance requirement, and the compensation paid from the hospital to the physician practice at Level I may be adjusted for failure to meet that expectation.

Step 2. Define Performance Expectations

Expectations are defined for at least the following:

- ► Entity, department, or division (e.g., time in clinic);
- ► Individual physician (e.g., production per CFTE, medical records or quality requirements, patient access); and
- ► Site level (e.g., attention to financial performance and role in cost management).

Step 3. Define Production and Cost Components and Pay Levels

Specific components (discussed below) are developed based on the basic assumptions that follow.

Level I Payment per WRVU

In a private practice setting, physicians do not receive the same amount of compensation (defined as money paid to the physician net of practice expenses for the physician's personal use) for both the first and last unit of service they provide. Instead, more of the first dollar of revenues must be used to pay practice overhead, because the practice generally has high fixed costs. As in other hospital-affiliated examples, this plan graduates the Level I payment amount per WRVU based on production levels in a manner that is more consistent with private practice realities. Accordingly, this plan requires production improvements by paying a lower level of compensation for low levels of production and by paying a premium level of compensation for production in excess of targets up to a certain level.

A "base dollar value per WRVU" (shown in Exhibit 14.30 at 85 percent of the estimated maximum) is determined based on the physician practice's *overall* (aggregate) WRVU production in relation to targets. The goal is to ensure that the physician practice as a whole (or alternatively, individual business units or entities, such as individual divisions or locations) have physicians that produce at some acceptable level by reference to benchmarks (e.g., median, 75th percentile, or otherwise).

Cost per WRVU

This variation *also* focuses on the management of controllable costs by measuring and awarding compensation based on improvements in performance to controllable operating costs per WRVU at the regional and local clinic levels. A smaller portion of the dollar per WRVU is determined based on the physician practice's success in managing controllable costs. This portion is measured at two levels: (1) regional; and (2) local

EXHIBIT 14.30   Production-Based Component – Base Dollar per WRVU Grid

	Percent of Maximum	Target WRVUs per CFTE	Base $ per WRVU Paid
Maximum	90%	4,600	$34.20
0.9		4,530	$34.01
0.8		4,460	$33.82
0.7		4,390	$33.63
0.6		4,320	$33.44
0.5		4,250	$33.25
0.4		4,180	$33.06
0.3		4,110	$32.87
0.2		4,040	$32.68
0.1		3,970	$32.49
Minimum	85%	3,900	$32.30

clinic levels as illustrated in Exhibits 14.31 and 14.32. These are measured by reference to improvements in "controllable costs per WRVU," effectively using an internal benchmark to assess improvements rather than using external benchmarking criteria. These cost-based measures require the physician practice to be divided into geographic regions for management purposes. Such a regional focus often provides practice physicians and hospital management with the incentive to work together to both improve production and control costs (e.g., consider site consolidation, review employee-sharing activities, etc.).

Step 4. Make Level I Payments from Hospital to Physician Practice

All Level I payments from the hospital to the physician practice under this example are based on a uniform methodology involving the combination of the base dollar value per WRVU, *plus* additional dollar value(s) per WRVU based on controllable costs per WRVU at the regional and local clinic levels. The combination of these factors results in the total amount paid from the hospital to the physician practice entities as a Level I payment.

EXHIBIT 14.31 Cost-Based Portion – Regional Controllable Cost per WRVU Grid

	Percent of Maximum		Target Controllable Cost per WRVU	Add'l $ per WRVU Paid
Maximum	95%		$52.09	$1.90
0.9			$53.40	$1.71
0.8			$54.70	$1.52
0.7			$56.00	$1.33
0.6			$57.30	$1.14
0.5			$58.60	$0.95
0.4			$59.91	$0.76
0.3			$61.21	$0.57
0.2			$62.51	$0.38
0.1			$63.81	$0.19
Minimum	90%	Current	$65.12	$ —

As with Example 8 discussed earlier, the Level II plan (that is, from the physician practice to physicians) is determined by physician practice leadership, although to further the underlying incentive structure, a substantial portion of Level II compensation (e.g., 30 to 50 percent) would generally be required to be linked directly to individual production.

The examples in Exhibits 14.30, 14.31, and 14.32 illustrate the basic approach for purposes of the Level I payments from the hospital to the medical practice under this example. Using the grid in Exhibit 14.30, if physicians within a particular medical practice have production equal to 4,123 per CFTE, the practice would be paid $32.87 per WRVU actually produced by those physicians as the Level I payment from the hospital. As with Hospital Example 8 above, these values could also be increased to reflect additional compensation to take into account salary, benefit, and malpractice costs in the physician practice. Such costs generally are in the range of 25 to 35 percent of total compensation. Using the grid in Exhibit 14.31, if the region in question had current (e.g., historic) controllable costs per WRVU of $65.12, and that region improved cost

EXHIBIT 14.32 Local Controllable Cost per WRVU Grid

	Percent of Maximum		Target Controllable Cost per WRVU	Add'l $ per WRVU Paid	Aggregate per WRVU (with amount)
Maximum	100%		$42.62	$1.90	$38.00
0.9			$43.92	$1.71	
0.8			$45.22	$1.52	
0.7			$46.52	$1.33	
0.6			$47.83	$1.14	
0.5			$49.13	$0.95	
0.4			$50.43	$0.76	
0.3			$51.73	$0.57	
0.2			$53.04	$0.38	
0.1			$54.34	$0.19	
Minimum	95%	Current	$55.64	$—	$36.10

control to $59.91 per WRVU, then the hospital would pay the practice an additional $0.76 per WRVU for all WRVUs generated by physicians in that region as part of the Level I payment. Using the grid in Exhibit 14.32, if the local practice site in question had current (e.g., historic) controllable costs per WRVU of $55.64, and that local site improved controllable costs to $45.22 per WRVU, then the hospital would pay the practice an additional $1.52 per WRVU for all WRVUs generated by the physicians in that particular practice location as part of the Level I payment.

Total Level I Amount Paid by the Hospital to the Medical Practice

The total amount paid by the hospital to the medical practice is determined based on the combination of the three different measures under an end-stage plan, as illustrated in Exhibit 14.33. This example assumes the application of concepts illustrated above related to the production and cost portions of the Level I payment. Payments due to performance in relation to quality and patient satisfaction factors would be in addition to the payments listed in Exhibit 14.33 from the hospital to the physician practice as a Level I payment. In Exhibit 14.33, the total amount paid from the hospital to the medical practice for Level I payments would equal the sum of:

► WRVUs for site 1 × $34.58

► WRVUs for site 2 × $35.34

► WRVUs for site 3 × $34.77

► WRVUs for site 4 × $35.34

► WRVUs for site 5 × $35.91

► WRVUs for site 6 × $34.77

An assessment of the strengths and weaknesses of Hospital Plan 9 is provided in Exhibit 14.34.

EXHIBIT 14.33   Level I Payment from Hospital to Medical Practice

Base Dollar per RVU	$33.25 (Based on Group-Level Production Measured vs. Target)					
Regional Controllable Cost per WRVU	Region A $.95 per WRVU		Region B $1.33 per WRVU		Region C $1.14 per WRVU	
	Site 1: $0.38 per WRVU	Site 1: $1.14 per WRVU	Site 3: $0.19 per WRVU	Site 4: $0.76 per WRVU	Site 5: $1.52 per WRVU	Site 6: $0.38 per WRVU
Total Amount Paid per WRVU (listed by local site)	$34.58	$35.34	$34.77	$35.34	$35.91	$34.77

EXHIBIT 14.34

Assessment of Hospital Example 9 – Indirect Hospital or Contracted Group Using WRVUs and Cost Control Plan

Dimension	Strengths	Weaknesses
Measure	Pays market levels for services performed, with production and cost components treated separately.	
Productivity	Promotes attention to enhanced productivity at multiple levels.	
Financial	Focuses physician and managerial attention on the effective management of *controllable costs,* as measured by improvements in the cost per unit of service (e.g., cost per WRVU). Allows for improvements in controllable costs by a combination of enhanced production and cost control. Couples cost of practice and production in determination of compensation.	Costs may receive excessive focus or productivity may become *the* primary focus to the exclusion of other important activities or behaviors.
Simplicity		Complex plan requiring significant administrative infrastructure. Intensity of data and analysis requires close attention to implementation and reporting.
Alignment	Creates an incentive for physician involvement in practice operations. Allows medical practice to determine underlying compensation system to allocate funds paid for services by hospital under indirect compensation arrangement. Establishes interorganizational goal alignment (e.g., hospital and medical practice).	Requires group practice orientation and greater levels of group cooperation. Focus on productivity and cost of practice may preclude attention to other areas (e.g., teaching, patient satisfaction, etc.).
"Fairness"	Does not link compensation to system revenues or receipts, thereby making physicians responsible only for activities within their control. Forces transparency of past and strategic decisions (e.g., expensive space that would not generally be acquired by a private practice).	Potential conflict between physicians and management related to operational choices.

© 2006 Johnson & Walker Keegan

The compensation plans for hospital-affiliated and hospital-employed groups generally differ from plans for bona fide Group Practices. The Stark law exceptions for direct employment, personal service arrangements, and others are typically used in these types of arrangements, and each of these exceptions imposes specific requirements. In particular, physicians may not receive "incident to" credit in determining "productivity bonuses" that may be paid under these exceptions to the Stark law, nor credit for DHS that are not personally performed.

As demonstrated by the hospital plan examples in this chapter, the plans range from simplistic to complex. In addition, variation of the individualistic to team-oriented plans discussed in Chapter 13 are available to hospitals as they craft the compensation to be paid under these arrangements, although, in all instances, appropriate modifications based on the applicable legal requirements are required.

In the next chapter, we provide examples of compensation plans used in the academic setting. Many of the plans illustrated in Chapter 13 and 14 may be adapted for use in academic settings, although the complexity and challenges of plan development and implementation are generally greater in the academic health care environment.

Notes

1. However, in many instances, the additional requirements and considerations related to FMV and reasonableness of compensation may also apply as an additional level of compliance requirements.

2. In reality, many physicians do consider such issues, but plans that look solely at individual physician revenues and expenses provide little or no real reason to consider such matters.

3. The final rule to the Stark law imposes specific requirements for the determination of such FMV hourly rates. As a general matter, those requirements involve averaging median national compensation data from specific compensation surveys for a specialty, and dividing the result by 2,000, or basing an hourly rate on the hourly rate paid to emergency room physicians in the market under defined circumstances. Consult the final rule 42 C.F.R. § 411.351 (definition of FMV) for more information.

4. When the plan is based on CFTE performance, the levels are uniform per CFTE being purchased, as measured by time. This type of approach generally works best when the group is a single specialty, or when the plan is further adapted and tailored to involve measurement per CFTE by specialty.

5. This notion is supported by data relating to practices that are better financial performers, which generally show higher operating costs (and higher revenue associated with these costs) per physician than in other practices. In the better financial performing practice, the additional cost is translated into a more efficient practice that can produce more revenues. It is clearly possible to "go overboard" in efforts to cut costs.

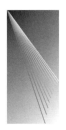

FIFTEEN

Compensation Plans in Academic Practices

ompensation plans in academic practices are among the most complex, as they not only attempt to measure and reward faculty engaged in clinical practice, but also recognize the faculty member's teaching, research, and service activities. While the clinical component of compensation may be determined by strategies as sophisticated as those embraced by many private medical practices, extending the performance and reward system to recognize the other parts of the academic mission – to create a compensation plan that is aligned with each component of that mission – is not an easy task.

The boundary line between private practice and academic practice is blurring. Many academic physicians "look like" their private practice counterparts by spending significant portions of their time in clinical pursuits. Likewise, many private practitioners resemble faculty (and may hold volunteer faculty appointments) and are involved in teaching and/or research. Academic practices will often look toward their private practice counterparts when designing methods to measure and reward clinical work and effort. Similarly, private practice physicians engaged in teaching and/or research will often look toward their academic colleagues to determine methods by which to measure and reward nonclinical activities.

The key for both academic and private practices is to craft a compensation plan that is aligned. In the case of faculty practice plans, internal alignment is needed among the multiple, diverse clinical, teaching, research, and service activities and also with the goals and future direction and strategy of the specialty, division, and department. The plan must also be aligned with key external entities, such as the school of medicine and the university as a whole, and with the academic practice's external environment.

FACULTY PRACTICE PLANS DEFINED

The term "faculty practice plan" is used to describe at least three different activities or entities. A faculty practice plan may refer to an administrative structure, a method by which compensation is determined in the academic setting, a collective faculty body, or potentially all three of these, depending upon the context.

1. **Administrative Structure.** Some use the term "faculty practice plan" to refer to the centralized billing operation and other support services of the clinical

enterprise, such as contracting with third-party payers, group purchasing, and other similar practice management support. When "faculty practice plans" are used in this context they generally refer to a structure that is not dissimilar to a management services organization in the private or hospital-affiliated practice worlds, which provide business support services to the clinical enterprise.

2. **Compensation Plan.** Alternatively, a faculty practice plan may refer to the method by which faculty are compensated. A faculty practice plan is comprised of the same three components as other compensation plans: (1) a funds flow model; (2) a compensation plan architecture; and (3) a compensation plan methodology(ies). In this context, the faculty practice plan may be established at the school level, the department level, or the division level, or, in some cases, all three. Many academic institutions have two compensation plans:

   ► An overall plan that outlines the architecture, funds flow, tithing requirements, base salary levels, maximums, and other key elements, combined with,

   ► A department's specific plan(s) that address(es) the technical methods by which faculty salary levels will be determined, such as how revenue and expenses are divided and distributed; expectations regarding faculty participation in teaching, research, clinical, and service activities; and other related details.

   Some academic institutions have even expanded to three broad compensation plans consisting of an overall plan architecture defined at the school or university level, department-specific plans, and divisional plans, with expectations of alignment among each of these layers.

3. **Collective Body.** Many will use the term "faculty practice plan" to indicate faculty who are party to a faculty practice plan. In this reference, the faculty practice plan is a collective body of faculty; essentially, a grouping of like-types of faculty.

   For purposes of this text, we will focus on the second definition – the faculty practice plan as a compensation plan consisting of a funds flow model, a plan architecture, and a plan methodology(ies).

CONTEXTUAL ISSUES IN ACADEMIC PRACTICES TODAY

It is important to understand some of the key contextual issues involved in academic practices today, as these issues play an instrumental role in influencing the type of faculty practice plan that is designed and/or available to an academic practice.

► KEY SUCCESS FACTORS FOR ACADEMIC PRACTICES

The key success factors for today's academic practices include issues regarding the business of medicine, such as clinical revenue generation and expense management. Equally important are access to patients in a competitive delivery environment for

EXHIBIT 15.1	Key Success Factors for Today's Academic Practices

➤ Clinical enterprise revenue generation and enhancement;

➤ Access to patients in a competitive delivery environment to ensure sufficient clinical exposure for medical student, resident, and fellowship training;

➤ Access to extramural funding support for basic science and clinical research;

➤ Management and accountability structures linked to strategic plans to guide research and service efforts;

➤ Flexibility to respond to change;

➤ Effective corporate compliance, business risk management, and expenditure controls; and

➤ Faculty compensation plans aligned with environment and internal organizational goals.

© 2006 Johnson & Walker Keegan

medical students, residents, and fellows, and access to extramural research funds from both federal contracts and grants and, increasingly, private sources. Today's academic practices are required to demonstrate flexibility in positioning themselves for the future. Alignment of the compensation and incentive system to promote a complex set of goals and objectives in the academic practice is a key element of faculty practice plan design. Exhibit 15.1 provides a list of these key success factors for today's academic practices.

➤ INCREASED FOCUS ON CLINICAL SERVICE PERFORMANCE AND PRODUCTION

Among the numerous changes that have occurred in the past few years in academic medicine is the increased focus on clinical service performance and production in the determination and payment of faculty compensation. This is required for a number of reasons, including the increased need for academic practices to rely on clinical service income to support components of the academic mission. Thus, today's faculty practice plans typically have a heightened focus on clinical productivity than those of the past.

➤ EVOLUTION OF FACULTY MEMBER COMPENSATION EXPECTATIONS

Equally apparent is an evolution of faculty member expectations of faculty practice plans. Historically, the compensation plan that was used to recognize and reward faculty served as a generally silent framework as the faculty worked to balance clinical, research, teaching, and service commitments. Today, many faculty are voicing desires for greater transparency in plan mechanics and greater linkage between work and compensation. Many faculty expect compensation levels for the clinical portion of their time that are more consistent with those of private practice physicians.

► EVOLVING ORGANIZATIONAL AND ADMINISTRATIVE STRUCTURES

Implicit in the design questions for a faculty practice plan are questions related to organizational and administrative structures within the faculty practice plan, and within the academic health care delivery system more generally. By organizational and administrative structures, we refer to the structural, financial, political, and other realities in the academic medical environment. Central to such issues are questions of legal structure and control, and the relationships between and among such parties as the medical school dean, the department chairs, and the academic hospital leaders. Also to be considered are the number of separate legal entities involved in the medical school and in resident education and training and ultimately, questions of autonomy and decision making regarding faculty salary and related issues.

Historically, although every setting for academic medicine is relatively unique, each system can generally be classified by reference to several basic structural models.

Centralized Models

In heavily centralized structures, the practice plan and the departments effectively constitute large, complex, multispecialty groups. Questions of autonomy and control between and among the centralized authority (whether that be a dean, a practice plan administrative body or board, or some other collective) and the department chairs typically ensue. In such centralized models, there is generally one (or a very few) legal entities that are involved in the delivery of clinical practice services and that house the faculty practice plan. Because of this, the practice plan's operations and funds flow are typically coordinated and managed via a centralized system. That "system" may, in fact, yield considerable autonomy to individual departments and their chairs when it comes to faculty compensation levels, compensation plans, and related issues, but the fact that a centralized system exists means that some level of centralized coordination and management authority is deemed to exist.

Federated Models

Just as individualistic compensation plans lie at the opposite extreme of what we've referred to as "team-oriented" plans, many academic medicine structures have historically involved "federated" structural models. In contrast to centralized models, in these models there frequently are multiple legal entities involved in the delivery of clinical services; therefore, there typically are multiple faculty practice plans. As a result, the questions of autonomy and control between and among the medical school dean, hospital leaders, and department chairs will also be more complex, with department chairs or other leaders of individual entities that are part of the federated model oftentimes exercising considerably greater power, autonomy, and control. In these models, although there may be some degree of centralized management and authority, that authority tends to be relatively weak. Thus, the centralized system's power and authority have generally been viewed as being granted rather than existing as a matter of right.

Mixed Structures

Between the centralized and federated models are numerous other "mixed" structures that tend to blend the characteristics of the two extremes. In these models, there is relatively greater understanding and appreciation of the relationships between the departments and centralized authority, and the negotiation regarding issues of finances, power, and autonomy is somewhere in between the two models referenced above.

We highlight the fact that different organizational structures exist because, just as in private medical practices where a practice falls on the continuum of compensation plan architectures will influence how the practice addresses issues of practice finances and culture, the nature of the compensation plans that will be used in the academic practice setting is influenced by where the institution falls on the structural continuum.

This means, for example, that when the academic institution uses a heavily centralized structure, and when changes to the compensation system are viewed to be required, the changes may result in relatively greater centralization and control (e.g., through the development of a uniform compensation plan architecture and a consistent system that applies in a uniform manner in every department). Or, the history of centralization may result in the development of a more federated model within the centralized practice plan as a means to promote greater autonomy, accountability, and responsibility at the level of individual departments or divisions. In either of these circumstances, the focus of change is likely to be both at the level of the underlying funds flow model *and* at the more specific compensation plan architectures that are used at the departmental, divisional, or other levels.

Likewise, where the academic institution has embraced a federated model, the change process will primarily be directed more at the funds flow issues – with the primary emphasis being on imposing relatively greater standardization and control over the tithing requirements and asking questions regarding the value of benefits received from such assessments. Some structural changes will also be made to reduce, if not eliminate, the federated structure (such as by making all of the otherwise separate practice plans part of a single physician organization). Even in such models, however, the primary focus will be on the level and degree of power and control that will be ceded to the centralized system, while considerable autonomy and authority will commonly be preserved at the departmental or other levels.

In an academic institution, the conditions "on the ground" at the time a new compensation plan is being considered will substantially influence the direction and nature of change from the current to future compensation plans and systems. For example, when the current system is heavily centralized but the centralized administrative body is perceived to be doing an inadequate job in certain areas (e.g., professional fee billing and collection performance), the focus may be on both improving that performance and allowing individual departments to structure their own arrangements. Conversely, when individual departments or divisions in a federated model are at deficit status, the focus may be on imposing additional requirements and management discipline on the departments through a centralized system or plan.

Likewise, in many public systems where financial support from the state is limited and frequently in decline, part of the solution to compensation-related questions will lie in dramatic changes to the underlying structures and traditions that have worked in the past. This will sometimes result in clinical faculty becoming employees of the academic teaching hospital or in the creation of other arrangements such that the fees for clinical faculty members' professional services will become hospital property, and the hospital can therefore receive "provider-based" reimbursement under the Medicare hospital outpatient prospective payment system (OPPS) as a means to provide additional funds to support the academic missions. In these systems, the change in compensation practices may involve the elimination of separate practice plan entities, coupled with a redefinition of the power and authority of departmental chairs as leaders of their respective academic departments and functions, and medical directors within the hospital environment.

Thus, the institution's current internal environment will influence the nature and direction of change that will occur in its faculty compensation systems, and, quite possibly, it will lead to changes in the structure of the system itself. In addition, the external environment in which the academic institution resides will also significantly influence changes that will occur. For the most part, in today's complex environment we tend to see greater rationalization of funds flow and faculty compensation practices primarily because of the financial challenges confronting medicine in general and academic medicine in particular. Yet, the degree and nature of change will tend to be influenced by both internal and external conditions affecting the practice plan and the system of medical education and resident training that is in effect.

► EVOLUTION OF FACULTY PRACTICE PLANS

The method by which faculty are paid in the academic setting has undergone significant fluctuation in the recent past. From a relatively predominant focus on fixed or straight salary levels, faculty practice plans now array their compensation methodologies along a wide continuum to ensure that the academic mission – which increasingly rests on clinical dollars generated by faculty – is met.

We are often asked what the "typical" faculty practice plan looks like or are asked to recommend two or three academic institutions that have the "best" plan. Unfortunately, there is no "typical plan," and what works for one academic institution may not work for another due to the complexity and variety of today's structures, encompassing health systems, academic medical centers, community teaching hospitals, schools of medicine, faculty practice plan organizations, and departments.

Some universities still require the majority of faculty to be "triple threat" physicians, while others have added clinical and teaching-track appointments to ensure a "triple threat" division, specialty, or department. Some schools of medicine have significant donor and/or extramural research support, while others rely heavily on revenue generated via the clinical enterprise. Some schools treat revenue generated from work differently if it is "private" as opposed to "departmental," while others include *all* work performed by the faculty in the compensation methodology, inclusive of expert witness fees and honoraria. Some schools are not even involved in the clinical enterprise; instead, a separate faculty practice plan is established to manage clinical services and associated revenue cycles.

Many universities will impose specific requirements related to the amount of compensation that may be earned and paid to any individual faculty member. These guidelines typically impose a cap that requires administrative approval at the school or university level for it to be waived. In addition to the application of such waivers, legal requirements governing tax-exempt organizations generally require that total compensation received by any faculty member may not exceed amounts that are reasonable based on the nature and scope of the services provided. In Chapter 16, "The Special World of Hospital and Academic Practices – Assessing Reasonableness and Promoting Compliance," we present a further discussion of these areas.

Despite the recent focus on faculty practice plan modification, in some academic settings the faculty practice plans are at best, rudimentary. And although the goals of a new plan might be to encourage greater clinical production, more closely align compensation with components of the academic mission, enhance transparency, and the like, a new faculty practice plan must be developed and implemented in light of the realities of the past. Those realities commonly include competition with community physicians for a defined patient population, limited faculty time devoted to clinical activities, financial deficits at the department and/or individual faculty levels, complex administrative infrastructures, the need for capital spending, and other challenges. Each academic institution and its clinical departments are uniquely situated among these realities, and this impacts the type of faculty practice plan that is, or may be, developed for an institution and its physicians.

APPROACH TO FACULTY PRACTICE PLAN DESIGN

The approach to compensation planning in an academic setting is the same as for other medical practices, and it is generally similar to the 12-step process we outlined in Chapter 2. A key difference, however, is the expanded design complexity of such a setting. Due to the complexities of academic medicine and the need to align the compensation plan with specific components of the academic mission, as well as the fact that each department is situated among many interorganizational units, the design phase in compensation planning typically is more complex and takes considerably longer than in other settings. It is not unusual for the full compensation planning process to take 6 to 12 months in the academic setting – if not more in some instances.

In developing a compensation plan for an academic practice, questions need to be asked and answered on a wide range of issues, including prioritization of goals, performance opportunities and requirements, methodological details and concerns, and issues related to current circumstances and opportunities. Key questions in each of these areas are summarized below.

Goal prioritization, such as:

- ▶ Achieve median levels of compensation based on academic surveys?
- ▶ Recruit and retain faculty through competitive salary offerings?
- ▶ Encourage more clinical productivity?
- ▶ Encourage more research?
- ▶ Encourage more teaching?
- ▶ Match work effort with funding sources?
- ▶ Encourage quality care?
- ▶ Ensure fiscal responsibility?
- ▶ Others?

Performance opportunities and requirements, such as:

- ▶ What level of autonomy should departments have in establishing department-specific compensation plans within an overall architectural framework?
- ▶ What revenue sources should be included in the compensation plan; e.g., clinical contracts, expert witness fees, honoraria, ancillary services, etc.?
- ▶ What financial performance is expected of departments (e.g., reserve levels, expenditure levels)?
- ▶ What behaviors and/or values within the organization should the compensation plan encourage, promote, and reward?
- ▶ Should the plan discreetly reward each component of the academic mission?
- ▶ How does compensation tie to faculty progression through the academic ranks?
- ▶ At what level should faculty be rewarded (e.g., individual, division, department, overall faculty practice plan, or in combination)?

Methodological details and concerns, including:

- ▶ How should the clinical component of compensation be aligned with the total compensation target for the faculty?
- ▶ What benchmark sources(s) should be used to target full compensation levels of faculty (e.g., Medical Group Management Association [MGMA], Association of American Medical Colleges [AAMC], specialty-specific surveys, blended measures, academic or private, others)?

▶ How should faculty be compensated for work conducted at outreach locations?

▶ How should faculty be compensated for work involved in new clinical programs?

▶ How should faculty be compensated for indigent care?

Issues related to current circumstances and opportunities, such as:

▶ Does a department have more faculty than would be required for teaching, research, clinical, and service requirements? If so, how will this affect compensation levels for faculty?

▶ Is there a differential productivity outcome between faculty within a given clinical full-time equivalency (CFTE) level and, if so, why?

▶ What is the financial state of a department and its ability to pay faculty members at median levels?

▶ Are clinical contracts and grants bringing in sufficient revenue when compared with the time, productivity, and directorship required for these arrangements?

▶ What approach to compensation should be taken for the faculty member who is a stellar researcher but who is less active in clinical service?

▶ Have historical or recent events created the need to use resources that might have been reserved or set aside for faculty compensation?

We can list many more questions that need to be addressed; however, this list demonstrates the sheer complexity of compensation planning in the academic setting.

KEY COMPONENTS OF FACULTY PRACTICE PLANS

Physician compensation plans in academic settings still must address the three key areas of any compensation plan: (1) the funds flow model that outlines revenue sources and treatment of those sources; (2) the plan architecture that provides the overarching framework for the plan; and (3) the plan methodology and its technical dimensions that are used to determine and pay faculty for their services. In the academic setting, there are additional issues in each of these areas that need to be taken into account, as further discussed below.

▶ FUNDS FLOW MODELS

By funds flow model, we mean how the academic institution has defined its revenue treatment, tithing requirements, and responsibilities for operating costs – with obvious impacts to compensation planning for its faculty. In practical terms, funds flow models address issues and treatment of funding support, to include support between and among various entities such as the health system, the university, the hospital, the school of medicine, the faculty practice plan organization, and others. They also address expenditure treatment, including taxation or tithing requirements and cost of clinical practice, divisions, and central department administration.

Some academic institutions have multiple avenues from which faculty are paid (e.g., the faculty practice organization and the university). In addition to these structures, specific fund categories are identified as restricted (e.g., research dollars, gift funds tied to specific purposes, or state funds that need to be used by year-end and may or may not "cover" faculty benefit expenditures).

We have seen some academic institutions err by approaching compensation planning as if it were simply a budgeting exercise or a method of redividing a finite pool of funds. In fact, the planning for a new faculty practice plan should be approached in the same way it is conducted in nonacademic practices – with a definition of goals, followed by design principles, and proceeding through a systematic process (see the 12-step process described in Chapter 2). Certainly the funds flow model, the compensation plan architecture, and the plan's methodology need to be aligned; however, equally important is the alignment of the plan with the academic mission. A budgeting approach to faculty compensation planning can be delimiting.

The differences in funds flow models among academic institutions generally relate to at least the following variations among institutions:

- ► Structural differences in organization;
- ► Market and political forces;
- ► Presence or absence of faculty practice plan organization;
- ► Presence or absence of a central billing office;
- ► Tithing or levels of taxation;
- ► Revenue sources and uses of funds (restricted and nonrestricted);
- ► External contracts and their related management;
- ► Reserves and their funding mechanisms;
- ► Level of subsidization granted to departments;
- ► Financial status of departments and the school of medicine; and
- ► Levels of autonomy granted to departments.

The funds flow models are generally designed with one or more compensation plan architectures in mind. However, funds flow models are needed whether the university has adopted a single school-wide compensation architecture and methodology, whether the university has encouraged department-specific compensation plans that are aligned within a common architectural framework, or any combination of these. Four basic examples of funds flow models are provided to demonstrate the variability of the models in use today.

Funds Flow Model 1 – Clinical Revenue Treatment with Central Business or Billing Office (CBO)

Funds Flow Model 1 is depicted in Exhibit 15.2. In this model, both direct and indirect expenses are subtracted from clinical revenue, generally defined as professional fee revenue generated by the faculty, prior to a determination of faculty compensation levels. This model is essentially a team-oriented expenditure model, with departmental expenditures subtracted from revenues before a determination is made regarding faculty compensation (which may be individual or team-oriented, as determined by the departmental compensation plan).

The steps in this model are listed below.

Step 1: Determine Professional Fee Net Collections at the Department Level

Net collections from professional services are determined for each department.

Step 2: Subtract "Indirect" Expenses

For purposes of this example, indirect expenses include:

- ▶ **Dean's tax.** Typically defined as a flat percentage of net professional fee (and potentially other) revenue.

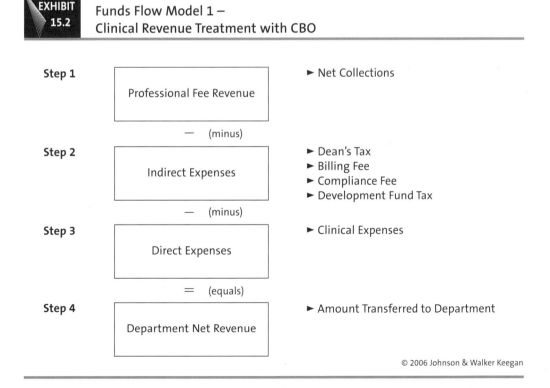

| | EXHIBIT 15.2 | Funds Flow Model 1 – Clinical Revenue Treatment with CBO |

Step 1	Professional Fee Revenue	▶ Net Collections
	— (minus)	
Step 2	Indirect Expenses	▶ Dean's Tax ▶ Billing Fee ▶ Compliance Fee ▶ Development Fund Tax
	— (minus)	
Step 3	Direct Expenses	▶ Clinical Expenses
	= (equals)	
Step 4	Department Net Revenue	▶ Amount Transferred to Department

© 2006 Johnson & Walker Keegan

► **CBO fee (billing and collection, contracting).** Typically defined as a flat percentage of net professional fee revenue to cover the cost of the CBO. Various approaches, however, can be taken with regard to the expense levels to be charged to departments, including equal share, percentage of net collections, percent to total claims volume, graduated threshold models, and others.

► **Compliance office fee.** Typically defined as a flat percentage of net professional fee revenue. Some academic institutions include this fee in the CBO fee above; others provide separate treatment.

► **Development fund tax.** Typically defined as a flat percentage of net professional fee revenue.

Step 3: Subtract Direct Expenses

In this example, direct expenses associated with clinical services are subtracted. These direct expenses include the typical practice overhead expenditures encompassing staffing and general operating costs of the clinical enterprise.

Step 4: The Balance Is Available to Departments

Many options exist to distribute the balance to faculty in the form of compensation. For example, the department may institute a departmental tax and then transfer money to divisions where division-specific compensation plans determine allocation to individual faculty. Alternatively, the department may manage finances centrally and implement a department-wide compensation plan that is mission-based or any number of plans that fall between these two extremes.

Funds Flow Model 2 – Full Revenue Treatment with Faculty Practice Plan Organization and Revenue Sharing

In this second funds flow model, a central faculty practice plan (FPP) organization contracts with the university and the hospital to provide clinical, teaching, and service activities. As shown in Exhibit 15.3, these contracted revenues flow through the faculty practice plan organization that is responsible for billing and collection, management of clinical practice sites, and administrative services and support. In this example, a revenue sharing model has been implemented between the faculty practice plan organization and the departments consisting of two elements: (1) a practice support fund; and (2) a practice development fund. The percentage of collections paid into each of these funds is determined on an annual basis. The practice support fund is used to subsidize – to some extent – departments in deficit status and/or those that are penalized due to a negative payer mix. The practice development fund is used for recruitment and retention, clinical programmatic development, and other growth and expansion activities for the practice plan as a whole.

The steps in this model include:

Step 1. Establish contracts with hospital and school of medicine;

EXHIBIT 15.3

Funds Flow Model 2 –
Full Revenue Treatment with FPP Organization and Revenue Sharing

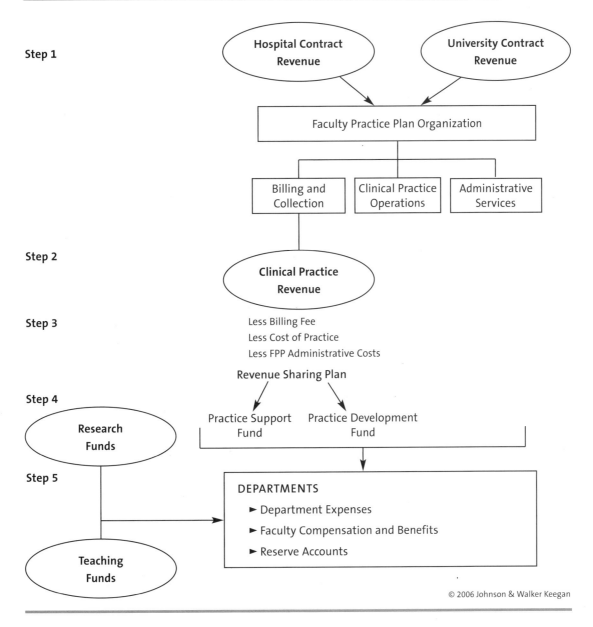

© 2006 Johnson & Walker Keegan

Step 2. Determine net collections from professional services;

Step 3. Deduct billing and collection expenses, cost of practice, and administrative services expenses incurred by the faculty practice plan organization;

Step 4. Deduct the amounts calculated as a percentage of net collections for two "revenue-sharing" funds: (1) the practice support fund; and (2) the practice development fund; and

Step 5. Allocate the balance to departments for distribution through department-specific compensation plans.

Funds Flow Model 3 — Full Revenue Treatment with Department-Based Billing

This example, depicted in Exhibit 15.4, reflects full revenue treatment assuming department-based billing and collection for clinical services. In this model, distinct revenue types are linked to their originating source; for example, university, school of medicine, hospital, community, or department. Outside earnings of faculty, such as expert witness fees, honoraria, and royalties, are addressed as part of the funds flow, with such earn-

EXHIBIT 15.4 Funds Flow Model 3 — Full Revenue Treatment with Departmental Billing

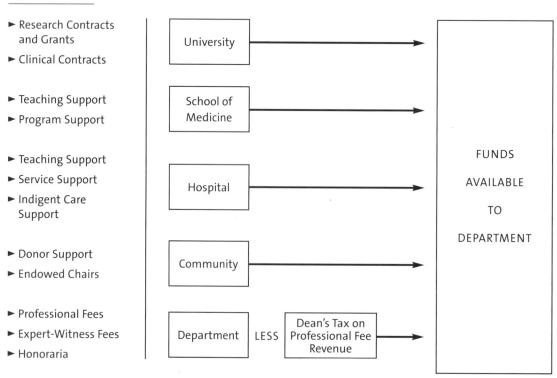

© 2006 Johnson & Walker Keegan

ings being allowed to be retained outside of the practice plan, or required to be brought into the plan. A dean's tax is applied to professional fee earnings (and potentially other fund sources). Since the department manages its own billing operation, it has latitude to decide on expenditure treatment for these services.

The steps in this funds flow model example include:

Step 1. Identify the sources of revenue;

Step 2. Identify the types of revenue and amounts;

Step 3. Assess the dean's tax on professional fee revenue;

Step 4. Allocate funds to the department; and

Step 5. Have the faculty self-report additional income earned and deposited outside the university.

Actual compensation paid to faculty will then be subject to the school, department, and/or division compensation plans. Typically, department-specific or division-specific plans are situated within an overall compensation plan architectural framework that has been developed for university-wide implementation.

Funds Flow Model 4 – Full Revenue Treatment: Mission-Based

To create viable financial structures in the academic setting, many universities have elected to pursue mission-based funds flow models. This model type is depicted in Exhibit 15.5.

Mission-based funds flow models link revenue sources with each part of the academic mission: research, teaching, clinical, and service. In mission-based models, it is assumed that research dollars fund research activities, teaching dollars fund teaching, service dollars fund service activities, and faculty are generally required to generate clinical revenue sufficient to not only cover the portion of their compensation that is not funded via other methods, but also to develop clinical programs, recruit faculty, and fund other key program areas.

The steps in this funds flow model include:

Step 1. Identify the components of the academic mission;

Step 2. Identify the sources and levels of funds for each mission;

Step 3. Assess the dean's tax on professional fee (and potentially other) revenue, and assess other associated costs (e.g., billing fees); and

Step 4. Identify funds that are available to the department.

▶ FACULTY PRACTICE PLAN ARCHITECTURES

After the funds flow model is determined and the funds available for faculty compensation purposes are identified, the compensation plan architecture needs to be determined. The basic compensation plan architectures that have been described in previous

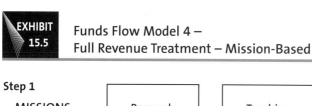

Funds Flow Model 4 –
Full Revenue Treatment – Mission-Based

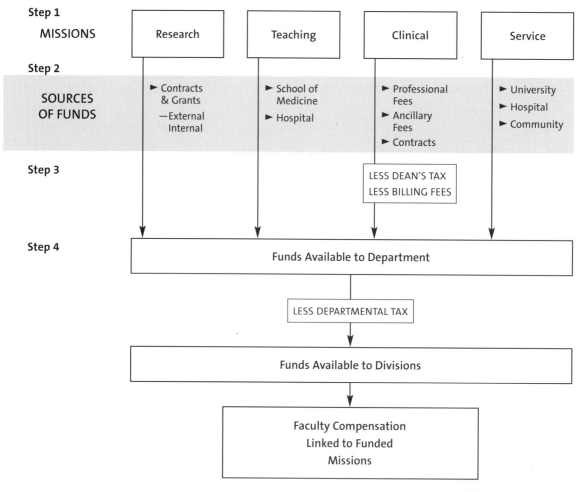

© 2006 Johnson & Walker Keegan

chapters can also be adapted to and used as faculty compensation plans. Thus, a faculty practice plan could, for example, adopt and implement a straight salary plan that uses unit-based compensation (Revenue Element 1 on the compensation plan matrix) and Architecture A on the array of compensation plan architectures, or a plan that uses a guaranteed share, base salary plus incentive compensation plan (Revenue Element 2) and Architecture B.

Likewise, within a single practice plan, a department, a division, or other subset, any of the more individualistic architectures, including those that use a pure production allocation of revenues, coupled with an allocation of cost of practice on a "strict" or "modified" cost accounting basis, through the use of a negotiated expense allocation system or the like, can also be used. In short, virtually all of the basic architectures described in the previous chapters can be used or adapted for use in an academic setting – with appropriate attention to the unique nature and requirements of the academic setting. The compensation plan matrix and array of basic compensation architecture are restated in Exhibits 15.6 and 15.7.

EXHIBIT 15.6   The Compensation Plan Matrix

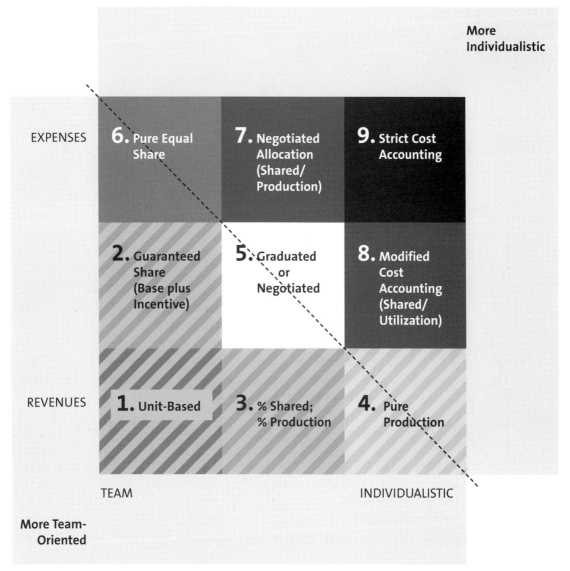

© 2006 Johnson & Walker Keegan

EXHIBIT 15.7 Array of Compensation Plan Architectures

Architecture	A	B	C	D	E	F	G	H	I	J	K	L	M	N	O	P	Q	R
Revenue Element	1	2	3	4	5	2	3	2	3	2	3	2	3	4	4	4	4	4
Expense Element						6	6	7	7	8	8	9	9	5	6	7	8	9
			TEAM					MIDDLE GROUND							INDIVIDUALISTIC			

© 2006 Johnson & Walker Keegan

A common body of compensation plans that are frequently used in academic settings involve plan architectures that are generally referred to as "XYZ plans." An XYZ plan is actually an extension of the base plus incentive architecture (using Revenue Element 2, guaranteed share of revenues or income) and Architecture B, as discussed in Chapter 13. It involves three distinct compensation segments.

1. Base Salary (X)

The base salary or X portion of compensation typically comprises the largest portion of the faculty member's compensation. This base salary may be tied to academic rank (e.g., assistant, associate, or professor level), linked to historical compensation levels of the faculty, tied to a percentage of market-based compensation levels, or linked to production levels (measured by professional services gross charges or net collections, WRVUs, some other measure, or in combination). Typically, the base salary is considered "guaranteed," with one-twelfth of this amount paid to the faculty each month. Faculty benefits are often calculated on the base salary level and/or on a combination of X plus Y. The same basic concepts outlined in connection with Architecture B in Chapter 13 apply to the base salary component in this context.

2. Supplement (Y)

The Y portion of faculty salary fluctuates to recognize teaching, research, and service efforts. The Y can be considered to be either: (1) additive; or (2) substituted. When it is additive, the Y is a supplement to the faculty member's base salary – additional money is paid to the faculty member to recognize his or her additional activities beyond the base level. For example, a faculty member asked to assume the role of division director, residency training director, or medical student clerkship director may receive a "stipend" to recognize these additional responsibilities, which is paid as a Y supplement.

When the Y component is considered to be substituted, base salary (X) may be reduced by the offsetting amount paid via the Y supplement. For example, the X plus Y portion of the faculty member's compensation would equal what he or she previously made via X alone, but the work activities associated with the Y replace some or all of those that are otherwise expected in connection with the base salary X payment.

The decision as to whether to treat the Y portion of salary as additive or substituted will depend on the funds flow model that has been embraced and the type of service for which the supplement is being paid. Two examples follow.

Example 1: Payment for Administrative Services

If the base salary for a faculty member is largely derived from clinical revenue and that faculty member is asked to take on an administrative role for the department, it is likely that the faculty member may devote less time to clinical activities. In this example, the Y supplement is likely to be treated in a substituted fashion. If, on the other hand, this same faculty member is asked to take on additional administrative tasks on top of his or her current responsibilities, then the Y supplement would likely be additive to recognize the additional work and effort required for the administrative assignment.

Example 2: Payment for Research Activity

If the faculty member generates extramural funding for his or her salary, that portion of salary payment is typically paid via the Y, or supplement component. In this case, base or X salary may be reduced by the Y amount. In general terms, the extramural dollars are used to fund some or all of the faculty member's base salary, yet the actual payment mechanism may be handled through the Y component.

3. Incentive (Z)

The Z portion of the XYZ plan typically consists of incentive or bonus payment based on individual, divisional, departmental, and/or institutional performance. The incentive is typically focused on clinical productivity; however, a number of institutions have implemented additional performance measures that move beyond simple production to recognize quality and service. Some have instituted incentives for "clinical" activity and separate incentives for "academic" activity, the latter rewarding research and teaching accomplishments.

The XYZ architecture can be used either as a single faculty compensation plan governing compensation for all faculty or as an overarching architecture in which department-specific and/or division-specific compensation plans are situated.

► FACULTY TIME SPENT IN CLINICAL ACTIVITY – CFTE LEVELS

In academic institutions, a fundamental measure for faculty compensation plans is a Clinical Full-time Equivalent (CFTE). This term is used in the academic setting to determine the portion of the faculty member's time that is spent in clinical pursuits. The

CFTE of a physician is distinguished from the physician's time spent performing research, teaching, and service activity. For example, some faculty have extremely low CFTE levels due to high levels of research activity, while others may be involved heavily in clinical activity such that a faculty member who spends 85 percent of his or her time in clinical pursuits will be considered a .85 CFTE.

It is admittedly difficult to parcel out a faculty member's time into discrete academic mission components – teaching, research, clinical, and service. No one day is "typical," and the boundary for each component is unclear. For example, if the faculty member supervises a resident in the clinic, yet also sees the patient and bills a professional fee for that service, should this time be counted as teaching or clinical, or should the time be apportioned in some fashion to both categories? Some institutions implement survey instruments, time studies, and other similar tools to attempt to quantify the time the faculty member spends in clinical work.

A common approach to determining CFTE levels by individual physicians is to calculate the CFTE based on the current production of the faculty member. In this method, the current WRVUs that are produced by a faculty member are identified. The WRVUs are then divided by the median academic survey benchmark for WRVUs (specialty-specific benchmark) to determine the faculty member's CFTE based on current clinical production. See Chapter 7 for an example of benchmarking related to CFTE levels.

A CFTE determination is needed when a faculty practice plan segments compensation into the component parts of the academic mission; for example, clinical vs. teaching vs. research. It is also useful in identifying opportunities to enhance the production of a faculty member or a department. For example, a faculty member could report 50 percent clinical time, yet his or her CFTE calculated on actual work outputs (e.g., WRVUs) may only be calculated at 25 percent. This would permit investigation and opportunities to explore enhanced clinical production (and/or efficiency) during clinical time.

FACULTY PRACTICE PLAN EXAMPLES

Faculty practice plans work in conjunction with funds flow models and plan architectures by defining the means to determine and pay faculty compensation, and by functioning as an incentive and feedback system regarding faculty expectations and performance. Well-designed compensation plans serve to encourage (or discourage) performance in furtherance of the academic mission. They address faculty compensation for teaching, research, clinical, and service activities. As with all compensation plans, regardless of the setting, the faculty compensation plan is typically designed and implemented with attention to two issues: (1) process related to plan design, modeling, education, and buy-in; and (2) technical methodology, mechanics, and implementation or transitional strategies of the plan.

No two faculty practice plans are exactly the same, and the options available to a particular academic institution will vary based on the contextual issues discussed earlier in this chapter. Chief among those are its legal designation, the centralized or decentralized nature of the institution, and the state of its current financial situation.

The compensation plans presented in the previous two chapters are candidates for faculty practice plans, with some variation and adjustment. In this chapter, we present two additional plan examples based on an XYZ plan architecture. We then build upon these examples with variations that can be used related to revenue and/or expenditure treatment, as well as recognition of the faculty member's activities beyond clinical production. As these additional plan examples demonstrate, a wide variety and complexity of compensation plans are used in the academic setting.

The two additional faculty practice plan examples include:

1. **Faculty Practice Example 1** – XYZ with direct faculty revenue and expense allocation plan; and

2. **Faculty Practice Example 2** – XYZ plan with Z based on a combination of departmental and individual incentives.

Following a description of each of these plans, we present variations of these two models, then provide an assessment of the plan based on the same dimensions identified in better-performing compensation plans and employed in the previous two chapters:

- ▶ **Measure:** Selection of a measure(s) that is clear and understandable;
- ▶ **Productivity focus:** Strength of the plan's focus on clinical productivity;
- ▶ **Financial:** Fiscal viability of the plan;
- ▶ **Simplicity:** Level of simplicity represented by the plan;
- ▶ **Alignment:** Alignment of the plan with the medical practice's goals; and
- ▶ **Fairness:** Issues of equity that may be of concern to physicians.

► FACULTY PRACTICE EXAMPLE 1-A – XYZ PLAN WITH DIRECT FACULTY REVENUE AND EXPENSE ALLOCATION
Revenue Element 4 (Production-Based) and Expense Elements 7 and 8 (Shared/Production and Modified Cost Accounting)

Overview

In Faculty Practice Example 1-A (illustrated in Exhibit 15.8), presented at the end of this section, we present a plan that directly links the faculty member's revenue and expenditures to his or her compensation. This model is generally used in a practice plan structure in which faculty compensation is allowed to be determined based on the performance of individual departments or divisions. Variations on this basic plan type are presented in Examples 1-B (Exhibit 15.9) and 1-C (Exhibit 15.10).

Goals

This type of plan has a number of goals, including: (1) encourage and reward clinical-service production; (2) promote responsibility and accountability for practice expenses and faculty member compensation; (3) use modified cost accounting to allocate expenses from the department's clinical service enterprise; and (4) promote openness and understanding regarding the financial realities of academic practice.

Methodology

The basic steps in Faculty Practice Example 1-A are listed below.

Step 1. Determine the Base Salary (X)

In this example, the base salary (X) is linked to 80 percent of each faculty member's historical compensation level. The base salary could also be linked to market rates, to a university or faculty practice plan specific salary scale, or determined using other means.

Step 2. Identify Supplement (Y) (If Any)

The supplement (Y) is discretionary and is not provided or guaranteed. It is administered and awarded by the department chair (or potentially by a division chief in conjunction with the chair) for specific administrative activities, including residency training director, division chiefs, and hospital unit heads.

Step 3. Determine the Incentive (Z) Compensation Method

The incentive (Z) component is paid only upon the existence of an individual financial surplus using the department's agreed upon revenue and cost allocation methodology. The incentive (Z) in this example is paid at a uniform percentage of each faculty member's calculated surplus, with the percentage recommended by the chair in conjunction with a departmental compensation committee comprised of a subset of departmental faculty members, and based upon the department's overall financial performance and funds availability.[1]

Step 4. Institute Uniform Treatment of Revenue

Two types of revenue are defined and addressed for taxation and practice plan purposes: (1) net clinical revenue; and (2) other revenue.

Net clinical revenue includes patient care revenues generated at the academic hospital and ambulatory care locations. This revenue is used to determine each faculty member's variable expense percentage (described below).

Other revenue includes patient care revenue from which overhead has already been deducted by a third party, and revenues for which there is little or no associated departmental overhead cost (e.g., Veteran's Administration [VA] clinical service revenues and medical director stipends). In Faculty Practice Example 1-A, "other revenue" is subject to the development fund assessment, but it is not used to determine variable expense percentages.

Step 5. Fund the Departmental Development Fund

In this example a departmental development fund is used to promote the department's goals as an academic department. This fund is paid for through a uniform assessment (e.g., 5 to 7 percent) on all revenues subject to the development fund assessment. The exact level of funding is determined based in the particular department. Moreover, in some departments, a graduated assessment might also be considered and used (e.g., 5 percent on the first $500,000 of revenues; 7 percent on the next $200,000 of revenues; and 2 percent on all revenues thereafter).

Step 6. Institute Uniform Allocation of Expenses

For expense allocation, any number of methods could be used, including those that use strict or modified cost accounting (Expense Elements 8 or 9), or other more negotiated cost allocation methods. In this example, it is assumed that overhead expenses are allocated on a direct, equal share and percentage of production basis (combining Expense Elements 7 and 8), in which expenses are classified and allocated into broad "bucket categories" as follows:

▶ **Direct Expenses.** Expenses that are directly allocated to the faculty member benefiting from the expense, such as support staff costs, faculty member travel, malpractice insurance, etc., plus the faculty member's base salary (X) and benefit costs.

▶ **Fixed (Equal Share) Overhead Expenses.** Overhead costs that are determined to be "fixed costs" are allocated among all clinical faculty members in the department. In this example, 35 percent of the total overhead costs are identified as "fixed costs" and are allocated on an equal share per CFTE basis.[2]

▶ **Variable (Production-Based) Expenses.** Overhead expenses that are determined to be "variable costs" are allocated among all clinical faculty members in the department. In this example, 65 percent of the total overhead costs are identified as "variable costs" and are allocated on the basis of each faculty member's share of total production (expressed as a percentage of net collections from professional services).

A number of other expense allocation strategies are available for use in the academic setting. See Chapter 13 for examples of expense allocation methods.

Step 7. Determine Minimum Overhead Assessment

Certain practice operating expenses continue to accrue regardless of faculty member productivity or presence or absence in the clinical setting. However, one common challenge faced by many academic departments is the absence of clinicians for extended periods of time due to attendance at conferences, research activity, or in connection with the performance of other activities. Although such activities may be consistent with the academic mission, the fixed costs of a clinical practice typically cannot fluctuate accordingly. Hence, the costs still need to be funded.

In this step, an overall assessment level is identified to cover the cost of practice. In this example, the department elects to use a minimum assessment of overhead equal to $150,000 per CFTE for a combination of direct expenses, fixed expenses, variable expenses, and combined fixed and variable expenses. By illustration, if a faculty member is a .5 CFTE, he or she would be responsible for a minimum of $75,000 of overhead expenses, regardless of the actual portion of overhead allocated to the faculty member under the overhead allocation portion of the plan.

Step 8. Determine Surpluses or Deficits and Pay Incentive (Z)

Under this example, each faculty member is expected to produce sufficient revenues to cover the faculty member's allocated share of expenses, including the faculty member's base salary (X) and benefits.

▸ If an individual surplus exists, the faculty member is eligible to receive incentive (Z) compensation.

▸ If an individual deficit exists, the faculty member is not eligible for incentive and, in fact, may be subject to a reduction of base salary (X) (subject to certain transitional rules).

Step 9. Determine Incentive Compensation

In this step, the portion of surplus to be paid as bonus to faculty is determined. In Faculty Practice Example 1-A, 50 percent of the total individual surplus is paid to the faculty member in the form of an incentive compensation or bonus.

Step 10. Determine Total Compensation

Total compensation consists of the sum of the base (X) plus the supplement (Y), plus the incentive (Z) compensation earned under the formula. The total amount of compensation paid to each faculty member would also be subject to any applicable university, school, or other compensation limits or guidelines, including requirements of fair market value (FMV) and tests of reasonableness of compensation.

Step 11. Reduce from Future Base Salary to Address Deficit

As depicted in Exhibit 15.8, two faculty members have net deficits, meaning that their allocated share of practice overhead plus direct expenses is greater than the revenues they generated from clinical activity. In many cases, a dollar-for-dollar reduction of the entire deficit amount will be taken from future earnings, although Faculty Practice Example 1-A assumes that this dollar-for-dollar reduction is capped at $30,000. Therefore, two physicians in this example have their future base salaries reduced by this deficit amount. Where deficits exist on a long-term basis, other modifications are generally required, including long-term reduction of base salaries.

➤ EXAMPLE 1-B – ADJUSTED STRAIGHT SALARY PLAN
Revenue Element 2 (Guaranteed Share)

In this variation of the basic plan (illustrated in Exhibit 15.9), the actual compensation that is paid to the faculty member is indexed to recognize academic rank or subspecialty; is linked to production; or is determined by some other method. In this plan variation, a total targeted compensation level is identified, with faculty receiving one-twelfth of the total X plus Y plus Z each month. The Z portion of compensation may fluctuate on a quarterly basis, however, depending upon actual net collections from professional services. In contrast to the previous faculty practice example, the department does not make a direct allocation of expenses. Instead, it pays all clinical practice expenses out of clinical service revenues and allocates the remaining amount to individual faculty members based on a percentage of clinical production to total clinical production. Each faculty member is evaluated in reference to the revenues actually generated by mission area. Those who generate a surplus of total revenues participate in an additional incentive payment; those who do not (e.g., Dr. B, Dr. C, and Dr. E) receive their full target compensation but do not participate in any additional incentive. This model, therefore, involves a greater level of sharing designed to ensure that faculty members are paid competitively at market levels, and it promotes a team focus.

➤ EXAMPLE 1-C – MISSION-BASED PLAN
Revenue Element 1 (Unit-Based)

In this example (illustrated in Exhibit 15.10), each component of the faculty member's compensation is directly aligned with its revenue source and with the percentage of time devoted by the faculty member to that mission element. A mission-based approach becomes the driver for determining the percentage of time the faculty member spends in various academic pursuits. For example, if Dr. B projects to receive $25,000 of salary support for extramural research and Dr. B's total compensation is $250,000, then 10 percent of Dr. B's time should be devoted to extramural research activities.[3] If the faculty member is not involved in teaching or service, then the rest of his or her time is expected to be devoted to clinical activity, including revenue-generating activities.

In this fashion, the revenue sources and percentages of faculty time in each mission area are linked with the objective to provide information for assessing the funding sources and their relationship to faculty member activities. That assessment may lead to an adjustment of faculty member activities; it may lead to a reassessment of priorities at the departmental or other levels (e.g., by identifying faculty who will have a greater dedicated focus on certain activities such as research or teaching, but not others); or, in many instances, it may lead to a combination of these.

In Example 1-C, although Dr. B was expected to obtain $25,000 in extramural salary support for research, he or she only received $5,000, resulting in a corresponding reduction in time assigned to research activities (from 10 percent to 2 percent). Example 1-C also shows that Dr. B's time commitment to clinical practice will most likely need to increase if he or she desires to receive the full targeted level of compensation by academic rank. The total targeted compensation of the faculty member can be linked to market rates, based on a single academic benchmark survey or a blend of multiple surveys.

In an ideal world, the revenue for each portion of the academic mission would be fully funded. For example, all of the medical student teaching activities performed by faculty would have a direct payment allocation to the faculty member based on courses, hours, combined student volume and contact hours, or some other quantitative method. If each of the mission categories were fully funded, it would be mathematically possible to take a given faculty member and allocate his or her time, as well as allocate associated funds from each of these categories. Unfortunately, such an ideal world is rarely found in the academic setting. Thus, the actual implementation of mission-based funds flow with direct linkage to faculty compensation plans can be complex. While alignment of the funds flow model and the compensation plan is optimal, such a directly aligned approach between mission-based funds flow and mission-based faculty compensation is not required. For example, the university could adopt a mission-based funds flow model as part of its overall plan architecture, with each department identifying its own compensation plan for the actual distribution of these funds.

Exhibit 15.11 provides an assessment of the strengths and weaknesses of Faculty Practice Example 1.

EXHIBIT 15.8

Faculty Practice Plan Example 1-A – XYZ with Direct Faculty Revenue and Expense Allocation Plan*
Revenue Element 4 (Production-Based) and Expense Elements 7 and 8 (Shared/Production and Modified Cost Accounting)

	Dept. Total	Dr. A	Dr. B	Dr. C	Dr. D	Dr. E	Dr. F	Dr. G
Step 1	**Determine base salary (X).**							
	Note: Assumes base equal to 80% of historic compensation levels.							
Rank		Instructor	Professor	Instructor	Assistant Professor	Assistant Professor	Associate Professor	Professor
CFTE	6.00	1.00	1.00	1.00	0.50	0.70	0.80	1.00
Base Salary (X)	$1,202,273	$218,326	$94,487	$189,013	$114,643	$232,976	$185,845	$166,983
Step 2	**Determine supplement (Y) (if any).**							
Supplement (Y)	$55,000		$30,000				$25,000	
Step 3	**Determine incentive (Z) allocation methodology.**							
	Assumes 50% of surplus of allocated revenues over expenses by physician							
	Actual percentage subject to funds availability, financial performance, and fair market value requirements							
Step 4	**Institute uniform treatment of clinical revenue.**							
Net Clinical Revenue (patient care fees)	$3,355,055	$596,787	$312,401	$522,302	$341,730	$458,720	$397,623	$725,492
% of Total Net Clinical Revenue		18%	9%	16%	10%	14%	12%	22%
Other Revenue (e.g., third-party medical director stipends)	$51,886	$28,010	$456	$600	$8,200	$120	$500	$14,000
Total Revenues before Development Fund and Overhead	$3,406,941	$624,797	$312,857	$522,902	$349,930	$458,840	$398,123	$739,492
Step 5	**Fund departmental development fund.**							
	Note: Assumes 7% applied to Net Clinical Revenue only	$(167,753)	$(29,839)	$(15,620)	$(26,115)	$(17,087)	$(22,936)	$(19,881)	$(36,275)
Net after Development Fund Assessment	$3,239,188	$594,958	$297,237	$496,787	$332,844	$435,904	$378,242	$703,217

	Total							
Step 6	**Institute uniform expense allocation.**							
Direct (base salary X plus benefit costs)	$(1,442,727)	$(261,991)	$(113,385)	$(226,815)	$(137,572)	$(279,571)	$(223,014)	$(200,380)
Total Overhead Expense	$(1,420,527)							
Fixed Expenses (35% of total) (equal per CFTE)	$(497,184)	$(82,864)	$(82,864)	$(82,864)	$(41,432)	$(58,005)	$(66,291)	$(82,864)
Variable Expenses (65% of total) (% of net clinical revenue)	$(923,343)	$(164,241)	$(85,976)	$(143,742)	$(94,047)	$(126,244)	$(109,430)	$(199,662)
Total Overhead (without minimum)		$(509,096)	$(282,225)	$(453,421)	$(263,051)	$(463,820)	$(398,735)	$(482,906)
Step 7	**Assess minimum overhead ($150,000 per CFTE).**							
	$(150,000)	$(150,000)	$(150,000)	$(150,000)	$(75,000)	$(105,000)	$(120,000)	$(150,000)
Step 8	**Determine surplus or deficit.**							
		$85,861	$15,013	$43,365	$59,792	$(27,916)	$(20,493)	$220,311
Step 9	**Determine incentive (Z) (assumed at 50% of surplus).**							
		$42,931	$7,506	$21,683	$29,896			$110,156
Step 10	**Determine total compensation (X + Y + Z).**							
		$261,256	$131,993	$210,695	$144,539	$210,845	$232,976	$277,139
Step 11	**Assess reduction from future base salary.**							
Note: Assumes dollar-for-dollar reduction of future compensation for deficit up to $30,000.						$(27,916)	$(20,493)	

* Hypothetical numbers presented for illustrative purposes only. Numbers may not total in all cases due to rounding.

EXHIBIT 15.9

Faculty Practice Plan Example 1-B – XYZ with Adjusted Straight Salary Plan*
Revenue Element 2 (Guaranteed Share)

Step 1   **Determine base salary (X).**
Note: Assumes base equal to 80% of historic compensation levels.

Rank	Department Total	Dr. A Instructor	Dr. B Professor	Dr. C Instructor	Dr. D Assistant Professor	Dr. E Assistant Professor	Dr. F Associate Professor	Dr. G Professor
Clinical FTE	4.50	0.80	0.60	0.80	0.30	0.70	0.80	0.50
Nonclinical FTE	2.20	0.20	0.40	0.10	0.50	0.30	0.20	0.50
Total FTE	6.70	1.00	1.00	0.90	0.80	1.00	1.00	1.00

Step 2   **Determine target total salary (X + Z) by academic rank.**

	Target per 1.0 CFTE
Professor	$250,000
Associate Professor	$225,000
Assistant Professor	$200,000
Instructor	$165,000

Step 3   **Determine target per faculty member based on academic rank.**

	Department Total	Dr. A	Dr. B	Dr. C	Dr. D	Dr. E	Dr. F	Dr. G
Base Salary (X) linked to academic rank and clinical service	$919,000	$132,000	$150,000	$132,000	$60,000	$140,000	$180,000	$125,000
Supplement (Y) from research, hospital, and other sources	$297,000	$10,000	$40,000	$10,000	$87,000	$20,000	$40,000	$90,000
Incentive (Z) from faculty practice plan and linked to target	$182,500	$23,000	$60,000	$6,500	$13,000	$40,000	$5,000	$35,000
Total Target Compensation Based on Rank	$1,398,500	$165,000	$250,000	$148,500	$160,000	$200,000	$225,000	$250,000
Incentive (Z) as Percent to Total		13%	33%	4%	7%	22%	3%	19%

Step 4   **Define target clinical service production by faculty.**

	Department Total	Dr. A	Dr. B	Dr. C	Dr. D	Dr. E	Dr. F	Dr. G
	$2,656,000	$420,000	$375,000	$480,000	$185,000	$420,000	$485,000	$291,000

Step 5 — Determine funds available for incentive (Z) (actual).

Item	Total							
Actual Clinical Practice Revenues (entire department)	$2,736,012	$487,550	$372,000	$475,021	$195,320	$411,202	$489,795	$305,124
Clinical Practice Overhead	$(1,162,783)							
Base Salary (X)	$(919,000)							
Faculty Benefit Cost	$(255,360)							
Departmental Development Fund (5% of net revenues)	$(136,801)							
Net Available for Incentive (Z)	$262,068							

Step 6 — Allocate incentive (Z) (percent of total basis) up to target.

Item	Total							
Target Incentive (Z) as Percent to Total Portion of Target		13%	33%	4%	7%	22%	3%	19%
Allocated Portion of Total Incentive	$262,068	$33,028	$86,159	$9,334	$18,668	$57,440	$7,180	$50,260
Target Incentive (Z) (from above)	$182,500	$23,000	$60,000	$6,500	$13,000	$40,000	$5,000	$35,000
Surplus (deficit) from Target for Additional Incentive	$79,568	$10,028	$26,159	$2,834	$5,668	$17,440	$2,180	$15,260

Step 7 — Allocate surplus between department and faculty.

Item	Total							
Department Share (50%)	$39,784							
Faculty Share (50%) Based on % of Clinical Production	$39,784							

Step 8 — Allocate faculty surplus on percent to total basis among faculty meeting target as additional incentive.

Item	Total							
Actual Production	$1,477,789	$487,550			$195,320		$489,795	$305,124
Percent of Total Clinical Service Production		33%	0%	0%	13%	0%	33%	21%
Share of Additional Incentive	$39,784	$13,126	$—	$—	$5,258	$—	$13,186	$8,214

Step 9 — Determine total compensation.

Base Salary (X)	$132,000	$150,000	$132,000	$60,000	$140,000	$180,000	$125,000
Supplement (Y)	$10,000	$40,000	$10,000	$87,000	$20,000	$40,000	$90,000
Target Incentive (Z)	$23,000	$60,000	$6,500	$13,000	$40,000	$5,000	$35,000
Additional Incentive (Z)	$13,126	$—	$—	$5,258	$—	$13,186	$8,214
Total Compensation	$178,126	$250,000	$148,500	$165,258	$200,000	$238,186	$258,214

* Hypothetical numbers presented for illustrative purposes only. Numbers may not total in all cases due to rounding.

EXHIBIT 15.10 Faculty Practice Plan Example 1-C – XYZ Mission Based Plan*
Revenue Element 1 (Unit-Based)

		Dr. A	Dr. B	Dr. C	Dr. D	Dr. E	Dr. F	Dr. G
Step 1	**Determine target salary based on academic rank.**							
	Rank	Instructor	Professor	Assistant Professor	Assistant Professor	Assistant Professor	Associate Professor	Professor
		Target per 1.0 FTE						
	Professor	$250,000						
	Associate Professor	$225,000						
	Assistant Professor	$200,000						
	Instructor	$165,000						
	Target Compensation by Rank	$165,000	$250,000	$180,000	$160,000	$200,000	$225,000	$250,000
Step 2	**Determine target funding by mission and projected FTE.**							
	Base Salary (X) Teaching (state funds)	$33,000	$75,000	$18,000	$16,000	$40,000	$—	$25,000
	Supplement (Y) Research and Other (external funds)	$—	$25,000	$—	$64,000	$20,000	$45,000	$100,000
	Incentive (Z) (surplus of revenues over allocated expenses)	$132,000	$150,000	$144,000	$48,000	$140,000	$180,000	$125,000
	Total Target Compensation	$165,000	$250,000	$162,000	$128,000	$200,000	$225,000	$250,000
Step 3	**Determine time by mission area based on expected funding support.**							
	Base Salary (X) Teaching (state funds)	20%	30%	10%	10%	20%	—%	10%
	Supplement (Y) Research (external funds)	0%	10%	0%	40%	10%	20%	40%
	Clinical (practice plan)	80%	60%	80%	30%	70%	80%	50%
	Total FTE	100%	100%	90%	80%	100%	100%	100%
Step 4	**Determine actual funding by mission (nonclinical only).**							
	Base Salary (X) Teaching (state funds)	$33,000	$75,000	$18,000	$16,000	$40,000	$—	$25,000
	Supplement (Y) Research (external funds)	$—	$5,000	$—	$10,000	$28,000	$30,000	$85,000

Step 5	**Determine actual FTE (nonclinical only) by funding support.**						
	Base Salary (X) Teaching (state funds)	20%	30%	11%	13%	20%	0%	10%
	Supplement (Y) Research (external funds)	0%	2%	0%	8%	14%	13%	34%
Step 6	**Determine actual clinical percentage of time based on funding support.**	80%	68%	79%	60%	66%	87%	56%
Step 7	**Determine clinical surplus required to meet target compensation.**						
	Incentive (Z) required	$132,000	$170,000	$144,000	$102,000	$132,000	$195,000	$140,000
	Difference from target†	$—	$20,000	$—	$54,000	$(8,000)	$15,000	$15,000
Step 8	**Determine compensation based on actual performance.‡**						

* Hypothetical numbers presented for illustrative purposes only. Numbers may not total in all cases due to rounding.

† Difference represents additional clinical service compensation required to achieve full target compensation level. Clinical practice income used to make up deficits in other funding sources.

‡ Actual clinical practice surplus (or deficit) would be determined for each faculty member in accordance with department-specific approach to revenue and clinical-practice expense allocation. Methods would include those illustrated elsewhere.

© 2006 Johnson & Walker Keegan

EXHIBIT 15.11   Assessment of Faculty Practice Plan Example 1

Dimension	Strengths	Weaknesses
Measure	Total compensation is linked to market rates based on academic rank. Faculty are rewarded for all revenue-generating activities (e.g., beyond clinical production). Promotes accountability for individual performance. In a mission-based approach, permits specific recognition of each portion of the academic mission.	Depending upon the method by which the total targeted compensation is determined, there may be insufficient linkage between individual performance and compensation level beyond academic rank.
Productivity	Faculty have incentive to generate clinical revenue due to individual profit or loss calculations.	May focus on clinical production to the exclusion of other components of the academic mission. If the plan variations are adopted, clinical productivity may be only indirectly addressed.
Financial	Close linkage between faculty revenue and expense.	Use of production-based component in expense allocation may be viewed as penalizing faculty with highest production levels. Variations on this plan may not effectively engage faculty with cost of practice issues or may allow faculty with low production to reduce the amount available to others.
Simplicity	Consistent with typical intuitive-based compensation models (i.e., revenues less expenses = compensation or mission-based approach).	Relatively complex plan design (depending upon plan variation adopted).
Alignment	Indirect to largely direct alignment with academic mission. Depending upon plan variation, may foster a group practice approach.	May place primary emphasis on clinical service production, to the detriment of other missions.
"Fairness"	The basic plan promotes attention to both practice revenues and expenses. Variations in the plan emphasize revenue and/or expense individually.	Faculty may question their ability to control expenditure levels. Faculty who work harder or who produce at higher levels in any of the mission areas are not directly rewarded for their efforts. May require "robbing Peter to pay Paul."

➤ Faculty Practice Example 2-A – XYZ Plan with Z Based on Combination of Departmental and Individual Clinical Performance

Overview

This second faculty practice example (illustrated in Exhibit 15.12) uses clinical production as a means to reward faculty Z portion of compensation. The department's funds are managed centrally, rather than being distributed to divisions (although this plan could be used with division-based budgeting). Restricted and unrestricted revenue sources, as appropriate, are used to compensate faculty for a base salary plus a supplement (X plus Y), with base salary levels determined by academic rank and level of state or other support assigned to each rank. Unlike Faculty Practice Example 1, in which individual faculty are assigned a portion of overhead that must be paid before incentive compensation is earned, this plan adopts a team-oriented approach to incentive compensation by requiring that the department must have a surplus before incentive compensation (Z) can be earned and paid. Thus, under this model, faculty in the department share in any overage of revenue after departmental operating expenses (including faculty member base plus supplement compensation) have been paid.

Goals

The goals of this plan are to encourage and reward individual clinical production and encourage a departmental focus on practice growth and expenditure management at the departmental level.

Methodology

The basic formulaic steps of the plan are listed below.

Step 1. Develop a Budget and Identify the Targeted Compensation Level by Faculty Member

Each faculty member's targeted compensation is based on the combination of base (X) plus supplement (Y) compensation, and the source of revenues is equal to this targeted compensation level. In this example, budgeted or expected levels of revenues to the department from different funding sources are shown (including state support linked to academic rank, school of medicine compensation for administrative services, extramural research funds allocated for salary support, clinical practice revenues, and others). The budgeting process also assumes compensation levels for each faculty member in addition to general overhead costs, departmental and other tithing, and other uses of departmental revenues. The budgeting process also includes a budgeted amount of incentive compensation (Z-1), although the amount that will be allocated within the department is set at only 75 percent (rather than 100 percent) of the full departmental surplus of revenues over expenses as part of sound budgeting and financial management practices. The level of individual incentive compensation is set using a 25 percent equal share/75 percent "percentage of production" methodology. The combination of X plus Y plus Z-1 compensation will then equal the faculty member's total budgeted or target compensation.

Step 2. Compare the Budget to Actual Performance

Faculty in this example will receive actual compensation as paid from state and other external (nonclinical) revenue sources. As a result, certain revenue sources, including state base salary support, hospital medical director and other services, school of medicine administrative compensation, and salary support from extramural research, are allocated directly to each respective faculty member.

Faculty in the department in this example share in incentive compensation (Z) in accordance with the budget. The budgeted amount of incentive compensation is awarded based on individual performance vs. the faculty member's revenue target. In this example, faculty member I fails to meet his or her revenue target; therefore, the difference between the budgeted and actual revenues ($19,200) is reduced from the faculty member's budgeted incentive compensation on a dollar-for-dollar basis. Despite the lower than expected revenue performance by one faculty member, the department as a whole achieved its target, such that a surplus of actual revenues over expenses exists. This amount is in excess of the budgeted surplus for the department as a whole.

Step 3. Allocate the Actual Surplus vs. Budgeted Surplus

At this step, the actual surplus is compared to the budgeted surplus, with an allocation methodology applied. In this example, the department is entitled to retain 100 percent of the surplus up to the budgeted surplus amount, after which it receives 80 percent of the actual surplus of revenues over expenses. This is designed to provide the department with the incentive to budget and manage revenue and expense performance as closely as possible and, in all instances, within the budget for the department as a whole. This surplus is allocated in the form of additional incentive (Z-2) compensation.

Step 4. Allocate the Surplus within the Department as Additional Incentive Compensation (Z-2)

In this example, of the portion of the surplus that is allocated to the department, 5 percent is allocated to the departmental development fund, and the remaining 95 percent is allocated to the individual faculty members based on a 10 percent equal share (based on FTE of the department), and 90 percent of clinical service production basis. The equal share portion for faculty member I is reduced by 50 percent, however, due to this faculty member's failure to achieve revenue targets. (The exact level of reduction would need to be determined as part of the plan.)

Indeed, some faculty practice plans impose a requirement that individual faculty members will not participate in such department-wide incentive compensation if they fail to meet the required production level. Although this example shows a distribution of 100 percent of the surplus, the more common approach is to distribute a reduced portion (e.g., 50 percent) through an additional incentive component. Moreover, while this model presents an allocation based on clinical service production, other measures and allocation methods can also be used to allocate incentive components, including those described in the examples that follow, those that use the emerging pay-for-performance (P4P) reimbursement systems, and others that consider factors other than clinical service in determining and paying compensation.

Step 5. Determine Total Compensation

Each faculty member's total compensation is the sum of the actual base salary (X) plus supplement (Y), plus budgeted incentive (Z-1) and additional incentive (Z-2).

Three variations of this plan are now outlined in Examples 2-B through 2-D to recognize alternatives related to Z distribution treatment.

➤ EXAMPLE 2-B — Z BASED ON INDIVIDUAL CLINICAL PRODUCTION ONLY

This variation of the basic plan (illustrated in Exhibit 15.13) uses clinical production as a means to reward faculty Z portion of compensation. Restricted and unrestricted revenue sources, as appropriate, are used to compensate faculty for base plus supplement (X plus Y), with base salary levels determined by academic rank and linked to market benchmarks. Faculty members pay a negotiated overhead rate that is determined as part of the budgeting process and expressed as a percentage of total overhead costs. This is designed to provide each faculty member with a target level of overhead costs that must be covered (while also creating an incentive for production in excess of the budgeted target). The use of a defined percentage of total overhead rather than a flat dollar amount, however, also recognizes that actual costs may differ from budget costs. Faculty receive direct payments of restricted funds and share in any surplus.

➤ EXAMPLE 2-C — Z BASED ON INDIVIDUAL POINTS AND WEIGHTS

Although the XYZ architectures previously shown allocate incentive (Z) largely based on individual or department-wide clinical practice performance, the Z component can be used to reward faculty members based on individual performance along a number of dimensions. For example, as illustrated in Exhibit 15.14, a point system may used to recognize faculty performance, and each dimension of performance is weighted depending on the faculty member's role in the department. Accordingly, a faculty member who is highly involved in research will have different weights assigned to research activity than a faculty member who devotes significant time to clinical activity. In this fashion, performance expectations are developed for each faculty member, and performance is linked directly to compensation. The goals of this approach are to ensure a direct relationship between the faculty member's performance and his or her compensation level. When properly designed, this plan encourages the development of a "triple threat" department, recognizing the specific role each faculty member performs in support of each component of the academic mission.

The total targeted compensation is linked to median benchmark sources. Performance categories are established for the department (or overall at the institutional level). In this example, the categories are clinical productivity, research, teaching, administration, and patient service. Points are assigned for specific activities in each of these categories, and weights are applied for each performance dimension for each faculty member.

An example of this approach is provided in Exhibit 15.14.

The actual total compensation under this model equals the sum of the base salary ($160,000) plus the incentive ($21,600), for a total of $181,600. Faculty practice plans that involve points and weight systems can be complex; however, their advantage lies in the direct relationships between performance expectations, outcomes in relation to these expectations, and the resulting compensation.

An alternative to the weights and points approach demonstrated in Exhibit 15.14 is to use a more subjective evaluation, such as "unsatisfactory," "satisfactory," and "more than satisfactory," or "low," "medium," and "high," then assign a quantitative score to these assessments (e.g., 1 for unsatisfactory or low, 2 for satisfactory or medium, and 3 for more than satisfactory or high). A weighted average score can then be computed. For an example, see Exhibit 15.15. In this example, total budgeted incentive compensation is determined by mission area, and weights are assigned within each mission area in relation to faculty member performance expectations and service time in Step 1. Faculty performance is evaluated using the above referenced one-to-three-point scale in Step 2, and weighted averages for each faculty member for each mission area are determined by multiplying each faculty member's assigned weights by the scores to yield a weighted value for each faculty member in Step 3. The weighted values are then used to award the incentive within each mission area, with each faculty member sharing in the incentive pool based on a percentage to total basis based on the faculty member's weighted value, expressed as a percentage of the total weighted values in the mission area. The incentive would be paid in addition to base salary.

An additional variation of this type of approach is described in Example 2-D below.

► EXAMPLE 2-D – USE OF CLINICAL AND ACADEMIC INCENTIVE POOLS

In Example 2-D, two incentive pools are used to reward faculty beyond their X and Y salary components: a clinical incentive pool and an academic incentive pool. The department assesses a tax for programmatic development prior to the determination of funds available for both incentive pools. It then determines the funding amounts available in each of the pools. The goals of this plan are to reward both clinical and academic activities while encouraging a group focus; hence the use of an incentive pool design as opposed to an individual performance approach.

The clinical incentive pool is allocated based on individual production as a percentage to total production using any number of production measures (e.g., net collections from professional services, WRVUs, or others).

The academic incentive pool is allocated based on individual faculty performance. A point system is employed to recognize faculty research, teaching, and service activities. The points each faculty member receives are totaled, and the academic incentive pool is awarded based on the individual faculty member's percentage to total points. Exhibit 15.16 presents an example of this approach using point values and weights for each category. When this approach is used, faculty are typically involved in the design of the point distribution and weighting factors. As demonstrated below, faculty are essentially internally competing for dollars in the academic incentive pool based on individual faculty points as a percentage of total points.

Assuming that the amount available for the academic incentive pool is $100,000, based on weights in Exhibit 15.16, $50,000 would be distributed based on research, $30,000 would be distributed based on teaching, and $20,000 would be distributed based on service. For illustrative purposes only, Exhibit 15.17 presents a distribution of the academic incentive pool based on faculty members A and B comprising the entire faculty of the department.

Exhibit 15.18 provides an assessment of the strengths and weaknesses of Faculty Practice Plan 2, including comments on the variations to the distribution of incentive compensation outlined above.

EXHIBIT 15.12

Faculty Practice Plan Example 2-A –
XYZ with Z Based on Combination of Department and Individual Incentive Plan*

Step 1 **Develop budget and identify targeted compensation by faculty member.**

Department – Budget Data

Faculty Revenue/Production Targets	Department Total	Faculty A	Faculty B	Faculty C
FTE of Department	9.50	1.00	1.00	1.00
Rank		Associate	Associate	Professor

Revenues

State Base Support by Rank	$747,500	$85,000	$85,000	$105,000
School of Medicine Administrative Compensation	$150,000	$—	$—	$—
Extramural Research (salary support only)	$170,000	$—	$10,000	$25,000
Clinical Service/Faculty Practice Plan	$6,390,000	$450,000	$500,000	$685,000
Other Revenues (e.g., consulting)	$210,003	$12,000	$10,000	$25,000
Total Revenues to Department	$7,667,503	$547,000	$605,000	$840,000

Expenses

Dean's Tax (7% of clinical and other revenues)	$462,000			
Practice Plan-Wide Revenue Share (fixed)[†]	$285,000			
Departmental Development Fund (5%)(fixed)[†]	$330,000			
Faculty Benefit Cost	$710,854			
Department Clinical Services Overhead Costs	2,492,100			

Faculty Compensation (targets)

Base (X)	$747,500	$85,000	$85,000	$105,000
Supplement (Y)	$320,000	$—	$10,000	$25,000
Incentive (Z-1) (budgeted) (75% of surplus)	$1,953,786	$155,953	$167,037	$211,948
Total Budgeted Compensation	$3,021,286	$240,953	$262,037	$341,948
Budgeted Department Surplus/Deficit	$366,262			

Step 2 **Compare budget to actual.**

Department – Actual Year-End Data

Faculty Revenue Actual	Department Total	Faculty A	Faculty B	Faculty C
FTE of Department	9.60	1.00	1.00	1.00
Rank		Associate	Associate	Professor

Revenues

State Base Support by Rank (actual)	$747,500	$85,000	$85,000	$105,000
School of Medicine Administrative Compensation (actual)	$150,000	$—	$—	$—
Extramural Research (salary support only) (actual)	$191,000	$—	$5,000	$31,000

Faculty D	Faculty E	Faculty F	Faculty G	Faculty H	Faculty I	Faculty J
0.50	1.00	1.00	1.00	1.00	1.00	1.00
Professor	Assistant	Assistant	Clinical	Clinical	Assistant	Associate
$52,500	$75,000	$75,000	$60,000	$60,000	$75,000	$75,000
$150,000	$—	$—	$—	$—	$—	$—
$50,000	$20,000	$40,000	$—	$—	$10,000	$15,000
$190,000	$590,000	$655,000	$900,000	$1,010,000	$760,000	$650,000
$80,000	$5,000	$75,000	$—	$—	$2,000	$1,000
$522,500	$690,000	$845,000	$960,000	$1,070,000	$847,000	$741,000

Faculty D	Faculty E	Faculty F	Faculty G	Faculty H	Faculty I	Faculty J
$52,500	$75,000	$75,000	$60,000	$60,000	$75,000	$75,000
$200,000	$20,000	$40,000	$—	$—	$10,000	$15,000
$125,563	$183,282	$212,904	$234,881	$255,903	$213,286	$193,028
$378,063	$278,282	$327,904	$294,881	$315,903	$298,286	$283,028

Faculty D	Faculty E	Faculty F	Faculty G	Faculty H	Faculty I	Faculty J
0.60	1.00	1.00	1.00	1.00	1.00	1.00
Professor	Assistant	Assistant	Clinical	Clinical	Assistant	Associate
$52,500	$75,000	$75,000	$60,000	$60,000	$75,000	$75,000
$150,000	$—	$—	$—	$—	$—	$—
$80,000	$10,000	$40,000	$—	$—	$10,000	$15,000

continued on next page

Exhibit 15.12 – *Faculty Practice Plan Example 2-A continued*

	Deptartment Total	Faculty A	Faculty B	Faculty C
Clinical Service/Faculty Practice Plan (actual)	$6,936,932	$606,878	$574,201	$709,213
Other Revenues (e.g., consulting) (actual)	$287,321	$18,000	$12,000	$55,000
Total Revenues to Department	$8,312,753	$709,878	$676,201	$900,213
Faculty Revenue Performance vs. Budget		$162,878	$71,201	$60,213
Expenses				
Dean's Tax (7% of clinical and other revenues)	$505,698			
Practice Plan-Wide Revenue Share (fixed)[†]	$288,000			
Department Development Fund (5%) (fixed)[†]	$330,000			
Faculty Benefit Cost (actual)	$714,968			
Department Clinical Services Overhead Costs	2,740,088			
Faculty Compensation Targets				
Base (X)	$747,500	$85,000	$85,000	$105,000
Supplement (Y)	$341,000	$—	$5,000	$31,000
Incentive (Z-1) (budgeted)	$1,953,786	$176,014	$170,078	$209,566
Total Compensation (before deficit adjustment)	$3,042,286	$261,014	$260,078	$345,566
Deficit Adjustment				
Adjusted Compensation (after deficit adjustment)	$3,023,086	$261,014	$260,078	$345,566
Budgeted Departmental Surplus/Deficit	$366,262			
Actual Departmental Surplus/Deficit	$710,912			
Step 3	**Allocate actual surplus vs. budget.**			
100% up to Budgeted Surplus	$366,262			
80% of Amount in Excess of Budget to Department	$275,720			
Total to Department	$641,982			
Step 4	**Allocate surplus within department (Z-2).**			
Departmental Development Fund (5%)	$64,198			
Faculty Additional Incentive (95%)	$577,784			
Share of Additional Incentive (FTE that shares in incentive is reduced for deficit)	9.00	1.00	1.00	1.00
Equal Share Portion (10%)	$57,778	$6,420	$6,420	$6,420
Production Portion (90%)	$520,005	$44,407	$42,300	$56,313
Step 5	**Determine total compensation.**			
Sum of Above	$3,620,070	$311,841	$308,798	$408,299

* Hypothetical numbers presented for illustrative purposes only. Numbers may not total in all cases due to rounding.

[†] Assumes tithing at fixed levels as determined in connection with annual budgeting process.

Faculty D	Faculty E	Faculty F	Faculty G	Faculty H	Faculty I	Faculty J
$225,621	$600,000	$690,000	$1,029,000	$1,012,019	$740,000	$750,000
$78,600	$5,321	$108,500	$—	$6,000	$2,800	$1,100
$586,721	$690,321	$913,500	$1,089,000	$1,078,019	$827,800	$841,100
$64,221	$321	$68,500	$129,000	$8,019	$(19,200)	$100,100
$52,500	$75,000	$75,000	$60,000	$60,000	$75,000	$75,000
$230,000	$10,000	$40,000	$—	$—	$10,000	$15,000
$133,953	$172,567	$211,908	$242,845	$240,909	$196,801	$199,146
$416,453	$257,567	$326,908	$302,845	$300,909	$281,801	$289,146
					$(19,200)	
$416,453	$257,567	$326,908	$302,845	$300,909	$262,601	$289,146
0.50	1.00	1.00	1.00	1.00	0.50	1.00
$3,210	$6,420	$6,420	$6,420	$6,420	$3,210	$6,420
$36,702	$43,183	$57,144	$68,123	$67,436	$51,783	$52,615
$456,365	$307,170	$390,472	$377,387	$374,764	$336,794	$348,181

EXHIBIT 15.13

Faculty Practice Plan Example 2-B – XYZ with Z Based on Individual Incentive Plan*

Step 1 Identify restricted and unrestricted funds via budget.

	Department Total	Faculty A	Faculty B	Faculty C
FTE of Department	9.50	1.00	1.00	1.00
Rank		Associate	Associate	Professor
Restricted Funds				
Base Salary (X) State Support by Rank	$747,500	$85,000	$85,000	$105,000
Supplement (Y) School of Medicine	$150,000	$—	$—	$—
Supplement (Y) (extramural research salary)	$170,000	$—	$10,000	$25,000
Unrestricted Funds				
Clinical Service/Faculty Practice Plan	$6,390,000	$450,000	$500,000	$685,000
Other Revenues (e.g., consulting)	$210,003	$12,000	$10,000	$25,000
Total Revenues to Department	$7,667,503	$547,000	$605,000	$840,000

Step 2 Negotiate expenses.

	Department Total	Faculty A	Faculty B	Faculty C
Restricted Funds				
Base Salary (X) State Support by Rank	$747,500	$85,000	$85,000	$105,000
Supplement (Y) School of Medicine	$150,000	$—	$—	$—
Supplement (Y) (extramural research salary)	$170,000	$—	$10,000	$25,000
Faculty Benefit Cost	$224,825	$19,550	$21,850	$29,900
Unrestricted Funds				
Dean's Tax (7% of clinical and other revenues)	$462,000	$32,340	$35,700	$49,700
Departmental Developmental Fund (5%)	$330,000	$23,100	$25,500	$35,500
Department Clinical Services Overhead Costs	2,492,100			
Fixed Cost (65% of total)	1,619,865	$170,512	$170,512	$170,512
Variable (35% of total) (% of production)	872,235	$61,056	$67,400	$93,831
		$231,569	$237,912	$264,343
% of Total Expenses (clinical enterprise only)		9%	10%	11%

Step 3 Determine actual performance.

Faculty Revenue (actual)	Department Total	Faculty A	Faculty B	Faculty C
FTE of Department	9.60	1.00	1.00	1.00
Rank		Associate	Associate	Professor
Restricted Funds				
Base Salary (X) State Support by Rank	$747,500	$85,000	$85,000	$105,000
Supplement (Y) School of Medicine	$152,500	$—	$—	$12,500
Supplement (Y) (extramural research salary)	$193,000	$—	$10,000	$2,000
Total		$85,000	$95,000	$119,500

Faculty D	Faculty E	Faculty F	Faculty G	Faculty H	Faculty I	Faculty J
0.50	1.00	1.00	1.00	1.00	1.00	1.00
Professor	Assistant	Assistant	Clinical	Clinical	Assistant	Associate
$52,500	$75,000	$75,000	$60,000	$60,000	$75,000	$75,000
$150,000	$—	$—	$—	$—	$—	$—
$50,000	$20,000	$40,000	$—	$—	$10,000	$15,000
$190,000	$590,000	$655,000	$900,000	$1,010,000	$760,000	$650,000
$80,000	$5,000	$75,000	$—	$—	$2,000	$1,000
$522,500	$690,000	$845,000	$960,000	$1,070,000	$847,000	$741,000
$52,500	$75,000	$75,000	$60,000	$60,000	$75,000	$75,000
$150,000	$—	$—	$—	$—	$—	$—
$50,000	$20,000	$40,000	$—	$—	$10,000	$15,000
$58,075	$21,850	$26,450	$13,800	$13,800	$19,550	$20,700
$18,900	$41,650	$51,100	$63,000	$70,700	$53,340	$45,570
$13,500	$29,750	$36,500	$45,000	$50,500	$38,100	$32,550
$85,256	$170,512	$170,512	$170,512	$170,512	$170,512	$170,512
$35,682	$78,633	$96,474	$118,941	$133,478	$100,703	$86,034
$120,938	$249,145	$266,987	$289,453	$303,990	$271,216	$256,546
5%	10%	11%	12%	12%	11%	10%

Faculty D	Faculty E	Faculty F	Faculty G	Faculty H	Faculty I	Faculty J
0.60	1.00	1.00	1.00	1.00	1.00	1.00
Professor	Assistant	Assistant	Clinical	Clinical	Assistant	Associate
$52,500	$75,000	$75,000	$60,000	$60,000	$75,000	$75,000
$140,000	$—	$—	$—	$—	$—	$—
$50,000	$20,000	$41,000	$45,000	$—	$10,000	$15,000
$242,500	$95,000	$116,000	$105,000	$60,000	$85,000	$90,000

continued on next page

Exhibit 15.13 – Faculty Practice Plan Example 2-B continued

	Department Total	Faculty A	Faculty B	Faculty C
Unrestricted Funds				
Clinical Service/Faculty Practice Plan (actual)	$6,936,932	$606,878	$574,201	$709,213
Other Revenues (e.g., consulting [actual])	$287,321	$18,000	$12,000	$55,000
Total	$8,317,253	$624,878	$586,201	$764,213
Total Funds (all sources)		$709,878	$681,201	$883,713
Expenses				
Restricted Funds				
Base Salary (X) State Support by Rank		$85,000	$85,000	$105,000
Supplement (Y) School of Medicine		$—	$—	$12,500
Supplement (Y) Extramural Research Salary Support		$—	$10,000	$2,000
Total Restricted		$85,000	$95,000	$119,500
Unrestricted Funds				
Dean's Tax (fixed)	$505,698	$32,340	$35,700	$49,700
Department Developmental Fund (fixed)	$288,000	$23,100	$25,500	$35,500
Faculty Benefit Cost (actual)	$249,039	$20,151	$19,582	$28,545
Department Clinical Services Overhead Costs (actual)	2,740,088			
Faculty Negotiated Percent of Clinical Overhead		9%	10%	11%
Faculty Overhead Expense		$254,612	$261,587	$290,648
Total Clinical Practice Expense (sum of above)		$330,203	$342,369	$404,393
Step 4 **Determine surplus (deficit).**				
Total Funds by Faculty Member (from above)		$709,878	$681,201	$883,713
Total Expenses by Faculty Member (from above)		$415,203	$437,369	$523,893
Individual Surplus (deficit)		$294,675	$243,832	$359,820
Step 5 **Allocate surplus.**				
30% to Department		$88,403	$121,916	$179,910
70% to Faculty Member		$206,273	$121,916	$179,910
Step 6 **Determine total compensation.**				
(sum of restricted plus unrestricted plus surplus)		$291,273	$216,916	$299,410

* Hypothetical numbers presented for illustrative purposes only. Numbers may not total in all cases due to rounding.

Faculty D	Faculty E	Faculty F	Faculty G	Faculty H	Faculty I	Faculty J
$225,621	$600,000	$690,000	$1,029,000	$1,012,019	$740,000	$750,000
$78,600	$5,321	$108,500	$—	$6,000	$2,800	$1,100
$304,221	$605,321	$798,500	$1,029,000	$1,018,019	$742,800	$751,100
$546,721	$700,321	$914,500	$1,134,000	$1,078,019	$827,800	$841,100
$52,500	$75,000	$75,000	$60,000	$60,000	$75,000	$75,000
$140,000	$—	$—	$—	$—	$—	$—
$50,000	$20,000	$41,000	$45,000	$—	$10,000	$15,000
$242,500	$95,000	$116,000	$105,000	$60,000	$85,000	$90,000
$18,900	$41,650	$51,100	$63,000	$70,700	$53,340	$45,570
$13,500	$29,750	$36,500	$45,000	$50,500	$38,100	$32,550
$54,241	$20,001	$27,584	$14,520	$17,542	$25,421	$21,452
5%	10%	11%	12%	12%	11%	10%
$132,973	$273,938	$293,554	$318,257	$334,240	$298,204	$282,075
$219,614	$365,339	$408,738	$440,777	$472,982	$415,065	$381,647
$546,721	$700,321	$914,500	$1,134,000	$1,078,019	$827,800	$841,100
$462,114	$460,339	$524,738	$545,777	$532,982	$500,065	$471,647
$84,607	$239,982	$389,762	$588,223	$545,037	$327,735	$369,453
$42,304	$119,991	$194,881	$294,112	$272,518	$163,867	$184,727
$42,304	$119,991	$194,881	$294,112	$272,518	$163,867	$184,727
$284,804	$214,991	$310,881	$399,112	$332,518	$248,867	$274,727

EXHIBIT 15.14

Z Based on Individual Points and Weights

Faculty Member Smith:		
	Total Targeted Compensation:	$200,000
	Base Salary:	$160,000
	Incentive to be "Earned"	$ 40,000

Category	Weight	Dollars Available	Activity	Dr. Smith	Award
Clinical Productivity	50%	$20,000	WRVUs: 2,500 – 3,000 = 25% 3,001 – 4,500 = 50% 4,501 – 5,000 = 75% 5,001 + = 100%	4,225 WRVU = 50% level	$10,000
Teaching	20%	$8,000	Available Point Total: 10 1. Evaluations (5 pts) 2. Mentor (5 pts) 3. Teaching Awards (10)	5 pts = 50% level	$4,000
Administration	10%	$4,000	Available Point Total: 100 Division Director (100) Section Chief (80) Residency Director (80) Med Student Director (60) Committees (10 each)	20 pts = 20% level	$800
Research	10%	$4,000	Available Point Total: Actual Number. Expectations Set in Advance Each Year: Grants Peer Journal Publications Nonpeer Journal Publications Books Book Chapters Editorial Boards Grants (Type & Level) Total: 7 (full level)	0 2 3 0 1 1 0	$4,000
Patient Service	10%	$4,000	Available Point Total: 10 Survey Scores (5) Time to Appointment (2) Waiting Time (2) Clinic Cancellations (1) Earned: 7 = 70% level	5 2 0 0	$2,800
Total	100%	$40,000			$21,600

EXHIBIT 15.15 Subjective Approach to Weighted Scores

Step 1 Assign weights by faculty member.

Faculty	Clinical	Teaching	Administration	Research	Patient Service	Total
A	0.50	0.20	0.10	0.10	0.10	1.00
B	0.40	0.30	—	0.20	0.10	1.00
C	0.60	0.30	—	—	0.10	1.00
D	0.60	0.10	—	0.20	0.10	1.00
E	0.50	0.40	—	—	0.10	1.00
F	0.20	0.10	0.10	0.50	0.10	1.00
G	0.90	—	—	—	0.10	1.00
Total Expected FTE	3.70	1.40	0.20	1.00	0.70	7.00
Total Budgeted $	$200,000	$100,000	$50,000	$100,000	$50,000	$500,000

Step 2 Assign scores based on individual faculty member performance.
Key: 1 = unsatisfactory or low; 2 = satisfactory or medium; 3 = more than satisfactory or high

Faculty	Clinical	Teaching	Administration	Research	Patient Service
A	3	3	1	1	2
B	2	2	0	2	2
C	1	3	0	3	1
D	2	3	0	1	2
E	3	3	0	0	2
F	3	2	2	2	2
G	2	0	0	0	3

Step 3 Determine weighted average (assigned weight x score).

Faculty	Clinical	Teaching	Administration	Research	Patient Service
A	1.5	0.6	0.1	0.1	0.2
B	0.8	0.6	0	0.4	0.2
C	0.6	0.9	0	0	0.1
D	1.2	0.3	0	0.2	0.2
E	1.5	1.2	0	0	0.2
F	0.6	0.2	0.2	1	0.2
G	1.8	0	0	0	0.3
Total Actual FTE	8.00	3.80	0.30	1.70	1.40	
Total Budgeted $	$200,000	$100,000	$50,000	$100,000	$50,000	$500,000

Step 4 Award incentive by category based on weighted averages.

Faculty	Clinical	Teaching	Administration	Research	Patient Service	Total
A	$37,500	$15,789	$16,667	$5,882	$7,143	$82,981
B	$20,000	$15,789	$—	$23,529	$7,143	$66,462
C	$15,000	$23,684	$—	$—	$3,571	$42,256
D	$30,000	$7,895	$—	$11,765	$7,143	$56,802
E	$37,500	$31,579	$—	$—	$7,143	$76,222
F	$15,000	$5,263	$33,333	$58,824	$7,143	$119,563
G	$45,000	$—	$—	$—	$10,714	$55,714
Total Awarded	$200,000	$100,000	$50,000	$100,000	$50,000	$500,000

EXHIBIT 15.16 Point System to Recognize Faculty Research, Teaching, and Service Activities

Category	Description	Point Value	Faculty Member A	Faculty Member B
Research	a. Peer review articles			
	First author	5	2 first author peer articles = 10	5 first author peer articles = 25
	Other author	2		
	b. Invited research presentations	4	1 invited presentation = 4	3 invited presentations = 12
	c. Books edited	3	1 book edited = 3	0 books edited = 0
	d. Book chapters	2	5 book chapters = 10	1 book chapter = 2
	e. Nonpeer review articles	2	4 nonpeer review articles = 8	0 nonpeer review articles = 0
	f. Abstracts	1	5 abstracts = 5	3 abstracts = 3
	g. Grant size-New grant		No grants	No grants
	Large (> $1M)	10		
	Medium ($500K-$1M)	5		
	Low (Less than $500K)	2		
	Research Weight	50%		
TOTAL			40	42
Teaching	Teaching awards	5	1 award = 5	0 awards = 0
	Course management	3	0 course = 0	1 course = 3
	Program management (e.g., Resident Paper Day)	3	1 program = 3	0 program = 0
	Consistently positive teaching evaluations	2	Yes = 2	Yes = 2
	Teaching Weight	30%		
TOTAL			10	5
Service	a. President of professional society	5	No = 0	No = 0
	b. Other officer of professional society	4	Yes = 4	Yes = 4
	Service Weight	20%		
TOTAL			4	4

EXHIBIT 15.17 Distribution of Academic Incentive Pool*

Point Category	Faculty A	Faculty B	Total
Research	40	42	82
Teaching	10	5	15
Service	4	4	8
Percent			
Research	48.78%	51.22%	100.00%
Teaching	66.67%	33.33%	100.00%
Service	50.00%	50.00%	100.00%
Dollars Awarded			
Research	$24,390	$25,610	$50,000
Teaching	$20,001	$9,999	$30,000
Service	$10,000	$10,000	$20,000
Total Awarded	$54,391	$45,609	$100,000

*For illustration purposes only.

EXHIBIT 15.18 Assessment of Faculty Practice Plan Example 2

Dimension	Strengths	Weaknesses
Measure	Recognizes balance of activities required for academic mission.	Performance expectations may be needed to ensure performance appropriate to base plus supplement compensation (X plus Y).
Productivity		Less direct recognition of clinical production, as funds may not be available for Z payment and/or dollars are shared among different pools (e.g., clinical and academic).
Financial	Fiscally appropriate; funds may or may not be available to fund incentive portion of compensation. Focuses management attention on all aspects of academic practice and creates incentives for strong performance in each area.	More likely to create perception that high producers are supplementing low producers. Less attention to expenditure controls since expenses are subtracted before compensation.
Simplicity	Builds on sound budgeting and financial management practices.	May require administrative infrastructure beyond current levels if point system is complex. Plan may be difficult to explain to faculty who may be adversely impacted.
Alignment	Aligned with academic mission via incentive reward in all mission areas. Depending on model selected, may promote view of department as a single economic unit with combination of team and individual incentive measures. May focus on individual and departmental performance in relation to budget target, and creates "win-win" situation when entire group meets financial targets. Recognizes financial funds flow.	Requires fairly sophisticated budgeting and financial management processes. Likely to work best in plan environment moving from largely straight salary arrangements to plans with larger portion of incentive compensation. When focus is on the individual only, may result in reduced focus on the division or department as a whole.
"Fairness"	Allows for advance determination of departmental support for clinical practice as a whole via tithing and other mechanisms. Faculty receive recognition for their academic activities.	Faculty may perceive that they have less control over expenditures. Faculty with high levels of revenue generation and production may suffer from poor performance of other departmental faculty or perceive that their efforts are undervalued. Junior faculty may be disadvantaged over senior faculty due to internal competition for the academic incentive pool.

The academic health care environment is one of the most complex in terms of compensation planning and alignment. The compensation plans and systems that may be used in a faculty practice plan are as varied as the academic settings and structures themselves. A faculty practice plan that provides incentives for only clinical production without also building in expectations and rewards for research, teaching, and service may indeed get what its asks for – faculty engaged in clinical practice at the expense of the other components of the academic mission.

On the other hand, a complex faculty practice plan that attempts to reward components of the academic mission at the individual level may miss the mark by creating imbalance at the divisional or departmental level, coupled with administrative complexity – and costs – that are not needed.

The faculty practice plans outlined here, along with those that build upon and incorporate the varied methodologies described in previous chapters, including those available for use in traditional group practices and those that may be used with hospital-affiliated medical practices, may be adapted for use in an academic setting.

Overall, the faculty practice plans that seem to work best are those that are aligned with the academic mission and with the unique setting of the particular academic practice. They are not overly complex, and they effectively integrate funds flow and expenditure treatment into their overall design. In most cases, changing the faculty practice plan is central and essential to changing the overall philosophy and mind-set regarding the academic clinical enterprise. Such a change often will be viewed as an essential means for changing the business and financial incentive model in the academic setting. As part of the process, other more fundamental structural adjustments and changes will frequently occur as the faculty practice plan and the overall academic institution adapt and change to today's challenging health care delivery environment.

Notes

1. Because compensation arrangements in academic settings typically occur in the context of tax-exempt enterprises, the level of surplus to be paid to faculty members and related decisions regarding the compensation plan are typically subject to decision making and approval by persons other than the faculty members themselves – such as a practice plan compensation committee or others. See Chapter 16, "The Special World of Hospital and Academic Practices – Assessing Reasonableness and Promoting Compliance," for more information on these issues.

2. Although most practice operating costs are fixed, in this example a lower percentage of actual fixed costs is allocated on an equal share basis because the expense allocation method is negotiated.

3. Note that some adjustment may be necessary to recognize research revenue and percent of time discrepancies due to maximum compensation levels and funding policies held by some agencies. In these situations, the actual percent of time to be devoted to the grant is used to reflect research time of faculty member (which may require another source of funding to supplement the grant award to fund the total compensation dollars this represents).

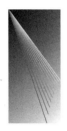

The Special World of Hospital and Academic Practices – Assessing Reasonableness and Promoting Compliance

The development, implementation, and maintenance of a compensation plan is challenging and complex in any setting. That complexity increases when a hospital or academic institution is involved because of the legal requirements applicable to physician compensation arrangements involving such organizations. Physician compensation relationships with these organizations are "special" for many reasons, including the following:

► Unique cultures of physicians and hospitals commonly make the two parties "strange bedfellows";

► Hospitals and health systems rely on physician referrals to fill their beds, creating a mutual dependency between hospitals and physicians; and

► Hospitals, health systems, academic medical centers, and similar organizations are often organized and operated for charitable, educational, and other tax-exempt purposes.

The basic requirements of the Stark, anti-kickback, and tax-exempt organization laws as applied to physician compensation were reviewed in Chapter 9, "The Legal Element." As discussed in Chapter 9, understanding the relationship between a physician and the organization that is the source of compensation paid to that physician is required in order to determine the legal requirements and standards that will apply to the particular compensation relationship. Because of that, we highlighted the importance of understanding the nature of the source organization (e.g., Group Practice or other organizational form), the nature of the compensation relationship (e.g., employment or independent contractor), and the taxable, for-profit, or tax-exempt character of the source organization.

This chapter focuses specifically on the special legal requirements that are implicated and that apply when the organization (e.g., a hospital, a health system, an academic medical center, or similar organization), which is the source of funds used to pay physician compensation, receives, benefits from, and is dependent upon physician referrals. This issue of physician referrals is important, because regardless of the nature of the compensation relationship, the legal requirements and prohibitions of the Stark and/or anti-kickback laws will typically apply.

This chapter also focuses on source organizations that are tax-exempt, because when the source organization is a tax-exempt hospital, health system, community health center, or even a group practice, the additional requirements governing tax-exempt organizations under sections 501(c)(3) and § 4958 of the Internal Revenue Code (IRC) will apply.

APPLICABLE STANDARDS

The Stark, anti-kickback, and tax-exempt organization laws impose different but similar legal standards on physician compensation levels. To comply with certain exceptions under the Stark and the anti-kickback laws, compensation must generally be consistent with "fair market value" (FMV) for the physician's services.[1] By illustration, the Stark law's final rule defines "FMV" in the case of services as:

> [t]he compensation that would be included in a service agreement as a result of bona fide bargaining between well informed parties to the agreement who are not otherwise in a position to generate business for the other party, at the time of the service agreement. Usually, the fair market price is the … compensation that has been included in bona fide service agreements with comparable terms at the time of the agreement, where the price or compensation has not been determined in any manner that takes into account the volume or value of anticipated or actual referrals.
>
> 42 C.F.R. § 411.351 (definition of FMV)

The rules and requirements under the IRC and applicable rules implementing the tax code use different terms. Under code section 501(c)(3), compensation levels must generally be reasonable, with the standards of reasonableness relating to those applicable under code section 162 (discussed in Chapter 9). Code section 4958, which provides for the imposition of intermediate sanctions on tax-exempt organizations under certain circumstances, states that "reasonable" compensation is:

> the amount that would ordinarily be paid for like services by like enterprises (whether taxable or tax-exempt) under like circumstances.
>
> Treasury Reg. § 53.4958-4(b)(1)(ii)(A)

As these definitions demonstrate, the legal standards imposed under the Stark and anti-kickback laws relating to federal health care programs, and those applicable under the tax code, are not precisely the same. Moreover, because the laws are typically implemented by different parties – usually the U.S. Department of Health and Human Services (HHS) in the case of the Stark and anti-kickback statutes, and the U.S. Department of Treasury in the case of tax laws – a compensation amount that satisfies one statutory requirement will not necessarily satisfy another. This has been noted by the HHS Office of Inspector General (OIG) and the Centers for Medicare & Medicaid Services (CMS). In the publication of anti-kickback statute safe harbors and the Stark law's final rule, and in other contexts, these agencies have indicated that compliance with Internal Revenue Service (IRS) and tax-exempt organizations requirements will not automatically result in Stark law or safe harbor compliance.[2]

In contrast, tax-exempt organizations are required to promote charitable purposes through activities that provide "community benefit." These requirements, when considered alone, might allow for relatively greater flexibility in terms of setting compensation levels that are "reasonable." Therefore, an exempt organization could potentially set compensation at a level that would be acceptable under reasonableness standards, but that may not be consistent with the requirements of FMV under the Stark and anti-kickback laws.

Yet in the practical world of hospitals, academic medical centers, and similar institutions, the process and activities that are used to assess whether compensation is consistent with FMV and reasonable will typically be similar: The level of compensation to be paid to a particular physician will be compared to market data in order to assess whether that amount is within a reasonable range of available market data. The market data will be used to help assess, evaluate, verify, and ultimately substantiate that the amount of compensation complies with the applicable legal requirements and, as a practical reference, to physician compensation planning and evaluation. And where the market data will not support the proposed level of compensation, the amount of compensation or plan methodology, and potentially both, will generally need to be adjusted in order to comply with the law. Because of this reality, it will be useful to briefly explore the nature, character, strengths, weaknesses, and uses of such market data.

UNDERSTANDING MARKET DATA

Numerous data sources exist for evaluating physician compensation. These include published surveys such as the Medical Group Management Association's *Physician Compensation and Production Survey Report*, the American Medical Group Association's *Medical Group Compensation & Production Survey*, and others. Each compensation survey is a self-reported survey of compensation levels earned by a subset of all physicians who happen to work in a subset of all physician practice organizations. And because the true universe of physicians and physician practices in the United States is not presently known, it is currently not possible to scientifically evaluate precisely how representative (or unrepresentative) any single survey is in relation to the physician population as a whole.

In light of the above, it is fair to say that every existing compensation survey has some level of bias and inherent weaknesses, because each is not truly "representative" of the entire population of physicians. By illustration:

► The MGMA survey is completed by MGMA member organizations who tend to be largely private practice medical groups ranging from the very small to the very large, although it does provide separate surveys for private practice and academic practice organizations.

► The AMGA survey focuses on very large medical groups, and it includes both academic and private practice organizations in the survey results.

Other proprietary surveys are conducted and maintained by other associations, recruiting firms, and consulting firms. These survey data may overrepresent newer physicians and starting salary levels, physicians who are only employed by hospitals or health systems, or physicians who are otherwise located in some other unique setting.

The physicians who are likely to be represented in each of these (and other) compensation surveys are likely to vary from one another in a variety of ways, including work levels and payer mix, access to income from ancillary services, different approaches to physician compensation, and legal designation of the practice. These variations will influence the level of physician compensation that the physicians receive. Thus, while there are numerous surveys of physician compensation, each has its own strengths and weaknesses, and no one survey will be perfect for all uses, or in all contexts.

EVALUATING THE DATA

Just as all surveys are not the same, not all compensation data or statistics have the same value or utility in assessing compensation levels. Given the inherent limitations of all survey data, the following rules of thumb tend to hold true in connection with evaluating most compensation survey data.

First, when it comes to survey data, drawing from many respondents is generally preferable to drawing from a select few. Until surveys employ a true random sample of the universe of potential survey respondents in order to ensure a representative sample, surveys with the largest sample or number of respondents will generally be preferred.

Second, three statistical measures will generally be important to consider and review: the mean, the median, and the standard deviation, as further described below.

The average or "mean" statistic measures the "average" data value of the data set. It is calculated by summing all data values and dividing by the number of individual values. In the context of physician compensation data, the mean may not be the most useful because it will be skewed by extreme values, as discussed below.

The "median" is typically the more helpful measure of central tendency. When a set of data values is arrayed from highest to lowest, the median will be the value in the exact middle or center of that array. Because it represents the value "in the middle," the median is not skewed by extreme values in the same way as the mean statistic.

The "standard deviation" measures the dispersion around the mean and therefore the level of variance or spread within the particular data set.

Most compensation surveys recommend the use of the median statistic because it is more "resistant" to the influence of extremely high or low values in the data set. The median is also important because the spread of physician compensation survey data rarely represents a "normal distribution" or classic "bell curve." In the normal distribution, the mean and the median are virtually the same – meaning that they are effectively in the center of the distribution of data. However, MGMA and most other survey data tend to be skewed to the right – meaning that the median is typically below the mean, and the data are generally influenced by extremely high values. In light of this skewing, the median is generally viewed as the more representative and appropriate statistic for use in assessing compensation levels and for other uses.

▶ MEASURING TO MEDIAN

As noted above, the median or midpoint of market data is the recommended measure or reference point, because the median is more resistant to extreme values. This is illustrated, for example, by the requirements of the final rule to the Stark law, which provides a "safe harbor" methodology for calculating compensation for hourly services. In the final rule, CMS indicates that one means to determine a presumptively "safe" and FMV hourly rate of compensation for physician services involves averaging median national compensation data values from four designated compensation surveys, and dividing that average by 2,000.[3] Thus, even the regulators recognize that the median is the strongest and most useful measure of central tendency.

The relative "resistance" of the median statistic and the value of that statistic are the reasons why many of the compensation plan examples illustrated in this book that incorporate market data into the plan methodology itself use the median as the standard reference or starting point to which percentages of median (e.g., 80 percent or 120 percent) are applied as part of the compensation plan methodology. This is in contrast to plans that link to specific percentiles as expressed in survey data. Linking to percentiles is certainly feasible, but such linkage will need to address the significant year-to-year variation and fluctuation that will commonly occur in connection with individual percentiles in the compensation benchmark surveys.[4]

COMPENSATION AND PRODUCTION RELATIONSHIPS IN THE MARKETPLACE

A review of market data illustrates that physicians with differing levels of production receive widely varying levels of compensation. Exhibit 16.1 reports MGMA data for a physician who practices family practice (without obstetrics). Exhibit 16.2 takes this information and depicts the range of compensation that is received by physicians with different ranges of production, as measured by collections from professional services. By illustration, family practice physicians who had production between the 51st and 60th percentiles received compensation that ranged from a low of $106,723 to a high of $218,448, resulting in a difference of $111,725 in aggregate compensation between the low and high values within this narrow range of production.

EXHIBIT 16.1

Data Example – Variability in Physician Compensation within Ranges of Collections
MGMA Physician Compensation Data for Family Practice (without Obstetrics)

Percentile	Collections Dollar Ranges	Count	Mean	Standard Deviation	COMPENSATION				
					Percentile 10	Percentile 25	Percentile 50	Percentile 75	Percentile 90
91 – 100th	≥ $458,265	159	$259,763	$98,211	$162,586	$189,882	$241,559	$308,072	$371,770
81 – 90th	$407,161 – $458,264	159	$212,980	$70,103	$140,000	$161,000	$200,486	$243,252	$318,078
71 – 80th	$365,647 – $407,160	159	$189,073	$53,916	$134,541	$149,676	$179,865	$212,543	$266,762
61 – 70th	$335,524 – $365,646	159	$166,252	$44,900	$119,056	$138,066	$159,039	$181,527	$205,937
51 – 60th	$310,109 – $335,523	159	$159,453	$46,388	$106,723	$130,682	$152,558	$178,185	$218,448
41 – 50th	$288,461 – $310,108	159	$156,393	$49,863	$111,244	$127,883	$147,164	$172,728	$211,422
31 – 40th	$264,278 – $288,460	159	$151,397	$40,783	$108,266	$127,088	$141,241	$172,773	$210,057
21 – 30th	$237,456 – $264,277	159	$149,054	$40,999	$107,873	$120,000	$136,599	$175,961	$210,906
11 – 20th	$199,227 – $237,455	159	$137,201	$40,693	$94,335	$108,477	$130,000	$162,277	$193,205
0 – 10th	≤ $199,226	159	$117,422	$36,256	$73,223	$91,873	$115,500	$135,907	$167,404

EXHIBIT
16.2

Data Example: Compensation and Production Relationships;
Range of Family Practice Compensation Based on Collections

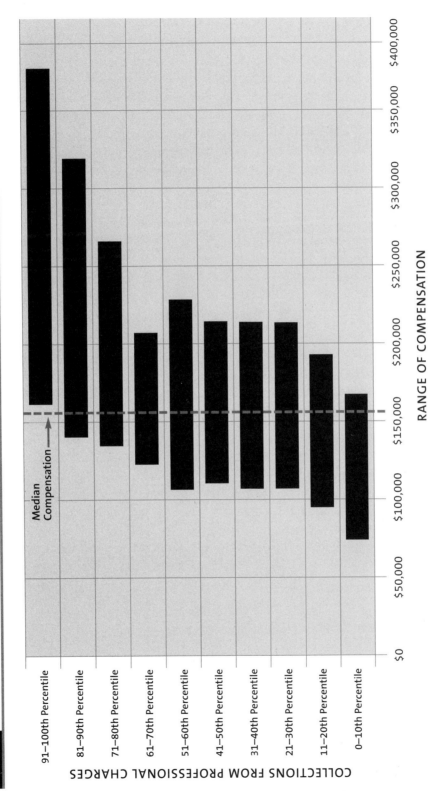

© 2006 Johnson & Walker Keegan

Source: MGMA Physician Compensation and Production Survey: 2005 Report Based on 2004 Data

Exhibit 16.2 illustrates a general relationship between compensation and production. It also illustrates, however, that as physician production levels increase (e.g., as the physicians move to the upper end of the range of production), the range of compensation that those higher producing physicians might receive for their services tends to widen and increase. Thus, a physician who has production that would place that physician at the 75th percentile, as measured by market data, could receive compensation that is below, at, or significantly above the 75th percentile of compensation data. As this example illustrates, arbitrary rules that require a direct correlation or linkage between market data compensation and production percentiles in evaluating compensation levels will generally not be appropriate.

Of course, Exhibit 16.2 does, in fact, indicate that compensation does vary somewhat in relation to production levels. But it also suggests that the range of variation in compensation levels that are paid to physicians with similar levels of production tends to increase as production increases, and that physicians with the highest levels of production tend to have the greatest range of variation in compensation levels. Moreover, as demonstrated in the exhibit, physicians who have production that is generally between the 20th and 80th percentiles will generally have compensation levels that fall within a defined range.

APPLYING MARKET DATA TO EVALUATE QUESTIONS OF FAIR MARKET VALUE AND REASONABLENESS

Market data are commonly used to both evaluate and verify that the compensation paid to a physician by a hospital, health system, faculty practice plan, or similar organization is consistent with FMV and reasonable. Yet, appropriate use of that market data will depend on a number of factors, many of which were discussed in Chapter 7, "Measuring Physician Work and Effort," in the context of benchmarking. These include ensuring that the data are applied on an "apples-to-apples" basis and understanding the bias inherent in small samples and skewed samples.

A variety of individual statistics may and commonly will be used to evaluate questions of reasonableness and FMV. The primary measures typically include:

▶ Actual compensation levels (to potentially include additional levels for employee benefit and retirement costs); and

▶ Compensation levels per unit of production, or "ratio" measures.

The use of these and potentially other measures will allow compensation to be assessed by reference to market norms. The use of actual compensation levels in comparison to market data provides a useful reference in raw dollar terms. The use of ratio measures focuses on the more specific issue of how much compensation the physician is receiving for each unit of production. Common ratio measures that are contained in the annual *MGMA Physician Compensation and Production Survey* reports and other surveys include physician compensation per total RVU and per WRVU, the ratio of physician compensation to professional services net collections, and the ratio of physician compensation to gross charges from professional services. In any compensation survey, there will be a distribution or range of values for each particular measure. However, as noted above, the median measure (e.g., the median value of compensation per WRVU) will generally provide a useful starting or reference point for evaluating questions of FMV and reasonableness.

It is important to note that no single statistic or reference point will definitively determine when compensation is, or is not, consistent with FMV or reasonable. The market data that are currently available for use in evaluating compensation levels are simply not of sufficient quality and consistency to allow for such black-and-white conclusions. Perhaps even more important, however, is the reality that the law does not require such black-and-white assessments. Indeed, under the law, the question of what level of compensation for a particular physician is FMV and reasonable will generally depend on consideration of the particular "facts and circumstances" related to a particular compensation relationship. Survey data will be important to that assessment, but they are by no means determinative.

Because there is certainly no single survey or survey statistic that will serve as the "gold standard" in evaluating reasonableness and FMV, multiple data sources and market data statistics should optimally be used in assessing physician compensation levels. The use of multiple measures – including actual raw compensation and production levels, as well as ratios such as those referenced above – will tend to provide useful perspective, both on the absolute level of compensation and on the amount of compensation paid for each unit of physician work. As noted above, no single statistic or measure is likely to be determinative. However, the combination of multiple measures, when taken together, will tend to help provide an assessment of whether the compensation level is within a reasonable range of what similarly situated physicians earn in the marketplace more generally.

Of course, market data consist of statistical information that can be used for legitimate and illegitimate purposes, and in both correct and incorrect ways. By illustration, one common fallacy related to market survey data holds that median compensation and median production levels as reflected in the survey data should correlate directly. This would mean, for example, that the physician who is compensated at median levels, as reflected on the compensation survey table, should have production that is also at median levels, as measured by a second survey table that reports production information.

The expectation of such a "direct correlation" between compensation and production based on survey tables may make intuitive sense, but it is actually not the case based on the survey data. This is because different tables in any one survey represent separate data sets and separate arrays of those unique sets of data. Because of this, the table providing compensation data might be based on a data set that contains data for several thousand physicians, while the table presenting production levels might be based on data derived from the same or different physicians, or from a data set with far greater (or fewer) respondents; or it may otherwise contain data that do not directly relate to the compensation data set. Each survey table should be recognized for what it is – a snapshot of data for a particular set of physicians, at a particular period in time.

The absence of a direct correlation between compensation and production levels as reflected in survey data should not be construed as saying that there is no relationship between compensation and production. There is, indeed, a relationship, but it is not reasonable to expect or require a direct correlation between compensation and production levels based on survey data. Instead, the data suggest that physicians who are "in the middle" in terms of physician production levels may actually receive compensation that spans a relatively wide range, as discussed below.

Because of the recognized importance of median levels in providing a compensation standard, many hospitals and other organizations have adopted the position that a physician may be paid at median compensation levels regardless of the physician's production. Organizations that take this position contend that even though the physician with low levels of production may be receiving a relatively high level of compensation, that compensation is likely to be acceptable, reasonable, and consistent with FMV because it does not exceed median levels.

Of course, many physicians will receive compensation that is in excess of median levels as measured by market data. And the fact that the physician's compensation is in excess of median levels does not automatically mean that the compensation is in excess of FMV or that it is not reasonable. As noted above, there clearly is a relationship between compensation and production levels; therefore, it is certainly possible that a physician is being paid compensation in excess of median levels for any number of entirely legitimate and appropriate reasons. For these physicians, additional questions are generally in order regarding why compensation is in excess of median levels. That additional inquiry may conclude that compensation is in excess of median levels for various reasons, including:

► Because the physician is working harder and has production levels that are in excess of the typical physician in the same specialty;

► Because the level of compensation for each unit of production is above expected levels; or

► Because of a combination of these or other factors.

When an individual physician's compensation is far above the compensation paid to similarly situated physicians, then questions may be raised whether that compensation is reasonable and/or consistent with FMV. In such a circumstance, additional information and inquiry into the reasons for that compensation will typically be essential in order to understand, for example, any other factors that may be impacting compensation levels (e.g., the mechanics of the particular compensation plan, compensation levels that are affected by recruitment challenges, and others). These last points highlight the fact, that while the data are clearly important and relevant to the assessment of compensation amounts, other factors will also be important and relevant to the question of legal compliance.

For example, the Stark and anti-kickback laws mandate that for compensation to be consistent with FMV, there must be no consideration of referrals or other business between the parties. A compensation plan that considers referrals to a hospital or another organization in the determination of compensation may therefore not be compliant.

Likewise, the standards applicable to tax-exempt organizations focus on the process and considerations associated with a particular compensation relationship. As noted above, whether a particular compensation level is appropriate will generally be subject to a "facts and circumstances" test, and as part of any such assessment, a number of factors other than market data will be relevant to the analysis, such as:

► Whether the compensation arrangement was developed through an arm's-length relationship, or whether the recipient of compensation has a level of control over the organization;

► The nature of the physician's duties and responsibilities for the organization;

► The physician's background, experience, and salary history;

► The individual's contribution to the organization's success in achieving charitable and other missions;

► The amount of time the physician spends in performing the duties for which compensation is paid; and

► The amount paid by similarly sized businesses in the same area to persons with equal qualifications for similar services.

THIRD-PARTY AND INTERNAL ASSESSMENTS

Other process issues will also be important to compliance. For many compensation arrangements, considerable compliance protection will be obtained through the use of third-party assessments to determine whether compensation levels are consistent with FMV and are, in fact, reasonable. For example, the rules governing the intermediate sanctions law contained in IRC § 4958 highlight the value of performing an objective assessment of "reasonableness" when a tax-exempt organization is involved in a compensation arrangement with certain "disqualified persons." Under rules implementing this law, when such an assessment is performed and certain other process-related issues are addressed, the managers of the tax-exempt organization will be entitled to benefit from a "rebuttable presumption" that the compensation level is reasonable.[5]

Unfortunately, such independent valuations do not determine compliance with the Stark and anti-kickback laws. Still, they can have substantial value in the event of a compliance challenge. Such an independent review process is commonly incorporated as part of structured compliance programs that are instituted as part of the standard practices of hospitals and other organizations to prevent potentially problematic compensation arrangements and transactions.

When an independent assessment of compensation is undertaken, close attention to certain core issues and assumptions will be helpful for ensuring that the assessment is as strong and useful as possible. Such issues include:

- ► Ensuring that certain core assumptions and requirements, such as the scope and focus of the opinion, are clearly addressed (e.g., whether the opinion considers questions of reasonableness only, whether it considers FMV standards under the Stark and anti-kickback laws, or both);

- ► Applying appropriate standards, such as external benchmark standards and consultant experience, to the question;

- ► Including valid comparability data as part of the valuation opinion in order to substantiate the data and methodology used in the assessment; and

- ► Indicating clearly in the opinion that, when assessments of FMV are undertaken, referrals have not been considered.

Legal counsel will, of course, play an important role in promoting legal compliance. In addition to the activities outlined in Chapter 9, legal counsel should optimally:

- ► Identify and assess compliance by reference to the appropriate Stark law exceptions, anti-kickback safe harbors, and standards applicable to tax-exempt organizations;

- ► Work in consultation with external and internal valuation consultants and other experts who assess the FMV and reasonableness of compensation;

- ► Monitor and manage the review process in a manner that promotes the appropriate use of protections provided by the attorney-client privilege; and

- ► Ensure that the findings and conclusions related to any assessment are contained in an appropriate file that can be accessed and used in the event of an external review.

Compensation relationships between hospitals, health systems, and academic medical centers and physicians will always be complex. These organizations depend on physician referrals, and many are also tax-exempt. Because of this, compensation arrangements that might "make sense" from a pure business perspective (e.g., pay physicians a premium) cannot be used, because they may likely result in violations of the Stark, anti-kickback, tax-exempt organization, and other laws.

Of course, these organizations must generally establish compensation relationships with physicians through any number of mechanisms, including direct employment and direct or indirect contractual arrangements. In every case, certain core threshold questions and themes will be pertinent as to whether the compensation arrangement is legal and appropriate. These questions relate to whether the compensation is consistent with FMV, whether the compensation paid by a tax-exempt organization is reasonable, and whether referrals were considered in determining the compensation amount. Hospitals, health systems, and other organizations will need to address these (and other) questions in connection with compensation arrangements. In doing so, they will inevitably consider and apply market data along with other facts pertinent to the particular relationship. As a result, the consideration and application of these standards will be important in developing an effective plan and compliance strategy.

Notes

1. As discussed in Chapter 9, the specific standards applicable to a particular compensation relationship will depend on numerous factors, including reliance on the particular exception to the Stark law. For the sake of brevity, this chapter contains only a general "high-level" discussion. Readers must consult with legal counsel to determine the particular standards and requirements applicable to a particular compensation relationship.

2. Importantly, the IRS has indicated that transactions that violate other federal laws (e.g., Stark or the anti-kickback statutes) will be inconsistent with charitable purposes; therefore, any greater flexibility under the tax code that may be theoretically available, is likely illusory at best.

3. The final rule implementing the Stark law provides that four of the following surveys can be used for such purposes: Sullivan Cotter & Associates, Inc. – *Physician Compensation and Productivity Survey*; Hay Group – *Physicians Compensation Survey Report*; Medical Group Management Association – *Physician Compensation and Production Survey*; and ECS Watson Wyatt – *Hospital and Health Care Management Compensation Report*.

4. For example, many of the plan examples described in earlier chapters linked compensation to market data. Although some plans are linked to specific percentiles as expressed in survey data, many plans are expressed as percentages of median values (e.g., 80 percent of median) as a means to help reduce the year-to-year variation and fluctuation that will commonly occur in connection with individual percentiles in the compensation benchmark surveys.

5. See Treas. Reg. § 53.4958-6 (rebuttable presumption that a transaction is not an excess-benefit transaction).

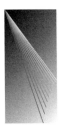

Conclusion

The compensation plan development process is not without its emotional challenges and legal minefields. Physicians need to be actively engaged in the process. They will obviously have a vested interest in the process and its outcome – after all, it does affect their livelihood. Consequently, the process of compensation plan development and its outcome are equally important in the design process.

We have provided a detailed blueprint to guide the compensation plan development process for a medical practice. From determining the need for a new compensation plan, to the compensation planning committee process, to defining compensation plan goals, to understanding the compensation plan matrix , to developing the plan's architecture, to addressing legal and human elements, to demonstrating plan technical components, to plan transition and implementation, the reader now has a set of tools and strategies to manage the compensation plan development process. The "science" of the process itself is relatively straightforward, and medical groups can adopt the blueprint to their own particular situation.

The "art" of the process, however, is the most challenging work of any medical practice. If the practice is to remain a viable entity, with physicians working together to further the practice's strategic and tactical goals, then it is vitally important that the process of plan development be conducted with equal attention and detail. We are aware of wonderfully crafted compensation plan architectures that simply did not get off the ground in the implementation phase. This was not due to intellectual capital being devoted to plan design; rather, it was due to a failure to pay attention and respond to the human element in the design process. A top-down approach rarely works well when it comes to physician compensation.

The authors have personally assisted private and academic medical groups, small and large, on their journey to a new compensation plan. From this work, we have learned a great deal from physicians and practice executives as they struggle with the art and science of compensation plan development. Perhaps the best compensation plan serves as a relatively "silent" framework that enables physicians to practice medicine and make a reasonable living in the process. In the successful medical practice, the compensation plan may not serve as the primary driver of performance, but neither does it serve as a significant barrier or impediment to individual or practice success. This is the challenge.

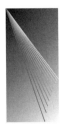

Additional Resources

This list of resources has been compiled for your reference and does not represent our commercial endorsement of any particular product. Readers may wish to investigate these and other resources as they embark upon the physician compensation planning process.

Websites

The Stark Law

The MGMA Stark Website ("Stark Compliance Solutions") authored by Bruce A. Johnson (www.stark compliance.com). This Website is a leading authority on the Stark law. To become a subscriber, contact MGMA at www.mgma.com.

Compensation Planning Tools

Online compensation tools are provided on the MGMA Website at www.mgma.com.

Benchmark Survey Instruments

Medical Group Management Association, Englewood, CO (www.mgma.com)

- ► *MGMA Physician Compensation and Production Survey* (available in both print and CD), published annually

- ► *MGMA Academic Practice Compensation and Production Survey for Faculty & Management,* published annually

- ► *MGMA Performance and Practices of Successful Medical Groups,* published annually

American Medical Group Association, Alexandria, VA (www.amga.org)

- ► *AMGA Medical Group Compensation & Financial Survey,* published annually

Association of American Medical Colleges, Washington, DC (www.aamc.org)

- ► *Report on Medical School Faculty Salaries*

Books and Book Chapters

Johnson B.A. "Medical Practice and Compensation Plans." In *Physician Practice Management: Essential Operational and Financial Knowledge*, edited by L.F. Wolper. Sudbury, MA: Jones and Bartlett Publishers, 2005, pp. 543–568.

Johnson, B.A. "Corporate Compliance in a Medical Practice Setting." In *Essentials of Physician Practice Management*, edited by B.A. Keagy and M.S. Thomas. San Francisco, CA: Jossey-Bass, 2004, pp. 195–210.

Johnson, B.A. "Better Performing Compensation Plans." In *Performance and Practices of Successful Medical Groups*. Englewood, CO: Medical Group Management Association, 2000, pp. 55–59.

Walker, D.L. "Managed Care Compensation Models." In *Physician Compensation: Models for Aligning Financial Goals and Incentives*, 2nd ed., edited by K.M. Hekman. Englewood, CO: Medical Group Management Association, 2002, pp. 47–62.

Walker, D.L. "Physician Compensation: Rewarding Productivity of the Knowledge Worker. *Journal of Ambulatory Care Management* 23:4 (October 2000): pp. 48–59.

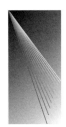

Index